Primary care Pediatrics

Pediatric Orthopedics in Clinical Practice

Second Edition

Pediatric Orthopedics in Clinical Practice

Second Edition

PETER V. SCOLES, M.D.
Director of Education
Department of Orthopedics
Assistant Professor
Departments of Orthopedics and Pediatrics
Case Western Reserve University
Cleveland, Ohio

YEAR BOOK MEDICAL PUBLISHERS, INC.
CHICAGO • LONDON • BOCA RATON

1 2 3 4 5 6 7 8 9 0 KC 92 91 90 89 88

**Library of Congress Cataloging-in-Publication
Data**
Scoles, Peter V.
  Pediatric orthopedics in clinical practice / Peter V.
Scoles.—2nd ed.
      p.   cm.
  Includes bibliographies and index.
  ISBN 0-8151-7585-X
  1. Pediatric orthopedia. 2. Pediatric orthopedia—
Diagnosis.
I. Title.
  [DNLM: 1. Bone Diseases—in infancy & childhood.
2. Muscular Diseases—in infancy & childhood.
WS 270 S422p]
RD732.3.C48S36 1988
617'.3'088054—dc19   87-34025
DNLM/DLC   CIP

Sponsoring Editor: James D. Ryan, Jr.
Associate Managing Editor, Manuscript Services:
  Deborah Thorp
Copyeditor: Sally J. Jansen
Production Project Manager: Nancy C. Baker
Proofroom Supervisor: Shirley E. Taylor

For Erica, Emily, Lindsey, and Lydia

CONTRIBUTORS

Stephen C. Aronoff, M.D.
*Associate Professor, Department of Pediatrics, Case
    Western Reserve University; Acting Chief,
    Division of Pediatric Infectious Disease,
    University Hospitals of Cleveland, Rainbow
    Babies and Childrens Hospital, Cleveland, Ohio*

Wilton H. Bunch, M.D., Ph.D.
*Professor, Department of Surgery and
    Orthopaedics, Dean of Medical Affairs,
    University of Chicago, Chicago, Illinois*

Victoria M. Dvonch, M.D.
*Assistant Professor, Department of Surgery,
    University of Chicago, Chicago, Illinois*

Peter V. Scoles, M.D.
*Director of Education, Department of Orthopedics,
    Assistant Professor, Departments of Orthopedics
    and Pediatrics, Case Western Reserve
    University, Cleveland, Ohio*

Angela D. Smith, M.D.
*Adjunct Professor, University of Delaware;
    Director, Division of Sports Medicine, Alfred I.
    DuPont Institute, Wilmington, Delaware*

PREFACE

The response to the first edition of *Pediatric Orthopedics in Clinical Practice* was quite gratifying. We expected that the text would be useful for family practitioners and pediatricians and were delighted at its reception by medical students, physical and occupational therapists, nurse clinicians, and beginning orthopedic residents. Musculoskeletal disorders constitute a large proportion of primary care, but as health care delivery shifts more to an ambulatory setting, the availability of the "curbside consult" is becoming limited. This text is designed to aid in evaluation and treatment of common musculoskeletal disorders in children.

As in the first edition, each chapter addresses those questions most frequently raised by primary physicians and nurse clinicians. Emphasis has been placed on identification of acceptable variations of normal. The signs and symptoms of common musculoskeletal disorders in children are emphasized, and treatment principles are outlined. We have indicated when we believe that referral is necessary, with the understanding that not all readers will agree. Concepts of orthopedic care of those conditions requiring referral are presented.

My colleagues in pediatric orthopedics have been very encouraging. Guided by their constructive comments, several areas of the first edition have been expanded and reworked. Drs. Wilton H. Bunch and Victoria M. Dvonch of the University of Chicago undertook revision of the chapter on congenital disorders of the hip. Dr. Stephen C. Aronoff of the Department of Pediatrics at Case Western Reserve University has revised and updated the chapter on infectious diseases. Dr. Angela D. Smith of the Division of Sports Medicine at the Alfred I. DuPont Institute added a much requested chapter on pediatric sports medicine. The chapters on trauma, lower extremity disorders, spinal deformity, and neuromuscular disease have been expanded and updated.

As in the first edition, space constraints and cost prohibit the inclusion of many topics of interest to both the authors and readers. Immunologic, neoplastic, and metabolic disorders of the musculoskeletal system are well covered in the standard texts in pediatrics, and are not discussed in this volume. We have attempted to limit discussion of other topics to practical lengths, and have provided suggestions for further reading for those who wish more detailed information.

A number of topics, such as the treatment of congenital hip disease, spinal deformity, and infectious diseases are controversial, even among pediatric orthopedists. We hope that we have presented a fair overview of opinion in these cases, but realize that our personal biases will be evident.

The encouragement and assistance of my colleagues, residents, and students have been invaluable in both editions of this text; their help is greatly appreciated. Jim Ryan and the staff at Year Book Medical Publishers, Inc., have once again gently but effectively pushed and prodded the manuscript to completion.

Finally, special thanks are once again due Rebecca J. Schieser, my secretary, for her patience and help.

Peter V. Scoles, M.D.

CONTENTS

1

Evaluation of the Musculoskeletal System

Abnormalities of form and function of the musculoskeletal system, both real and perceived, are among the most common problems in the daily care of children and adolescents. A wide variety of congenital, developmental, inflammatory, and traumatic disorders can affect the growing musculoskeletal system. Fortunately, most problems are minor and not difficult to identify or treat.

In most cases accurate evaluation is straightforward; a thorough history and systematic physical examination will disclose most abnormalities. Attention to detail and careful observation are the principal diagnostic skills required. A few words of caution are necessary, however, before beginning a discussion of musculoskeletal physical diagnosis. At times, abnormalities seem obvious, and careful investigation may be neglected before treatment is started; this is perhaps best illustrated in the primary evaluation and treatment of musculoskeletal trauma. At other times, subtle signs of early musculoskeletal disease may be overlooked in the routine examination of the otherwise healthy child. Unfortunately, hastily drawn conclusions are often incomplete and sometimes entirely incorrect. Systematic evaluation will prevent such errors.

There are several general categories of musculoskeletal physical examination. At times musculoskeletal evaluation is conducted as part of the overall evaluation of a child with a primary problem involving another organ system. At other times, the examination is conducted as part of a screening evaluation of an apparently otherwise normal child; the neonatal screening examination and adolescent scoliosis screening examinations are examples. Finally, examinations may be performed for the evaluation of primary complaints involving the trunk or extremities. The focus and depth of examination in each of these circumstances is different, but in each case, a systematic approach prevents errors of oversight.

In this chapter, general principles of musculoskeletal physical diagnosis in children will be discussed and specific examinations outlined. Pertinent regional topographic and functional anatomy will be presented first. Next, since physical examination of the musculoskeletal system is composed of a series of regional examinations, normal and abnormal findings will be presented region by region. Finally, guidelines for examination of the hand and for neonatal, childhood, and adolescent screening examinations will be given. More detailed discussions of specific problems will be presented in subsequent chapters.

GENERAL PRINCIPLES

Evaluation of musculoskeletal structure and function is best performed as a series of regional examinations. The detail with which examination of each region is conducted varies with the purpose of the examination and the nature of the chief complaint. Healthy children undergoing routine physical examination usually require only brief screening, with special attention to areas of the musculoskeletal system at risk in their age group. Comprehensive examination is essential for children with suspected metabolic, neoplastic, or inflammatory diseases. Trauma victims require detailed examinations of the central nervous system, thorax, and abdomen, in addition to the extremities.

Examination of the trunk and extremities should be conducted in a series of steps. In most instances, symmetry of size, configuration, and motion can be used as a reference for evaluation. The physician first inspects the area in question, noting absence or duplication of parts, obvious differences in size, cutaneous lesions, joint swelling, limb or trunk deformity, or muscle wasting. Next, the extent of areas of tenderness or inflammation identified in the history or suggested by inspection should be determined by gentle palpation. The size of soft tissue or bony masses should be estimated. The adequacy of blood flow to an injured extremity should be determined by checking peripheral pulses and capillary refill (more extensive tests may be necessary if these suggest vascular compromise). If sensory impairment is suggested by the history or the initial steps of examination, its extent should be outlined.

Next, the range of voluntary active motion of joints in the region under examination should be tested. In most instances, the contralateral limb can be used for reference. When limitation of active motion exists, the limits of comfortable passive motion should be noted. Excessive joint laxity or motion in abnormal planes suggesting joint instability should be noted.

Finally, those specific tests suggested by history, primary evaluation, or age group of the patient should be performed.

TOPOGRAPHIC AND FUNCTIONAL ANATOMY

Before beginning a presentation of normal regional anatomy and joint function, it is necessary to define several conventions dealing with angulation, range of motion, and muscle testing. The terms *varus* and *valgus* are often used to describe angular deformity of the extremity in the frontal plane. They can be quite confusing. In varus deformity, the extremity distal to the joint in question is tilted toward the midline of the body. In valgus deformity, it is tilted away. The terms are most commonly used in reference to the knee, ankle, and elbow joints. Genu valgum refers to knock-knee, genu varum to bowlegs. About 5 degrees of valgus angulation is ordinarily present at the knee joint in males; slightly more valgus is present in females. Valgus deformity of greater than 10 degrees is usually perceived as knock-knee. Varus deformity of the heel is the deformity of clubfoot, while heel valgus is found in children with severe flatfoot. About 5 degrees of valgus angulation is normally present in the elbow in men; slightly more valgus angulation is present in some women. Accentuated valgus alignment, termed *cubitus valgus*, may follow fractures of the lateral humeral condyle. Decreased elbow valgus with a reverse deformity, *cubitus varus*, may follow malunion of the fractures around the elbow.

A uniform system of grading muscle strength is important in recording the results of muscle testing. Zero strength implies no palpable or visible contraction in a tested muscle. Trace or grade I function implies a flicker of palpable contraction that produces no joint motion. Poor function (grade II) is present when the affected muscle can produce motion in its respective joint with gravity eliminated (appropriate positioning of the limb is necessary to eliminate the effects of gravity). Fair function (grade III) indicates the ability of muscle to move its joint against gravity but without added resistance. Good muscle function (grade IV) implies no deficit.

TRUNK AND NECK

Topographic Anatomy

In anatomical position, the anterior surfaces of the trunk and limbs are termed *ventral surfaces* (Fig 1–1). The pos-

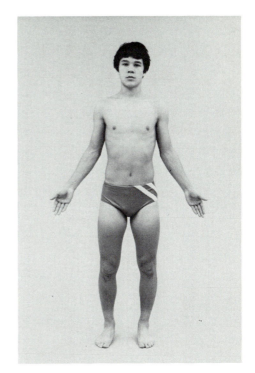

FIG 1–1.
Ventral surface, anatomical position. Note symmetry of body parts and limb alignment. The clavicles are symmetric, and the acromioclavicular prominences are evident. Valgus alignment of the elbow joint is normal. This young man has mild varus alignment of the knees (bowlegs).

terior surfaces are termed *dorsal surfaces* (Fig 1–2). The anterior and posterior surfaces of the normal neck and trunk are symmetric. Viewed from behind, shoulder height is equal, and the bulk of the trapezius muscles is symmetric. The tips and spinous processes of the scapular bones are clearly visible and at the same levels on both sides of the body. The posterior aspects of the iliac crests are at the same level, and slight depressions overlying the superior sacroiliac joints are evident. A prominence overlying the spine of the seventh cervical vertebra and a linear bony ridge extending from the spines of the upper thoracic to the spines of the lower lumbar vertebrae can be seen.

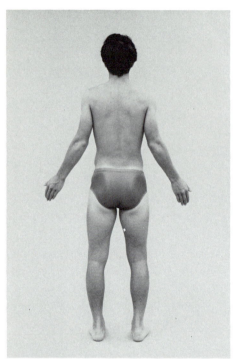

FIG 1–2.
Dorsal surface, anatomical position. Shoulder height is equal, and the iliac crests, marked in this case by the upper border of the bathing suit, are level. Note normal valgus alignment of the elbow and slight varus alignment of the knees.

If the patient is asked to bend forward at the waist with the hands hanging freely downward, the posterior aspects of the rib cage should be equal in height.

Viewed from the front, the bony ridges of the clavicles are obvious. The sternoclavicular notch is visible and the sternocleidomastoid muscles can be seen as oblique straps running from the occipital region of the skull to the sternoclavicular joints. The prominences of the shoulders overlying the acromioclavicular joints should be equal in height. The anterior chest wall should be symmetric and nipple height should be equal. The anterior aspects of the iliac crests are normally level.

Range of Motion

Cervical and Thoracolumbar Spine

Most children can flex the cervical spine far enough forward to touch the chin to the chest and can extend the neck far enough to look directly overhead (Fig 1–3). Symmetric lateral rotation and lateral bending of approximately 45 degrees are possible for most children. The orientation of the joints of the thoracic spine and the attached ribs prevents significant motion of the thoracic region of the spine. Flexion and extension as well as lateral bending and rotation occur primarily at the thoracolumbar junction and in the lumbar spine. Apparent flexion and extension of the lumbar spine usually involves flexion and extension at the hip joints as well. It is difficult to isolate pure flexion and extension of the spine, but for practical purposes most children can bend forward far enough to touch their fingertips to the floor. Lateral bending and lateral rotation are also complex motions. If the pelvis is stabilized to prevent pelvic motion, most patients can laterally bend approximately 20 to 30 degrees in the thoracolumbar spine and can laterally rotate a similar amount.

Muscle Testing

Testing of the strength of the major muscle groups of the spine is indicated when observation or palpation disclose muscle wasting or tenderness or when patients report pain or weakness. Patients with normal strength in the flexor muscles of the neck can touch the chin to the chest while the examiner applies contrapressure over the forehead. If neck flexor function is not normal, patients may be asked to touch their chin to the chest from the supine position. Inability to flex the neck against gravity implies poor neck flexor muscle function. The ability to sit with the head upright and unsupported

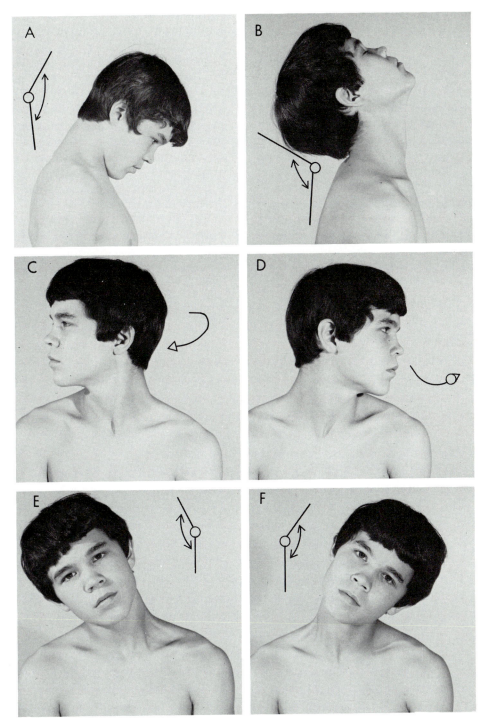

FIG 1–3.
Normal range of motion, cervical spine. **A,** flexion. **B,** extension. **C,** right rotation. **D,** left rotation. **E,** right lateral bend. **F,** left lateral bend.

implies at least fair neck extensor muscle function. Resistance can be added by asking the patient to extend his neck while the examiner applies backward pressure over the occiput. Patients with trace or poor neck extensor muscle function are unable to sit in the upright position unless their head is supported.

Function in the trapezius muscle can be assessed by asking the seated patient to shrug his shoulders, first against gravity and then against added resistance. Function in the supporting muscles of the scapula can be assessed by asking the standing patient to press his extended arm firmly against a wall. Winging of the scapula implies weakness in the serratus anterior muscle group and is a sign of injury to the long thoracic nerve.

Common Abnormalities

Back pain and resultant restriction of motion is uncommon in children. Most commonly it implies soft tissue injury resulting from recent trauma or overuse. Spontaneous improvement is the rule. Chronic or severe back pain, or pain associated with neurologic abnormalities is strongly suggestive of inflammatory or neoplastic lesions of the spinal column or enclosed neural elements. Passive motion should not be forced past comfortable limits, and under no circumstances should patients with suspected spine injury be moved for physical examination before careful radiologic examination.

At the time of initial inspection, asymmetry in trunk configuration, cutaneous lesions, and muscle atrophy or spasm should be noted. Dimpling, hairy nevi, and open defects suggest underlying spinal column abnormality. Café-au-lait spots or hemangiomas may be associated with generalized disorders such as neurofibromatosis or arteriovenous malformation.

Scoliosis screening should be an inte-

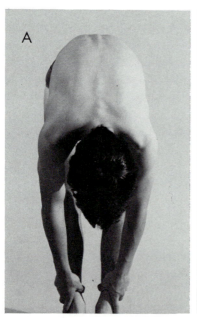 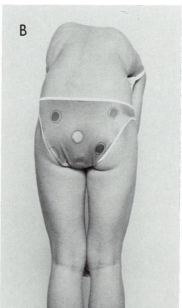

FIG 1–4.
Forward-bending test for scoliosis. **A,** rib height should be symmetric. **B,** asymmetry indicates probable underlying spine deformity.

gral part of routine musculoskeletal examination. The forward bend test is the most sensitive determinant of the presence of underlying spine deformity in juvenile and adolescent patients. The standing child is asked to bend forward at the waist, allowing the hands to hang freely (Fig 1–4). Asymmetry of the posterior ribs in this position is highly suggestive of underlying spine deformity. The child should next be asked to turn sideways and bend forward. Sharp angular deformity in the thoracic region indicates the presence of kyphotic deformity.

UPPER EXTREMITY

Topographic Anatomy

The topographic anatomy of the upper extremity is illustrated in Figure 1–5. The deltoid muscle arises from the clavicle, acromion, and scapular spine and inserts into the deltoid tuberosity of the humerus; it gives bulk to the shoulder. Most of the bulk of the anterior aspect of the upper arm is formed by the biceps muscle. At the elbow, the bony prominences of the medial and lateral epicondyle are obvious. When the elbow is flexed, the point of the olecranon process is visible. Immediately below the lateral epicondyle, a slight prominence formed by the radial head can be seen. A shallow depression between the two bony prominences is usually present.

The styloid process of the distal end of the ulna is prominent on the ulnar side of the dorsal aspect of the wrist. The pisiform bone is palpable on the volar aspect of the ulnar side of the wrist at the base of the hypothenar eminence. The anatomical snuffbox at the base of the thenar eminence on the lateral aspect of the wrist is bordered by the thumb abductor and extensor tendons (tenderness in this region after a fall on the outstretched hand may indicate either distal radial or navicular fracture). The pulse of the radial artery is palpable at the base of the thenar eminence on the volar aspect of the wrist; the ulnar artery can sometimes be palpated proximal to the pisiform bone on the ulnar side of the wrist. Separate proximal and distal palmar creases are normally present on the anterior aspect of the hand. The distal palmar crease overlies the metacarpophalangeal joints. On the dorsal aspect of the wrist, the extensor tendons of the fingers and thumb are evident. Transverse creases overlie the interphalangeal joints on the anterior and posterior surfaces of the hand. Slight fusiform widening at the interphalangeal joints is common; tapering of the fingers between the joints is normal.

The digits of the hand are best named rather than numbered to avoid confusion. Hence, thumb, index, middle, ring, and small are properly used in referring to the fingers rather than first, second, third, etc. Little confusion arises when the small finger is referred to as the fifth finger, but "the first digit" might be taken to mean either the index finger or the thumb, unless carefully specified.

In general, *abduction* is motion away from the sagittal plane of the body and *adduction* is motion toward the sagittal plane (see Chapter 3). In the hand and foot, abduction and adduction are used relative to motion toward or away from the central digit. *Opposition* is the term applied to the complex motions required to bring the pulp of the thumb into contact with the pulp of the fingertips (Fig 1–6).

Range of Motion

Shoulder

The wide arcs of motion normally present around the shoulder can be broken down into six components (Fig 1–7).

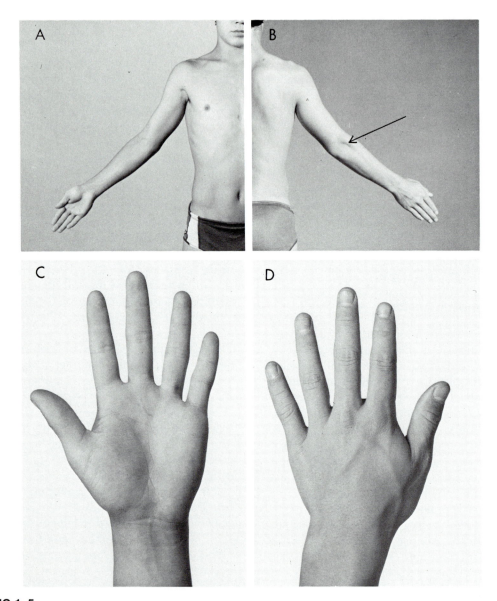

FIG 1–5.
Topographic anatomy of the upper limb. The anterior surface of the upper limb is referred to as volar, the posterior surface as dorsal. **A** and **B,** the trapezius muscle, sloping downward and outward from the cervical spine to the spine of the scapula, marks the upper border of the shoulder girdle. The acromioclavicular joint at the junction of the distal end of the clavicle and acromion process of the scapula is obvious in this subject. The deltoid muscle provides the rounded contour of the shoulder; the biceps muscle provides the bulk of the anterior portion of the upper arm; the triceps muscle underlies the skin of the posterior surface of the upper arm. A shallow recess overlies the junction of the radial head and lateral condyle of the distal humerus *(arrow)*. Obliteration of this fossa is a sign of elbow joint effusion. The extensor muscles of the wrist arise from a common origin immediately above it. The ulnar nerve passes in a shallow groove behind the medial epicondyle of the humerus and is easily palpated there. **C,** the proximal palmar crease overlies the carpus. The radial pulse is palpable at the base of the thenar eminence; the ulnar pulse is palpable at the base of the hypothenar eminence. The distal palmar crease overlies the metacarpophalangeal joints. **D,** the ulnar styloid is palpable on the ulnar border of the wrist. Transverse creases overlie the interphalangeal joints.

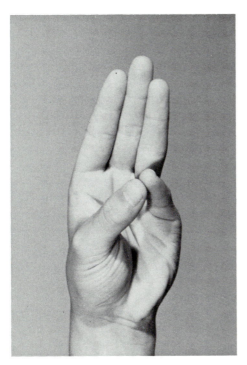

FIG 1–6.
Opposition of the thumb and small finger.

Abduction and adduction are motions parallel to the frontal plane of the body. In full abduction, the arm is in a straight overhead position, termed 180 degrees. To achieve this, the scapula must rotate on the chest wall posteriorly, and the greater tuberosity of the humerus must rotate below the acromioclavicular joint. To adduct the humerus across the midline, slight flexion or extension of the shoulder joint is necessary. Flexion and extension are motions parallel to the sagittal plane. Full flexion is said to be present when the long axis of the humerus is at a right angle to the long axis of the body. The end point of extension is that at which further posterior motion of the arm cannot be obtained without trunk flexion. This usually occurs at about 45 degrees. Medial and lateral rotation are motions parallel to the transverse plane; 60 to 90 degrees of rotation in each direction is normal.

Elbow

The normal active and passive ranges of motion of the elbow are from full extension, or 0 degrees of flexion, to 130 degrees of flexion (Fig 1–8). Many individuals are capable of several degrees of hyperextension. In full extension, 5 to 8 degrees of valgus alignment of the elbow is normal. When the elbow is flexed to 90 degrees and the thumb is held in a vertical position, 90 degrees of pronation (medial rotation) and 90 degrees of supination (lateral rotation) are usually present.

Wrist

The wrist can normally be flexed 70 to 80 degrees from a neutral position and extended to approximately 70 degrees (Fig 1–9). Ulnar deviation of approximately 25 degrees in the frontal plane is normal. Radial deviation of 5 to 10 degrees is usually present.

Hand

Flexion and extension of the metacarpophalangeal joints and interphalangeal joints permit the hand to clasp and open fully (Fig 1–10). The metacarpophalangeal joints of the index through small fingers normally extend approximately 10 degrees and flex to 90 degrees. The proximal interphalangeal joints move from 0 degrees of flexion (full extension) to 100 degrees of flexion. The distal interphalangeal joints move from 0 degrees of flexion to approximately 80 degrees of flexion. The ability to touch the fingertips to the palm is a rapid screen for full finger flexion.

A complex series of motions at the carpometacarpal, metacarpophalangeal, and interphalangeal joints of the thumb permit the tip of the thumb to be opposed to the tips of any of the fingers. Opposition requires normal joint mobility and coordinated function of extrinsic and intrinsic thumb muscles (see Fig 1–6). It is often difficult to test opposition specifically in a

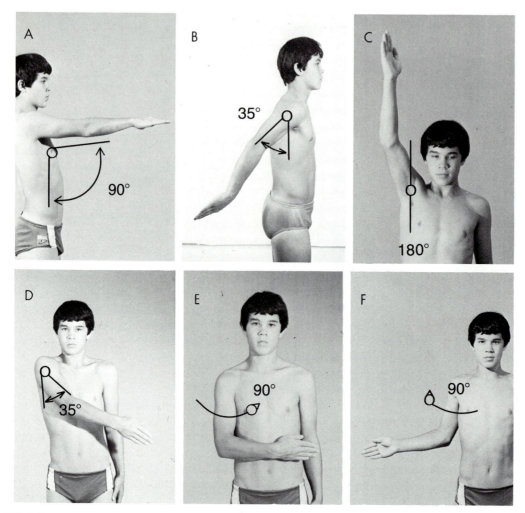

FIG 1–7.
Normal range of motion of the shoulder joint. **A,** 90 degrees of flexion. **B,** 35 degrees of extension. **C,** 180 degrees of abduction. **D,** 35 degrees of adduction. **E,** 70–90 degrees of medial rotation. **F,** 90 degrees of lateral rotation.

young child; the ability to pinch small objects such as keys or raisins is evidence of normal function.

Muscle Testing

Tests for muscle function in the upper extremity are indicated when there is evidence of muscle atrophy or wasting on visual inspection or palpation. Deltoid function (axillary nerve, nerve roots C-5, C-6) may be tested by asking the patient to ab-duct the arm, first against gravity and then against added resistance. Biceps muscle function (musculocutaneous nerve, roots C-5, C-6) may be tested by asking the patient to flex the forearm, first against gravity and then against added resistance. The biceps tendon reflex may be elicited by percussion over the biceps tendon in the antecubital fossae. Triceps muscle function (radial nerve, roots C-5, C-6, C-7, C-8) may be tested by asking the patient to actively extend the elbow

FIG 1–8.
Normal range of motion of the elbow. **A,** full extension (0 degrees of flexion). **B,** 135 degrees of flexion. **C,** 90 degrees of supination. **D,** 80–90 degrees of pronation.

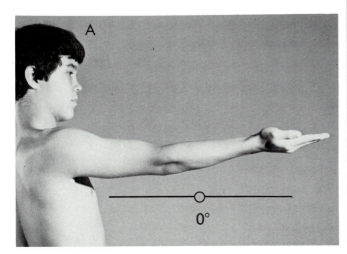

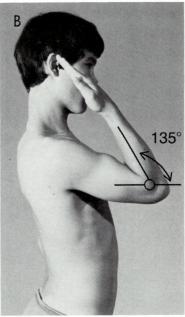

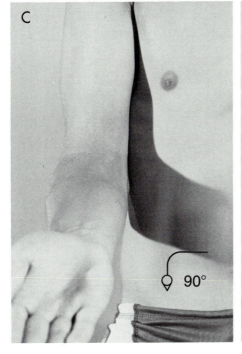

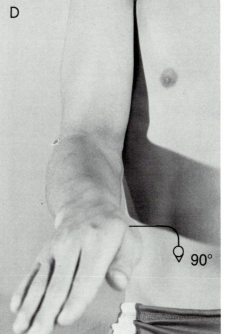

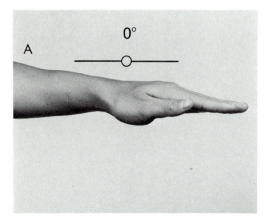

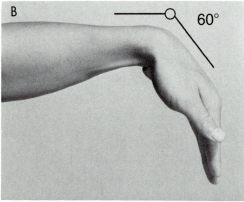

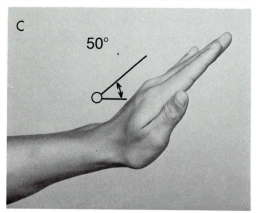

FIG 1–9.
Normal range of flexion and extension of the wrist. **A,** neutral position. **B,** full flexion (60–70 degrees). **C,** full extension (50–70 degrees).

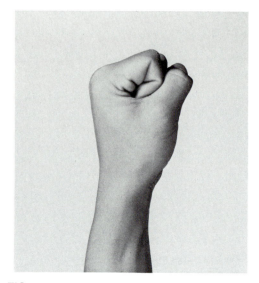

FIG 1–10.
Full flexion of the metacarpophalangeal and interphalangeal joints.

against gravity and then against added resistance. The triceps tendon reflex may be elicited by percussion over its tendon at the elbow. Function in the wrist extensors (radial nerve and posterior interosseous nerve, roots C-6, C-7, C-8) may be tested by extension of the wrist. Wrist flexor function (median and ulnar nerves, roots C-5 through T-1) may be tested by the ability to flex the wrist against gravity and then against added resistance.

Common Abnormalities

Any congenital abnormality, inflammatory disease process, or injury to the bony, ligamentous, or muscular components of the shoulder girdle will interfere with shoulder motion. In the neonate, limited active or passive motion may indicate malformation, fracture, infection, or nerve injury. It may be difficult to identify the cause on examination alone; radiologic evaluation and appropriate laboratory studies usually permit diagnosis.

In older patients, the history is a valuable clue.

Limitation of motion of the elbow is present in patients with congenital bony abnormalities of the proximal radius or ulna and in patients with inflammatory diseases or injuries around the elbow. If active motion is restricted, gentle, passive motion of the elbow joint should be carried out. The most common cause of acute, painful limitation of elbow motion in young children is radial head subluxation (nursemaid's elbow). This is discussed in detail in Chapter 2.

LOWER EXTREMITY

Topographic Anatomy

The topographic anatomy of the lower extremity is illustrated in Figure 1–11. The upper borders of the lower limb are formed laterally by the anterior superior iliac spine and medially by the pubic tubercle. The inguinal ligament stretches between the two points. The femoral nerve, artery, and vein pass beneath the inguinal ligament near the median border. The associated inguinal lymph nodes are often enlarged and tender in children with inflammatory disorders of the lower extremity. The ischial tuberosity is palpable in the buttock beneath the gluteal fold. The greater trochanter of the femur can be felt at the lateral aspect of the hip, just distal to an imaginary line drawn between the ischial tuberosity and the anterior superior iliac spine.

The anterior mass of the thigh is formed by the quadriceps muscle. Distally, the quadriceps tendon tapers to insert into the superior aspect of the patella; the patellar tendon continues downward to insert into the tibial tuberosity. Shallow depressions are normally present on the medial and lateral aspects of the knee at the upper and lower poles of the patella;

obliteration of these recesses is an early sign of intra-articular swelling (see Chapter 4).

The posterior aspect of the knee, called the popliteal fossa, is bordered medially and laterally by the hamstring tendons. Through the popliteal fossa pass the major neurovascular structures of the lower leg. The pulse of the popliteal artery is palpable within the popliteal fossa. The fibular head is visible on the lateral aspect of the knee; just beneath the fibular head, the peroneal nerve winds around posteriorly to anteriorly to supply the muscles of the anterior compartment.

The medial and lateral malleoli are prominent at the ankle; the medial malleolus normally lies slightly anterior to the lateral malleolus. A shallow depression is usually present on the lateral aspect of the ankle just anterior to the lateral malleolus. Swelling in this region is an early sign of inflammation within the ankle joint. The posterior tibial pulse is palpable behind the medial malleolus; the dorsalis pedis pulse is palpable on the dorsum of the foot.

Range of Motion

Hip

The hip joint is a ball-and-socket that permits motion in three planes. Although motion is more constrained than in the shoulder, the other major ball-and-socket joint, stability is much greater. Flexion and extension of the hip occur parallel to the sagittal plane of the body; abduction and adduction occur parallel to the frontal plane. Medial and lateral rotation occur in the transverse plane. Care must be taken to separate apparent hip motion from hip motion combined with pelvic rotation or trunk flexion. Because the joints of the lumbar spine allow motion parallel to the sagittal plane, hip flexion and extension are easily confused with trunk flexion.

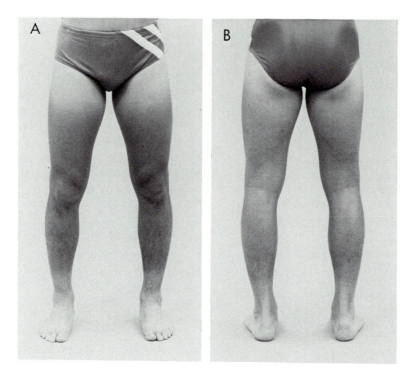

FIG 1–11.
Surface anatomy of the lower limb. **A,** anterior surface. The inguinal ligament forms the upper border of the lower limb. The mass of the thigh is formed by the quadriceps muscle, which inserts through its tendinous aponeurosis into the superior border of the patella. Shallow depressions are normally present medially and laterally above and below the patella. The anteromedial surface of the tibia is subcutaneous from the knee to the ankle. The medial malleolus of the tibia and the lateral malleolus of the fibula are prominent. **B,** the gluteus maximus muscle forms the mass of the buttock. The medial and lateral hamstring muscles form the muscle mass of the posterior aspect of the thigh; their tendons form the medial and lateral borders of the popliteal fossa. The gastrocnemius and soleus muscles form the mass of the calf and taper into the Achilles tendon at the back of the heel.

Minor restrictions of hip motion are easily masked.

Hip flexion should be tested in the supine position. Both hips should be fully flexed simultaneously to eliminate trunk flexion and to stabilize the pelvis (Fig 1–12,A). While one hip is held in the flexed position, the other is slowly extended (Fig 1–12,B). The process is then reversed to test the opposite hip. Zero degrees flexion is defined as the point at which the long axis of the femur is parallel to the long axis of the body; the hip can usually be flexed at least 120 degrees. Often contact of the surface of the thigh with the ante-

rior surface of the trunk is the limiting factor for hip flexion.

Hip extension is best tested in the prone position (Fig 1–13). From a position of 0 degrees flexion, the hip can usually be extended 20 to 30 degrees. Medial and lateral rotation of the hip joint also can be readily evaluated in the prone position. With the knee flexed to a right angle, the lower leg serves as a protractor to estimate hip rotation. Lateral rotation of the hip joint occurs as the lower leg is rotated toward the midline of the body; the angular deviation of the lower leg from vertical is an indication of the amount of lat-

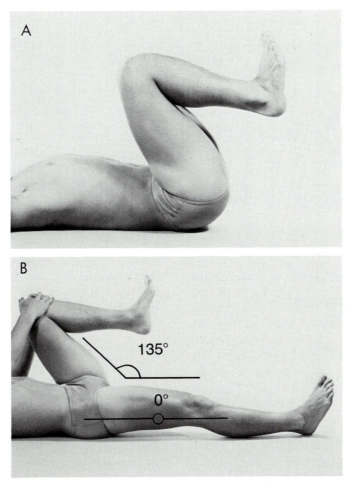

FIG 1–12.
Hip flexion. **A,** both hips are flexed simultaneously to eliminate lumbar lordosis and stabilize the pelvis. **B,** while one hip is held flexed, the hip in question is extended.

eral rotation possible. Medial rotation of the hip joint can be tested by reversing the process and moving the lower leg laterally. Medial and lateral rotation are age dependent; in the neonate, lateral rotation normally exceeds medial rotation. During early childhood medial rotation frequently exceeds lateral rotation. By the time skeletal maturity is reached, symmetric arcs of medial and lateral rotation are present.

Abduction and adduction of the hip are best tested in the supine position. Ab-duction is lateral motion away from the midline in the frontal plane of the body; 45 degrees of abduction is usually possible. Adduction is motion toward the midline; 30 degrees of adduction is usually possible.

Knee

The knee is not a simple hinge joint. Although flexion and extension are the principal motions present at the knee joint, internal and external rotation of the tibia on the femur are also possible. The

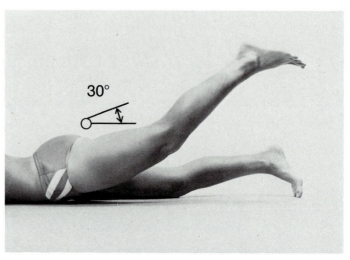

FIG 1–13.
Extension of the hip joint.

normal range of extension of the knee joint is from 0 to 130 degrees of flexion (Fig 1–14,A and B). Internal and external rotation of 10 degrees each around the long axis of the tibia are usually present when the knee is flexed 90 degrees. The range of motion of the knee is usually tested with the hip either extended or slightly flexed. When the hip is flexed more than 90 degrees, hamstring tightness may interfere with the ability to fully extend the knee joint.

Ankle

The ankle is considered to be in the neutral position when the long axis of the foot makes a right angle with the long axis of the leg in the midsagittal plane. The ankle can normally be dorsiflexed 20 degrees and plantar flexed 30 to 50 degrees from this neutral position (Fig 1–15). About 5 degrees of inversion (sometimes termed supination) and 5 degrees of eversion (sometimes termed pronation) are possible in the subtalar ankle joint. Ankle motion may be quickly tested by asking a patient to walk first on his toes to test for plantar flexion and then on his heels to test for dorsiflexion. Inversion may be tested by asking the patient to walk on the lateral borders of the foot; eversion may be tested by instructing the patient to walk on the medial borders of the foot.

Muscle Testing

The major flexor of the hip joint is the iliopsoas muscle (femoral nerve, L-1, L-2, L-3). Iliopsoas function is usually tested with the patient in the seated position with the hip and knee flexed to 90 degrees. The patient should be asked to flex the thigh, first against gravity and then against added resistance. The major extensor of the hip joint is the gluteus maximus muscle (inferior gluteal nerve, S-1). Gluteus maximus function should be tested with the patient in the prone position with the hip in full extension and the knee flexed 90 degrees to relax the hamstring muscle. The patient is then asked to further extend the hip by lifting the thigh off the examining table, first against gravity and then against added resistance. The major abductors of the hip are the gluteus medius and gluteus minimus muscles (superior gluteal nerve, L-5). Abductor function is tested with the patient lying on the side opposite that to be tested. The patient is asked to abduct the leg, first against gravity and then against

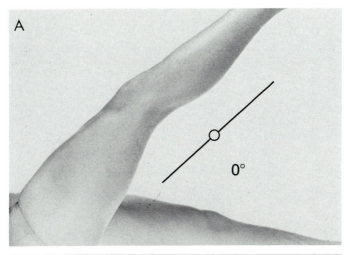

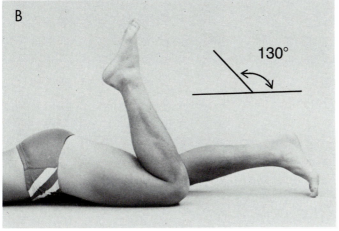

FIG 1–14.
Flexion and extension at the knee joint. **A,** full extension of the knee. **B,** full flexion.

added resistance. The primary adductor of the hip is the adductor longus (obturator nerve, L-3, L-4). Function of the primary adductor and the secondary adductors (adductor brevis, magnus, pectineus, and gracilis) can be tested by asking the patient to adduct his legs against the resistance of the examiner's hands.

Trendelenburg's Test

The abductor muscles of the hip, the gluteus medius and minimus, support the pelvis in the single-stance phase of gait. Abductor weakness, whether caused by nerve injuries or by functional shortening as a result of alterations of the bony archi-

tecture around the hip, results in a characteristic lurching gait. To test for abductor competence, the child is asked to stand unsupported and to sequentially flex first one hip and knee, then the other. When the abductor muscles are weak, the pelvis opposite the affected hip will dip downward during single-leg stance (see Fig 5–4).

The primary extensor of the knee is the quadriceps muscle (femoral nerve, L-2, L-3, L-4). Quadriceps function is usually tested in the seated position with the hip and knee flexed to 90 degrees. The patient is asked to extend his knee, first against gravity and then against added re-

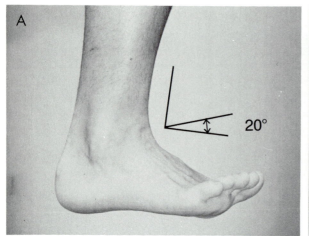

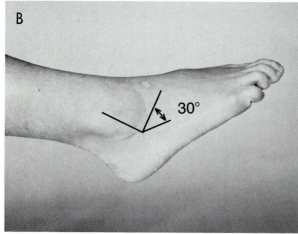

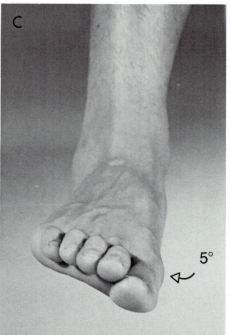

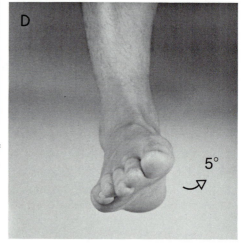

FIG 1–15.
Normal range of motion of the ankle joint. **A,** 10–20 degrees of active dorsiflexion. **B,** 30–50 degrees of active plantar flexion. **C,** 5–10 degrees of eversion. **D,** 5–10 degrees of inversion.

sistance. The hamstring muscles, semi-membranous and semitendinous muscles, and biceps femoris are the primary flexors of the knee joint. They are innervated by the tibial portion of the sciatic nerve, L-5 and S-1. Hamstring function may be tested by asking the prone patient to flex his knee, first against gravity and then against added resistance.

The major dorsiflexors of the foot are the tibialis anterior muscle, extensor hallucis longus muscle, and extensor digitorum longus muscle (deep peroneal nerve, L-4, L-5). Dorsiflexor function can be quickly tested by asking the patient to walk on his heels. The anterior tibial muscle may be isolated for testing by asking the patient to dorsiflex and invert his foot against gravity and then against added resistance. The extensor hallucis longus muscle may be isolated by asking the patient to extend his great toe against resistance. In a similar manner, the extensor digitorum longus muscle may be tested by asking the patient to dorsiflex his other toes against resistance. The plantar flexors of the ankle are the gastrocnemius and soleus muscles (tibial nerve, S-1, S-2), the flexor hallucis longus muscle (tibial nerve, L-5), flexor digitorum longus muscle (tibial nerve, L-5), and tibialis posterior muscle (tibial nerve, L-5). Plantar flexion function may be tested by asking the patient to walk on tiptoe. The tibialis posterior muscle may be isolated by asking the patient to plantar flex and invert his foot. The flexor digitorum longus and flexor hallucis longus muscles may be tested in similar fashion. The evertors of the foot are the peroneus longus and brevis muscles. Function may be tested by asking the patient to evert his foot, first against gravity and then against added resistance.

SPECIAL EXAMINATIONS

Neonatal Examination

A careful evaluation of the musculoskeletal system should be part of every newborn examination. Early diagnosis and prompt referral are essential elements of care in many of the orthopedic problems of infancy and early childhood. Review of the history of pregnancy and identification of possible familial musculoskeletal disorders should precede examination. Systematic evaluation of the head, neck, trunk, and extremities will disclose most of the common disorders of the musculoskeletal system. The following outline is offered only as a guide for neonatal neuromusculoskeletal examination; format is less important than thoroughness.

I. History
  A. Significant findings
    1. Family history of musculoskeletal disease
    2. Exposure to teratogenic substances, irradiation, or infections during pregnancy
    3. Bleeding during pregnancy
    4. Lack of normal fetal movement
    5. Breech position
    6. Traumatic delivery, birth asphyxia, neonatal sepsis
II. Physical examination
  A. Head and neck
    1. Skull symmetric and normally shaped
    2. Neck normal in configuration; no torticollis
    3. Normal range of passive motion
  B. Trunk
    1. Anterior and posterior surfaces closed; no signs of neural tube defects
    2. No cutaneous dimpling, nevi, or hairy patches over spine
    3. Trunk symmetric, with no evidence of underlying spinal deformity
    4. Both clavicles present
  C. Upper limbs
    1. All parts of both extremities present; both limbs equal length
    2. Spontaneous motion present at shoulders, elbows, wrists, and hands in both limbs
    3. Full range of passive motion present at shoulders, elbows, wrists, and fingers
  D. Lower limbs
    1. All parts of both limbs present; limbs equal in length, thigh folds symmetric
    2. Spontaneous motion present at hips, knees, ankles, and in feet
    3. Symmetric passive abduction possible at both hips in both flexion and extension

4. No instability with Barlow's or Ortolani's test (see Chapter 5)
5. No intrinsic foot deformity present

Examination of the Hand

Examination of the hand is often difficult in young patients. Injured and apprehensive children cooperate poorly, and many of the diagnostic tests useful in older patients are impossible to perform. Fortunately, a reasonable assessment of hand function can be made by observation alone. The position of the hand at rest frequently offers clues to the nature of acute injuries, and the opportunity to watch the child at play permits assessment of function in congenital anomalies and remote injuries.

At rest, the flexor and extensor tendons combine to curl the hand into a loose fist with increasing amounts of flexion at the metacarpophalangeal and interphalangeal joints from the index through small fingers. Nerve injuries that affect the extrinsic or intrinsic muscles of the hand and tendon lacerations in the forearm, wrist, or hand upset the balance of the flexor and extensor muscles. As a result, affected fingers may lie slightly above or slightly below their uninjured neighbors. Lacerations of extensor tendons result in flexor muscle overpull. The corresponding metacarpophalangeal joint drops into more flexion than the adjacent digits. Often some voluntary extension of the metacarpophalangeal joint remains present through the action of tendinous interconnections on the extensor surface of the hand. Interphalangeal joint extension, a function of intrinsic hand musculature, remains intact.

Flexor tendon lacerations result in extensor muscle overpull. When the flexor digitorum superficialis tendon alone is cut, the involved finger will lie in slightly more extension than its neighbors. Flex-

ion of both the interphalangeal joints remains present through the action of the flexor digitorum profundus muscle. When both tendons are cut, interphalangeal joint flexion is impossible, but flexion of the metacarpophalangeal joints resulting from intrinsic hand muscle function remains present.

In older and more cooperative patients, function of the flexor tendons of the fingers may be more accurately assessed. Function of the profundus flexor tendons may be tested by holding the proximal interphalangeal joints in extension and asking the patient to flex the distal interphalangeal joints. Because the flexor digitorum superficialis muscle and flexor digitorum profundus muscle combine to produce flexion of the proximal interphalangeal joint, the profundus tendon must be blocked to test superficialis function. To isolate the flexor digitorum superficialis muscle for testing, the distal interphalangeal joints of the adjacent fingers should be held in extension while the patient is asked to flex the proximal interphalangeal joint of the finger in question. Because the flexor digitorum profundus muscle functions as a unit, profundus function in a single finger can be blocked by stopping profundus function in the adjacent fingers.

The intrinsic muscles of the hand provide flexion of the metacarpophalangeal joint and extend the distal and proximal interphalangeal joints. They are responsible for positioning the hand in grasp while the extrinsic muscles provide power. In addition, the intrinsic muscles abduct and adduct the fingers toward and away from the central ray. Intrinsic muscle function can be quickly assessed by asking the patient to abduct and adduct the fingers toward and away from the midline.

The principal vascular supply to the hand is provided by anastomotic branches of the radial and ulnar arteries. The radial

pulse can be felt at the base of the thenar eminence just lateral to the palmaris longus tendon. The ulnar pulse can be felt on the anterior and ulnar aspect of the wrist just proximal to the prominence of the pisiform bone. Competence of the anastomotic network can be tested by performing Allen's test. The patient is first asked to flex the fist tightly; the examiner then palpates firmly over both the radial and the ulnar arteries to occlude blood flow temporarily. The palm should blanch when the fist is relaxed. If the ulnar artery is competent, circulation will return to the hand when pressure is released over the ulnar artery with the radial artery still occluded. The test may be reversed to check the competence of radial blood flow. This should be done whenever radial artery catheterization is contemplated.

Sensation in the hand is provided by branches of the radial, median, and ulnar nerves. The radial nerve supplies most of the dorsal surface of the hand to the level of the proximal interphalangeal joints. The ulnar nerve provides sensation to the ulnar aspect of the dorsal surface of the hand as well as to the small finger and the ulnar half of the ring finger. The remainder of the hand is supplied by the median nerve.

In children old enough to cooperate, light pinpricks can be used to chart areas of sensory loss. This is impossible in younger patients. Sometimes an otoscope with a magnifying lens can be used to determine areas of nerve damage. Microscopic beads of moisture are usually present in the creases of the fingertips. When digital nerves are divided, sympathetic

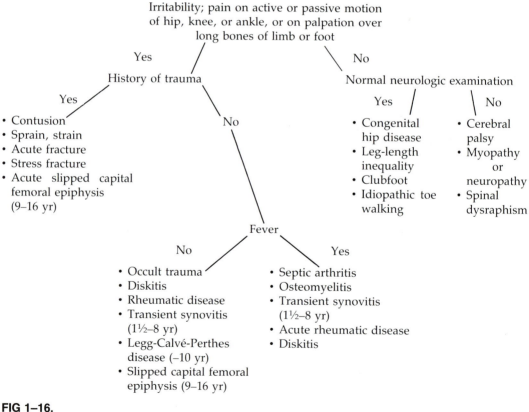

FIG 1–16.
Differential diagnosis of a limp in childhood.

function is disrupted as well, and the affected area is dry. This is, however, a crude test at best.

Evaluation of Limp

Refusal to walk, hip pain, and limping are common occurrences in childhood. They may be the common clinical manifestations of a variety of disorders. A screening guide for evaluation of the child with leg pain or who limps is presented in Figure 1–16. The specific disorders are covered elsewhere in this text.

Examination of the Knee and Foot

Because of the frequency and importance of knee injuries and foot deformities, physical diagnosis of these regions is covered in more detail in subsequent chapters.

SUGGESTED READINGS

Enneking WF (ed): *Manual of Orthopedic Surgery*, ed 4. Chicago, American Orthopedic Association, 1972.

Bates B: *A Guide to Physical Examination*. Philadelphia, JB Lippincott Co, 1979.

Hoppenfeld S: *Physical Examination of the Spine and Extremities*. New York, Appleton-Century-Crofts, 1976.

2

Musculoskeletal Trauma

Contusions, sprains, strains, fractures, and dislocations are common consequences of many routine childhood activities. Data gathered by the Massachusetts Department of Public Health indicate that injuries account for approximately 15% of all hospitalizations in children; in children older than 6 years, extremity fractures are a more common cause of hospitalization after injury than any other cause, including intracranial injury. Injuries resulting in emergency room visits occur 10 to 20 times more commonly than those requiring hospitalization. It has been estimated that as many as one child in five will sustain an extremity injury serious enough to require emergency room evaluation in a given year. Fortunately, most childhood mishaps are minor, and

few result in permanent sequelae. It is, however, extremely important to carefully evaluate all children with extremity injuries for other more threatening conditions.

Because of the ability of the growing musculoskeletal system to adapt and remodel, many fractures in children can be treated much more simply than similar fractures in adult patients. Anatomical alignment is rarely necessary, healing occurs rapidly, and little formal rehabilitation is usually required.

The generally good prognosis after childhood musculoskeletal injury is not absolute, however, and there is no room for complacency in the management of trauma. The immediate potential complications of open fractures and of vascular

compromise are as severe in children as in adults. In addition, injuries to the active growth plate may produce late sequelae not obvious at the time of fracture; shortening and angular deformity may follow injuries that appear initially minor. Furthermore, serious extremity injuries may be associated with damage to other organ systems. An obvious fracture is only the tip of the iceberg; in addition to local soft tissue damage, occult intracranial, thoracic, or abdominal injury may be present.

Every trauma patient, regardless of age, requires rapid systemic evaluation before attention is directed to the musculoskeletal injuries. A preliminary history should be obtained while a screening examination is conducted. Certain information is of immediate importance in planning treatment:

1. Respiratory and cardiovascular function immediately after injury and during subsequent transport.
2. Level of consciousness at the time of and subsequent to injury.
3. Extremity weakness or loss of sensation at injury or during transport.
4. Estimated blood loss, if any.
5. Current medications and drug allergies.
6. Preexisting serious illnesses.
7. Time of the patient's last meal.
8. Immunization status.

Other information, including the detailed mechanism of injury, can be obtained with the remainder of the history after resuscitation has been completed.

At the time of initial evaluation, the airway, thorax, abdomen, and neurologic systems should be examined in rapid sequence. Treatment of extremity wounds seldom takes precedence. Local pressure will control bleeding, and splintage will provide pain relief and prevent further soft tissue damage until more pressing problems have been solved. The conscious, cooperative patient with no neck or back pain, no signs of trauma around the head or neck, and no neurologic abnormalities on screening examination may be safely moved during initial examination. The unconscious patient or the patient with back or neck pain or maxillofacial trauma must be assumed to have spinal column injury and must not be moved until splinted on a backboard. A normal initial screening examination in patients with other signs that suggest the possibility of injury to the cervical spine does not eliminate the need for careful radiographic examination and repeat clinical evaluation of the cervical spine.

Competency of the upper airway can be established by looking and listening. The thorax should be carefully inspected for signs of blunt or penetrating injury. Bruising across the sternum is a warning sign of mediastinal injury. Gentle lateral chest compression produces pain in conscious patients with rib fractures; careful palpation localizes the injury. Dullness to percussion and decreased breath sounds at the bases of the lungs suggest the presence of hemothorax; increased resonance and decreased breath sounds imply pneumothorax.

Abdominal contusions should be noted. Bruises around the lower rib margins may indicate renal injury. Discoloration over the symphysis pubis or swelling in the groin are signs of possible lower genitourinary tract injury. Bowel sounds are often decreased after injury and are not reliable indicators of visceral injury. Guarding, rigidity, and rebound tenderness are more consistent signs.

Contusions around the head and neck are important signs of possible intracranial injury. They may be the only signs in unconscious patients, and they signal the need for careful neurologic evaluation. Pupillary reflexes and ocular motility should be tested; funduscopic examina-

tion should be performed. Sensation and weakness in the extremities may be quickly tested to complete the initial neurologic examination.

Musculoskeletal evaluation should begin after preliminary examination has been completed and after steps necessary to ensure the patient's overall safety have been taken. The sites of contusions, lacerations, and open fractures should be noted. Peripheral pulses, capillary refill, and sensation in injured extremities should be evaluated without moving the limb. Open wounds should be cultured and covered with dry sterile dressings. Bleeding should be controlled by local pressure; tourniquets should not be used. Attempts to probe wounds and to clamp bleeding vessels with hemostats in the poorly lighted and unsterile emergency room usually further compound soft tissue damage and may irreversibly injure a vessel that could have been repaired.

Before roentgenograms are obtained, suspected fractures should be splinted to decrease discomfort and prevent further soft tissue damage. Deformed limbs should be splinted where they lie; reduction should be attempted before roentgenographic examination only when blood flow distal to the fracture is in jeopardy. Padded wooden, aluminum, or temporary plaster splints are best; folded blankets are also useful. Air splints must be used with caution since they may further compromise impaired circulation by compressing the soft tissues of the limb. Ice packs must not be placed under air splints since they may cause local frostbite.

X-ray examination of the suspected fracture and of the joints proximal and distal to it should be obtained. Roentgenograms must be made in two planes, at a right angle to each other without moving the injured extremity, if at all possible. If necessary, the physician should accompany the patient to the x-ray department to assist in positioning and to ensure that proper views are obtained.

CHILD ABUSE

Incidence

The characteristic soft tissue and bone injuries in abused children have been reported frequently since the mid-19th century; Kempe and co-workers in 1962 used the term "battered child syndrome" to refer to the association of soft tissue, bone, and psychological injuries suffered by these unfortunate patients. It is difficult to determine the exact incidence of child abuse since many cases probably escape attention. The magnitude of the problem is enormous; estimates run between 60,000 and 5 million incidents per year in the United States. More than 2,000 children per year die from deliberately inflicted injuries. Child abuse is second only to sudden death syndrome as a cause of death in infants and second only to true accidental death in children between 1 and 5 years of age. Throughout history it has probably accounted for more children's deaths than any other causes except famine and plague.

Manifestations

It is usually impossible to obtain a clear history in suspected cases of child abuse. Parents are often reluctant to discuss the cause of injury and frequently alter the details of the history on repeated inquiry. Conflicting explanations may be offered by those in contact with the child, and often the alleged mechanism of injury does not correlate with physical findings. This pattern should immediately raise suspicions of abuse.

Contusions, lacerations, and burns in various stages of healing are the most common external signs of repeated abuse.

At times, the imprint of the object with which the child was injured is present. Rope burns and strap marks, andiron and fist imprints do not occur accidentally. Multiple cigarette burns on the back and buttocks do not occur by chance; burns of varying ages on the hands are evidence of neglect, if not abuse. Human bites on extremities are always deliberate.

Contusions on the trunk may indicate serious abdominal trauma. The possibility of visceral rupture must be considered and carefully evaluated. Death from hypovolemic shock may occur with hepatic or splenic rupture. Blunt trauma to the paraspinal area may injure the kidneys; hematuria indicates the urgent need for intravenous pyelography.

Intracranial bleeding is a common cause of death in abused children. Those who recover from chronic subdural hematomas often have residual intellectual and neurologic impairment. Contusions around the eyes and nose, on the scalp, and around the base of the skull are signs of potential intracranial injury. Immediate neurosurgical consultation is mandatory if the level of consciousness is altered or if findings on the peripheral neurologic examination are abnormal.

Fractures are important manifestations of abuse. Often children present for treatment after the acute soft tissue signs of injury have subsided, and radiologic findings may be the only objective evidence of suspected abuse. Important findings include:

1. Spiral fractures of long bones of the limbs in infants less than 1 year old. The twisting loads required to produce such injuries do not often occur accidentally in prewalkers (Fig 2–1,A and B).

2. Hypertrophic callus formation and florid periosteal elevation. These are manifestations of incomplete immobilization and delay in obtaining help after injury (Fig 2–1,C).

3. Multiple fractures in various stages of healing in children without evidence of metabolic bone disease.

4. Multiple rib fractures or vertebral compression fractures.

Management

Skull, spine, rib, pelvis, and long-bone roentgenograms should be obtained in all suspected cases of physical abuse. In infants, a "babygram" can be obtained. In larger children, specific x-ray examinations are necessary. At times a bone scan may be helpful in identifying multiple fracture sites.

Suspected abuse victims should be hospitalized immediately to break the cycle of repeated abuse. Careful, complete medical evaluation is essential to identify all potential injuries. Injuries should be carefully documented, and photographs of contusions, burns, and lacerations should be made for later reference. Adequate medical records help greatly if subsequent court appearances are necessary.

Prompt and thorough medical evaluation and treatment may be lifesaving for abused children. Family counseling and outside support often successfully break the cycle of repeated abuse and are an important part of treatment of the patient and his family. At times, however, counseling is unsuccessful, and a child must be removed from the home to prevent further injury.

SOFT TISSUE INJURIES

The trunk and extremities are composed of materials with different mechanical properties. During use, normal and abnormal forces are distributed between bone and soft tissue. Skin, fascia, ligaments, and muscles undergo greater de-

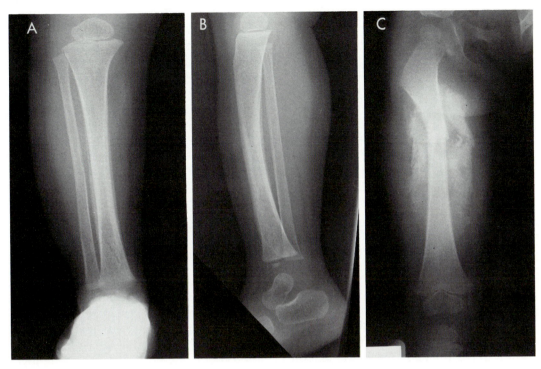

FIG 2–1.
Roentgenographic signs of child abuse. **A** and **B,** anteroposterior and lateral views of spiral tibial fracture in a 2-year-old toddler, with periosteal new bone formation at time of initial examination. **C,** hypertrophic callus formation in a femur fracture not immobilized after injury.

formation in response to loading than does underlying bone; areas of increased stress may develop where soft tissues are tethered to bone by vascular or neural connections. When applied forces are too great to be absorbed by temporary deformation, damage to soft or hard tissues occurs. In general, the nature and extent of any injury depend both on the characteristics of the injuring force and on the mechanical properties of the tissues that absorb it.

Contusions

Bruises are probably the most common musculoskeletal injuries of childhood. Injuring forces produce local increases in stress, with disruption of the microcirculation to the affected region.

Bleeding into surrounding soft tissues gives rise to the familiar black-and-blue discoloration. Most contusions are of little consequence and can be treated with ice packs and rest. At times, however, contusions signal more serious underlying injury. Children with bruises around the head and neck must be carefully evaluated for intracranial or cervical spine injury. As previously mentioned, contusions on the thorax or abdomen may be associated with serious visceral damage. Multiple poorly explained contusions in various stages of healing may be signs of neglect or abuse. In each of these instances, the occult problems are of much greater importance than the obvious contusions. Hospitalization and thorough evaluation are justified if any possibility of underlying injury exists.

Ligament and Tendon Injuries

Serious ligament and tendon injuries are uncommon in children. Forces sufficient to cause ligament or tendon failure in adults more often result in greenstick fracture or fracture through the growth plate in children. Ligament and tendon injuries become more common in adolescence as closure of the growth plate occurs.

The nomenclature of ligament and tendon injury is confusing. The terms *sprain* and *strain* are often used interchangeably to apply to both ligament and tendon damage. Furthermore, strain is not usually used in its strict mechanical sense of change in length resulting from applied load. In an attempt to minimize confusion, the American Medical Association Committee on Sports Medicine has recommended that the term strain be used to refer to tendon or muscle-tendon unit injuries and that the term sprain be reserved for ligament injuries.

Ligaments and tendons in vivo exhibit complex mechanical behavior. The site of failure, extent of damage, and energy absorbed before failure depend on both the magnitude and the rate of application of the applied load. Experimental work indicates that ligaments absorb more energy before failure when loaded rapidly than when loaded slowly. Deformation occurs sequentially, first by elastic displacement of individual fiber bundles, then by failure of isolated fibers of the ligament, and finally by ligament rupture. Experimentally, loads applied slowly tend to cause failure at the bone-ligament junction, while loads applied more rapidly cause failure within the substance of the ligament.

Sprains and strains vary in clinical severity. In minor or grade I sprains or strains, the injured ligament or tendon appears intact when tested manually.

Pathologic studies show only disruption of local microcirculation and failure of a few fibers of the involved ligament or tendon. Pain, tenderness, and discoloration may be present at the site of injury, but muscle strength is normal, and joint instability is not present. Rest, ice packs, and mild analgesics provide symptomatic relief. Functional return may occur in a few days, although it takes some weeks for the damaged tendon or ligament to regain full strength.

In more severe injuries, partial failure of the involved ligament or tendon occurs. This failure is manifested respectively by joint laxity or muscle weakness. This is sometimes termed grade II injury. Pain and tenderness at the site of injury are more pronounced, and joint effusion may be present. Permanent laxity and weakness of the injured ligaments and tendons may result unless the extremity is protected while healing occurs. Immobilization for 4 to 6 weeks may be necessary for recovery of strength in the injured tissues.

Rupture of a ligament is marked by frank instability of the involved joint on examination. This is called grade III injury. Traumatic joint effusion is the rule when damage to the joint capsule accompanies failure of the supporting ligaments. Pain may be severe, and local tenderness will usually be present at the site of ligament failure.

Tendon failure results in the inability of the involved muscle to produce its usual effect. Hematoma formation is common, and a bulge in the affected muscle is often seen. Tenderness at the site of tendon rupture is present, and spasm of the involved muscle is severe. Such injuries are uncommon in children.

Joint dislocation is a special case of soft tissue failure. Rupture of supporting capsular ligaments and/or tendons permits partial or complete displacement of articular surfaces. *Luxation* or *dislocation* are terms applied to complete displacement of the bony elements of a joint. *Subluxation* is the term applied to partial displacement of joint surfaces.

Traumatic dislocation and subluxation may occur alone or in combination with fractures of the involved bone. In addition, vascular injury and nerve damage sometimes accompany dislocations of a major joint. A careful search for associated neurologic and vascular damage must be made as soon as the patient's general medical condition permits. Roentgenograms should be obtained before reduction is attempted because of the danger of impaling soft tissues on sharp fracture fragments or trapping articular fragments within a joint. Fractures, vascular deficits, and nerve injuries must be carefully documented before reduction for both medical and legal purposes. Disloca-

tions should be reduced as promptly as possible; dislocations associated with vascular or nerve compromise are orthopedic emergencies.

FRACTURES IN CHILDREN

Failure of bone under load indicates that the ability of the bone to store energy by temporary deformation has been exceeded. Bone may fail in either tension or compression, but few fractures in vivo are the result of pure compressive and tensile loads. Ordinarily, bending loads result in compressive stress on one side of the bone and tensile stresses on the opposite side of the bone. In children, the result may be an incomplete or greenstick fracture, with disruption of the bone cortex on the tension side and deformity of the cortex on the compression side (Fig 2–2). Loads of higher magnitude or longer du-

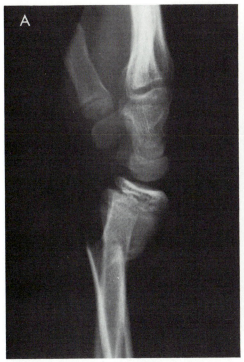
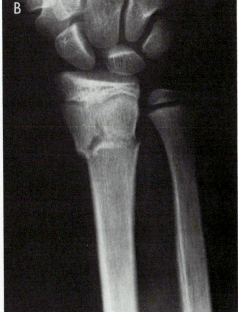

FIG 2–2.
A and **B,** greenstick or incomplete fractures of the distal radius and ulna.

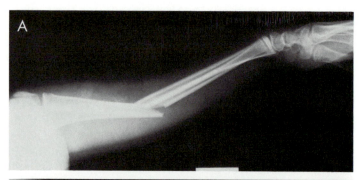

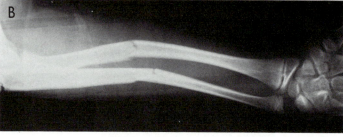

FIG 2–3.
Complete radial and ulnar shaft
fractures. **A,** lateral view. **B,**
anteroposterior view.

ration may produce complete fractures
(Fig 2–3). Axial loading may produce
buckling of one or both cortices, repre-
senting compression failure (Fig 2–4). The
addition of twisting forces to tension and
compression forces produces spiral or
oblique fracture surfaces (Fig 2–5).

The number of fracture fragments
produced at the time of failure is related
to the magnitude and rate of application
of the deforming load. Like ligaments and
tendons, bone absorbs more energy before failure when loaded rapidly than
when loaded slowly.

Fractures with two principal fragments are termed *simple fractures* and result from low-magnitude, slowly applied
loads (Fig 2–6,A). Fractures wth three or
more fragments are termed *comminuted
fractures* and result from more rapidly ap-

FIG 2–4.
Compression or buckle fracture of
distal radial metaphysis, sometimes
referred to as a "torus" fracture.

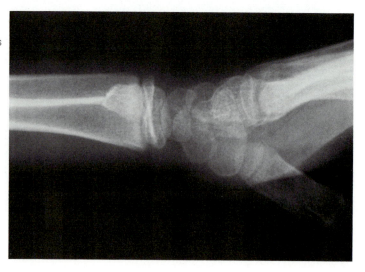

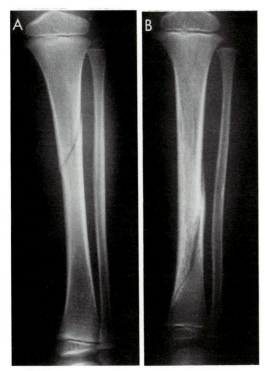

FIG 2–5.
Minimally displaced tibial shaft fractures resulting from torsional loads. **A,** short oblique fracture of proximal diaphysis of tibia. **B,** long spiral fracture of distal tibial diaphysis. In children too young to walk, such fractures are often evidence of deliberately inflicted injury.

plied, higher-magnitude loads (Fig 2–6,B). Comminution of a fracture surface implies increased damage to soft tissues surrounding the fracture site.

Fractures in which there is no break in the skin over the fracture site are said to be *closed fractures*. In *compound* or *open fractures*, the skin over the fracture site has been broken. In some cases, penetration occurs from within, as a small spike of bone punctures the skin; in other instances, the skin may be broken by the object that produces the fracture. In the most severe instances, large, open skin defects are present over the fracture site. All open fractures, regardless of degree, must be considered contaminated. Gas

gangrene, sepsis, and death so often followed open fractures in the pre-Listerian era that for centuries amputation was considered appropriate primary treatment. The combination of thorough surgical debridement under sterile conditions, open wound management, and effective antibiotic therapy has dramatically changed the prognosis of open fractures in this century.

Open fractures are orthopedic emergencies. Primary treatment in the accident ward should consist of wound culture and application of sterile dressings. The child's immunization records should be reviewed and tetanus toxoid administered, if necessary. Passive immunization with human tetanus immune globulin is rarely necessary but must be considered individually for each patient based on

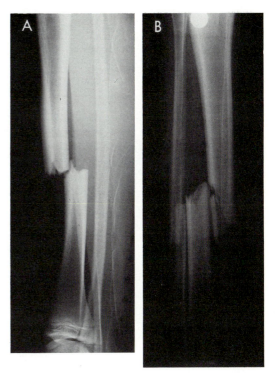

FIG 2–6.
A, simple fracture of tibial mid-diaphysis. **B,** comminuted tibial diaphyseal fracture with associated fibular fracture.

wound characteristics and the previous immunization status of the patient. It is not indicated in individuals who have ever received two or more injections of tetanus toxoid. It may be necessary in patients with grossly contaminated wounds who have not received prompt care and whose immune status is unclear. An intravenous line should be established, and broad-spectrum antibiotic therapy with semisynthetic penicillin or cephalosporins should be started. Surgical debridement of the fracture site should be carried out in the operating suite as soon as the patient's overall condition is stable. Open fractures should not be managed in the emergency room.

Fractures that involve the growth plate are unique problems of childhood. Although many growth plate fractures heal rapidly without permanent sequelae, others may be complicated by partial or complete growth arrest with resultant late deformity. The outcome of growth plate injury depends to a great extent on the location of fracture planes within the physis.

The growth plate can be divided into a number of distinct histologic regions (Fig 2–7). Longitudinal growth occurs

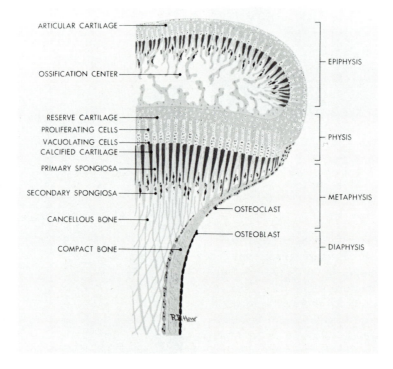

FIG 2–7.
Anatomy of the end of a growing long bone. The *diaphysis* or shaft of a long bone separates the centers for longitudinal growth at each end of the bone. The *metaphysis* is that segment in which calcified chondroid is replaced by enchondral bone. *Physis* is the term most correctly applied to the active cartilage growth plate; it is often but less precisely called the epiphyseal plate. The *epiphysis* is that portion of a long bone that caps the physis. It contains a secondary center of enchondral ossification, and its cartilaginous covering contributes to the growth of the joint surface. The physis itself is divided into zone of resting cartilage, proliferating cells, vacuolated cells, and calcified chondroid bars. An area of weakness exists in the lower layers of the physis, where the chondroid matrix is undergoing provisional calcification. (From Rubin P: *Dynamic Classification of Bone Dysplasias,* Chicago, Year Book Medical Publishers, 1964, p 4. Reproduced by permission.)

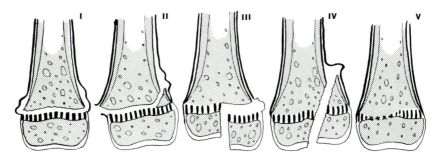

FIG 2–8.
Classification of physeal and epiphyseal fractures. Type I physeal fractures occur through the region of provisional calcification. The proliferating portion of the physis remains attached to the epiphysis and is not damaged. Type II fractures include a segment of the metaphysis. Again, the proliferative portions of the physis are intact. Type III fractures extend through a segment of the provisional calcification zone, then cross through the epiphysis to the articular surface. Type IV fractures extend obliquely from the metaphysis across the physis and into the epiphysis. They, too, are articular fractures. Type V fractures are crush injuries of all or a portion of the physis. The proliferative zones of the physis sustain irreversible damage. (From Salter RB, Harris WR: Injuries involving the epiphyseal plate. *J Bone Joint Surg* 1963, 45A:587. Reproduced by permission.)

through a process of chondrocyte replication, intercellular matrix production, provisional calcification, and endochondral remodeling. A zone of weakness exists in the region where chondroid matrix is undergoing provisional calcification. This area resists shear poorly and is a consistent site of fracture when loaded abnormally. From this zone, fracture lines may extend into the metaphysis, epiphysis, or both.

Physeal and epiphyseal fractures occur in a number of well-defined patterns. The studies of Poland, Aitken, Salter, Harris, and others have produced a logical classification system for growth plate fractures that permits estimation of prognosis for fracture healing and potential growth disturbance (Fig 2–8). In general, fractures through the zone of provisional calcification, with or without an accompanying metaphyseal fragment, can be expected to heal promptly without growth disturbance if adequate alignment is attained. Fractures that involve both the physis and the epiphysis have a more guarded prognosis since they have crossed the germinal layer of the growth plate. Bridging between the epiphysis and

the physis may occur if anatomical reduction is not achieved. Late angular deformity and articular incongruity may occur.

Crushing injuries of the growth plate have a poor prognosis. Damage to the germinal layers of the growth plate may permanently alter or arrest longitudinal growth. Shortening, angular deformity, or both are consistent sequelae.

Basic Treatment Principles

Children's fractures are often treated quite differently from the same types of fractures in adults. Prompt union is the rule in most fractures, and prolonged immobilization is usually unnecessary. Anatomical alignment of metaphyseal and diaphyseal fractures is rarely necessary in children. Many fractures need no reduction at all; immature bone has remarkable remodeling potential. Within certain guidelines, angular deformity can be expected to correct spontaneously with growth. In general, residual angulation in the plane of motion of the adjacent joint will remodel. Angulation close to the joint will remodel more than midshaft angulation, and younger children have much more remodeling potential than adolescents. After growth plate closure, little remodeling can be expected. Rotational malalignment and angulation not parallel to the plane of motion of the adjacent joints will not remodel and should not be accepted.

Overriding and side-to-side contact of diaphyseal fracture fragments is often desirable. Fracture usually stimulates bone growth in children, and end-to-end apposition or overdistraction may result in undesirable lengthening. One to 2 cm of override is usually acceptable in femoral shaft fractures in children over age 2 years and under age 10 years.

Anatomical alignment is necessary only in specific fractures in children. Fractures that involve an articular surface must be accurately repositioned, or joint incongruity will result. Late degenerative arthritis is a potential complication. Type III and type IV growth plate fractures also must be anatomically reduced to prevent late deformity. In these instances, open reduction and limited internal fixation are sometimes employed.

Extremity ischemia is an important potential complication of certain fractures and dislocations. Injuries around the elbow and knee and fractures of the forearm and lower leg particularly may be associated with vascular impairment. Unfortunately, the full extent of vascular compromise may not be immediately obvious. Irreversible soft tissue damage often occurs before circulatory impairment is recognized.

Interruption of the blood supply to the limb distal to the site of fracture or dislocation may occur in several ways. Avulsion of a major arterial branch may occur at the time of fracture or dislocation in an area where the vessel is tethered by soft tissue attachments. In other cases, sharp fracture fragments may partially or completely lacerate nearby vessels. In some instances, critical arteries may sustain intimal damage during the deformation that occurs at the time of fracture or dislocation. Displaced fracture fragments or dislocated articular surfaces may on occasion occlude vascular structures by direct pressure. Finally, swelling within a closed fascial compartment or under a tightly applied circular cast may gradually elevate interstitial pressure above capillary pressure, decreasing tissue perfusion. Unless such swelling is decompressed, tissue death will ensue.

Extremity ischemia is an absolute emergency. Irreversible soft tissue damage begins within 6 to 8 hours of vascular occlusion and progresses rapidly. Muscle and nerve necrosis resulting in paralysis, contracture, deformity, and occasional amputation are predictable consequences of delay in diagnosis and treatment. The symptoms and signs of vascular compromise vary with the nature of the lesion. Complete interruption of arterial supply at the instant of injury produces a cold, pallid or cyanotic, and pulseless extremity. Capillary occlusion due to swelling within a compartment may be more subtle. Pulses distal to the fracture site may be present, and pallor or cyanosis may not be obvious. Capillary refill in nail beds is not a reliable index of vascular adequacy. Pain is a consistent sign, however, of impending ischemia. After splintage, the pain associated with fracture or dislocation usually diminishes. Persistent, progressive pain following splintage, accentuated by attempts to actively or passively move fingers or toes distal to the site of injury, is a cardinal sign of ischemia. Paresthesia and paralysis distal to the injury site are frequent additional findings in ischemia.

Treatment of suspected ischemia must be immediate. Irreversible damage may occur during observation and deliberation periods. If reduction of a displaced fracture or dislocation does not immediately improve circulation, emergency surgical consultation is necessary. Prompt arteriography and surgical repair can salvage an otherwise hopeless situation.

UPPER EXTREMITY FRACTURES AND DISLOCATIONS

Injuries of the bones of the upper extremity are the most common fractures of childhood. They vary greatly in complexity and prognosis. In some cases, a great deal of displacement can be accepted. In other cases, anatomical alignment must be obtained for satisfactory results. Some fractures are appropriately treated by the primary physician; others should be promptly referred for orthopedic care. In the following section, upper extremity fractures will be discussed in detail, both to provide guidelines for primary care and to acquaint the primary physician with the principles of subsequent management.

Clavicular Fractures

Clavicular fractures are common in infancy and childhood. They may occur through lateral compression during the course of a difficult delivery or may result from force transmitted across the glenohumeral joint during a fall on the outstretched arm. Most fractures involve the midportion, although fractures at either end are occasionally seen in older children and adolescents (Fig 2–9). Incomplete or greenstick fractures are common in infants and toddlers. Complete fractures are more common in older children.

Pain, tenderness, and deformity at the fracture site are common clinical findings in older children. Younger children at times sustain incomplete clavicle fractures with few associated symptoms, and a diagnosis may be made only when a parent notes the lump associated with callus formation. In neonates and infants pseudoparalysis of the upper extremity on the affected side and crepitation on palpation over the fracture site may be present. An anteroposterior roentgenogram of the shoulder will confirm the diagnosis.

Neurovascular complications are rarely associated with clavicular fractures but may occur with injuries produced by large-magnitude, high-velocity forces. Sharp, comminuted fracture surfaces may pierce overlying skin or damage the subclavian vessels. Damage to the brachial plexus or underlying lung is another potential complication. The initial evaluation of patients with clavicular fractures should include careful assessment of neurologic and vascular function in the injured extremity.

Most clavicular fractures can be treated quite simply. In infants and young children, reduction is usually unnecessary. A flannel-filled, figure-of-eight bandage or commercial clavicle strap provides sufficient immobilization for comfort and healing. Union will occur in 10 to 14 days in infants and 4 to 5 weeks in toddlers and young children. A palpable mass of callus may appear during healing. This usually remodels within 2 to 3 years.

Clavicle fractures in older children and adolescents may be more difficult to manage. Fractures in good alignment may be placed in a clavicle strap without reduction for 4 to 8 weeks. Sharply angulated or grossly displaced clavicle fractures may heal slowly and produce an undesirable prominence in adolescents. Such fractures must at times be treated by closed reduction before application of a figure-of-eight bandage. Open reduction is rarely if ever necessary.

Incomplete clavicle fractures can be appropriately treated by primary care physicians. With complete fractures, especially those accompanied by marked angulation or displacement, patients should be referred for treatment after ini-

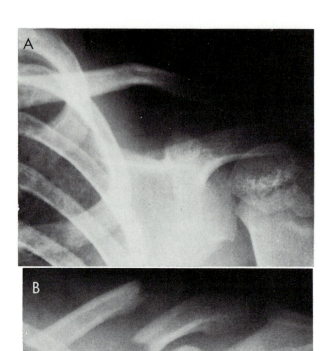

FIG 2–9.
A, incomplete fracture of the distal third of the clavicle in a 3-year-old child. **B,** complete fracture of the clavicle in a 12-year-old girl.

tial splinting. Even though most such fractures do well with no further treatment, delayed union or excessive callus formation may be alarming to the patient and his or her parents. Consultation should be obtained immediately when neurovascular complications are present.

Proximal Humeral Physeal Fractures

The radiologic appearance of the proximal humerus varies with age. A secondary ossification center for the humeral head is usually present by age 6 months but may be present at birth. An ossification center for the greater tuberosity usu-

ally appears by age 2 years and unites with the head by age 7 years. A separate ossification center for the lesser tuberosity is occasionally seen and usually unites with the humeral head by age 5 to 7 years (Fig 2–10). The humeral shaft is ossified at birth. The proximal growth plate closes between ages 17 and 22 years.

Proximal humeral physeal fractures are uncommon. They occur most often in late childhood and early adolescence. The usual mechanism of injury is a fall on the outstretched arm while the shoulder is in extension. Adduction and external rotation create a shearing force across the proximal humeral growth plate, resulting

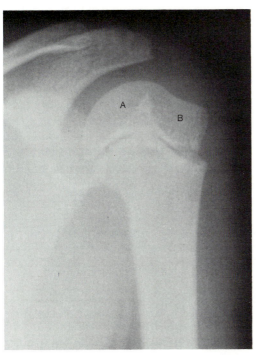

FIG 2–10.
Proximal humeral growth plates in an 8-year-old child. The centers for the humeral head *(A)* and greater tuberosity *(B)* have united. The growth plate between the head and the shaft remains open.

in type I or II physeal fractures (Fig 2–11). Type III, IV, and V injuries are uncommon.

Pain and tenderness at the fracture site, and resistance to attempts at passive motion are consistent findings. Good quality anteroposterior and lateral roentgenograms of the shoulder are necessary to confirm the diagnosis and to distinguish it from glenohumeral dislocation. Manipulation should not be performed before roentgenograms are obtained; damage to the brachial plexus or axillary vessels could occur.

Minimally displaced proximal humeral fractures require no reduction and can be treated by the primary physician. The involved arm should be supported in a sling and bandaged to the trunk with a loose elastic wrap or commercial immobilizer. Union occurs within 4 to 6 weeks. Rough play and contact sports should be restricted for an additional month.

More displaced fractures should be referred for evaluation and treatment. Closed reduction and spica cast immobilization are required for some displaced fractures, and at times open reduction may be necessary to remove interposed soft tissues.

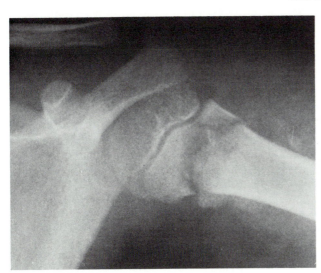

FIG 2–11.
Type II fracture of the proximal humeral growth plate. A metaphyseal fragment remains attached to the humeral head.

Shoulder Dislocation

The shoulder joint is not intrinsically stable and so requires the support of the joint capsule and surrounding muscles for proper function. The remarkable range of motion of the glenohumeral joint depends on smooth and synchronous interaction of both intrinsic and extrinsic shoulder musculature. Shoulder dislocation is usually the result of damage to the supporting capsular structures and muscles of the glenohumeral joint.

Traumatic shoulder dislocation is rare in children. Abnormal loading usually produces physeal fracture rather than dislocation prior to closure of the growth plate. Traumatic dislocation becomes more common in late adolescence and may occur throughout adult life. Although the shoulder may dislocate in any direction, in most cases the proximal humerus moves anteriorly and inferiorly in response to forced abduction, lateral rotation, and hyperextension. Damage to the neurovascular structures of the axilla may occur at the time of dislocation or during forceful manipulative reductions. The nerve supply to the deltoid muscle is especially at risk. Careful neurovascular examination should precede and follow reduction attempts.

Radiologic evaluation of suspected glenohumeral dislocation is strongly advised before treatment (Fig 2–12). Fracture of the proximal humerus may be confused with or may accompany shoulder dislocation, and attempts at reduction may impale major neurovascular structures on the jagged surface of the proximal humeral shaft (Fig 2–13). Follow-up roentgenograms are essential to document reduction.

Closed reduction of shoulder dislocations is almost always possible. A wide variety of manipulations has been proposed. Adequate muscle relaxation is a prerequisite. Although in most cases in-travenous drugs can be used, on occasion general anesthesia is necessary. Forceful manipulation may fracture the proximal humerus or damage the brachial plexus and axillary artery. In most cases, reduction can be obtained by applying traction to the arm in the line of deformity. Countertraction can be applied with a sheet passed through the axilla and led to the opposite side. Steady traction combined with gentle internal and external rotation usually achieves reduction. Immobilization in a sling and swathe bandage or a commercial shoulder immobilizer is necessary for 3 to 4 weeks to permit healing to occur. Surgical repair may be necessary to prevent late degenerative joint disease in patients with recurrent traumatic dislocation.

Some adolescents experience partial or complete spontaneous dislocation of the shoulder. The dislocations are usually painless, although often alarming, and may occur during sleep or routine athletic activities. This spontaneous dislocation probably represents a disturbance in the force couples produced by the shoulder muscles and can occur even in adolescents who have no history of prior shoulder injury. Some adolescents can voluntarily sublux the glenohumeral joint.

Voluntary shoulder dislocation can be quite refractory to treatment. In some patients it may be a manifestation of underlying psychological disturbance. In most cases, a concerted trial of strengthening exercises should be employed before consideration is given to other forms of treatment. Surgical repair is usually reserved for patients who continue to dislocate despite genuine attempts at nonoperative treatment.

Humeral Metaphyseal and Diaphyseal Fractures

Fractures of the proximal humeral metaphysis may result from the same forces

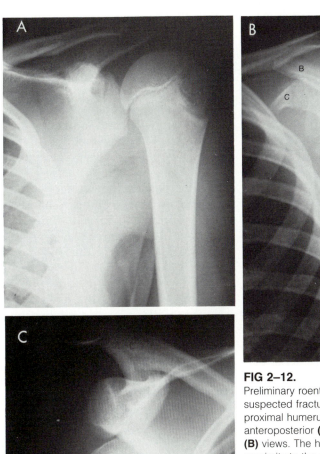

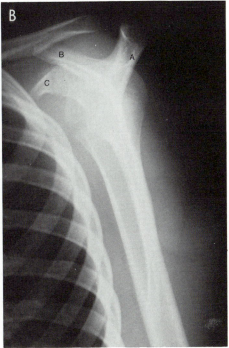

FIG 2–12.
Preliminary roentgenograms of a patient with suspected fracture or dislocation of the proximal humerus should consist of anteroposterior **(A)** and transscapular lateral **(B)** views. The humeral head should lie in close proximity to the glenoid fossa of the scapula on the anteroposterior view. On the transscapular lateral view, the humeral head normally lies centered beneath the acromion *(A)*, scapular spine *(B)*, and coracoid process *(C)*. Dislocation is manifested by displacement of the humeral head from its normal position **(C).**

that produce proximal humeral physeal fractures and may be confused clinically and radiologically with physeal fractures. Diaphyseal fractures may result from transverse loads, torsional loads, or combinations of both. As in other fractures, comminution at the fracture site implies more severe associated soft tissue injury. The radial nerve is particularly at risk in distal humeral fractures, as it spirals close to the bone on its lateral aspect. Injury to the radial nerve at this level results in wrist drop and paralysis of finger extensors.

Minimally to moderately displaced proximal humeral metaphyseal fractures require no reduction. Immobilization for 3 to 4 weeks in a sling and swathe bandage usually suffices. Patients with humeral shaft fractures may require more formal treatment and should be referred for treatment. Closed reduction and immobilization in a plaster splint or hanging cast are often needed (Fig 2–14). Open reduc-

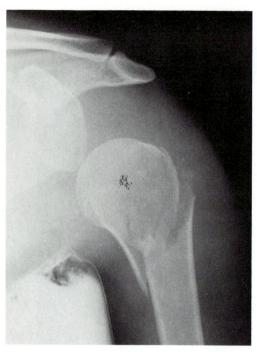

FIG 2–13.
Fracture dislocation of the shoulder in an 18-year-old woman. The inferior dislocation of the humeral head was not recognized at the time of initial evaluation; open reduction of the shoulder was subsequently required.

tion and internal fixation are rarely necessary in children.

Elbow Injuries

Elbow injuries are common in children and range in severity from uncomplicated sprains to open, comminuted fractures with associated neurovascular damage. Careful evaluation of sensation, motor function, and vascular status of the forearm and hand are essential first steps in assessment of elbow injuries. Flexor weakness and paresthesia in the hand, with pain on active or passive motion of the fingers, may indicate secondary ischemia in the forearm.

The soft tissues and bones of the el-bow are complex, and radiographic anatomy can be quite confusing. Normal growth plates may be mistaken for fracture lines, and minimally displaced fractures are often overlooked. Six separate secondary ossification centers contribute to the formation of the elbow joint, and there is considerable individual variation in the times of their first appearance and subsequent closure (Figs 2–15 through 2–17).

The distal humerus has four separate ossification centers and is composed of articular and nonarticular portions. The medial and lateral epicondyles are outside the synovial cavity of the elbow joint and serve as sites of origin for the flexor and extensor muscles of the forearm. The medial and lateral condyles, often referred to as the trochlea and capitulum, respectively, form the articular surface of the humeral side of the elbow joint. The secondary ossification center for the lateral condyle appears at about age 1½ years and fuses with the distal humerus at about age 15 years. The secondary center of the medial epicondyle appears at about age 5 years and unites with the humerus between ages 16 and 20 years. The secondary center of the medial condyle appears between 8 and 10 years and is often quite irregular in contour. Its growth plate closes between ages 17 and 20 years. The lateral epicondylar epiphyseal center develops around age 10 years. It may appear as a small flake of bone on the lateral side of the elbow and is often confused with an avulsion fracture. It fuses at around age 20 years.

The secondary ossification center for the radial head appears between ages 4 and 6 years and usually fuses with the proximal radial shaft by age 16 to 17 years. The secondary center at the proximal end of the ulna is one of the most confusing of the elbow epiphyses. It usually appears between ages 10 and 12 years

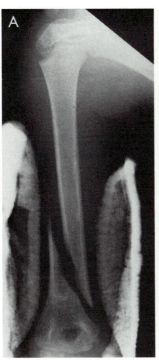
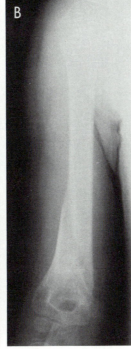

FIG 2–14.
A, long oblique fracture of the humeral shaft in an 18-month-old girl. A plaster splint has been applied for immobilization. Spiral fractures such as this occur uncommonly during routine activities of toddlers; the possibility of abuse or neglect must be considered. **B,** healing has occurred after one month of immobilization in a plaster splint and sling. Anatomical reduction is unnecessary; with growth and remodeling the normal configuration of the humeral shaft will be restored.

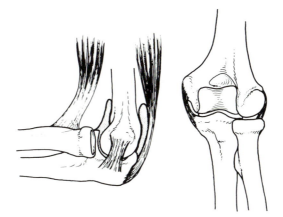

FIG 2–15.
Left, anterior view of the bones of the elbow. The medial and lateral condyles, referred to as the trochlea and capitulum, are intra-articular and covered with hyaline cartilage. The medial and lateral epicondyles are extra-articular and serve as attachment points for the ligaments of the elbow and common flexor and extensor muscle origins. *Right,* lateral view of the bones of the elbow. The sigmoid fossa of the ulna articulates with the trochlea of the distal humerus. The radial head articulates with the capitulum. Support for the joint is derived from medial and lateral collateral ligaments and from the muscles that power the joint. (From Enneking WF (ed): *Manual of Orthopedic Surgery,* ed 4. Chicago, American Orthopedic Association, 1972, p 136. Reproduced by permission.)

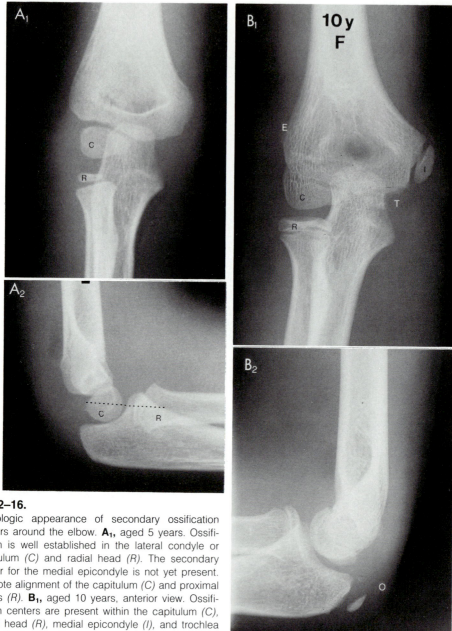

FIG 2–16.
Radiologic appearance of secondary ossification centers around the elbow. **A₁,** aged 5 years. Ossification is well established in the lateral condyle or capitulum *(C)* and radial head *(R)*. The secondary center for the medial epicondyle is not yet present. **A₂,** note alignment of the capitulum *(C)* and proximal radius *(R)*. **B₁,** aged 10 years, anterior view. Ossification centers are present within the capitulum *(C)*, radial head *(R)*, medial epicondyle *(I)*, and trochlea *(T)*. A fleck of ossification can be seen in the region of the lateral epicondyle *(E)*. **B₂,** the olecranon secondary ossification center *(O)* is evident on the lateral view. Irregularity of this ossification center is common.

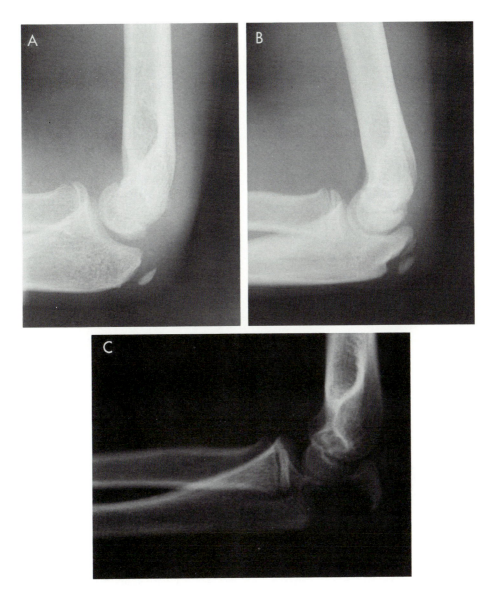

FIG 2–17.
Secondary ossification center or fracture through proximal ulna? **A,** normal olecranon ossification center. **B,** normal olecranon ossification center. Irregularity is common. **C,** olecranon fracture. Note wide displacement produced by pull of triceps muscle.

and closes between ages 14 and 16 years. In the interval, it is often mistaken for a fracture of the proximal ulna.

Injuries around the elbow joint are often the result of combinations of transverse and torsional loads. Both intra-articular and extra-articular fractures may occur, and fracture dislocations are common. Accurate early diagnosis is important since delay in treatment may result in malunion or nonunion with significant late deformity. Severely displaced fractures are not difficult to recognize clinically or radiologically. More minimally displaced fractures can be troublesome. Comparison views of the opposite elbow can be helpful in distinguishing growth plates from fracture lines.

Small collections of fat are present in the olecranon and coronoid fossae of the distal humerus, between the bone and the synovial lining of the joint. Injuries that cause extra-articular bleeding may displace these fat pads, creating a zone of relative radiolucency (Fig 2–18). The fat-pad sign seen on lateral roentgenograms may be a subtle sign of underlying injury. It is not always present, however, and it is sometimes seen as an incidental finding in children with no history of elbow injury.

Supracondylar Fractures

Fracture of the distal humeral metaphysis just above the epicondyles is termed *supracondylar fracture* (Fig 2–19). This common injury usually results from forced hyperextension or hyperflexion of the elbow. Posterior and medial displacement of the distal fracture fragment with respect to the proximal humerus is the most common finding, although displacement in any direction may occur. The neurovascular structures of the antecubital space may be damaged by sharp fracture fragments at the time of injury or during reduction attempts. Subsequent swelling may occlude the brachial artery or block perfusion of the volar forearm compartment during the course of treatment, with resultant signs and symptoms of ischemic paralysis.

Supracondylar fractures are best treated by an experienced orthopedist. Accurate reduction is essential. Rotational or angular malalignment predictably results in late deformity and cannot be accepted. A number of methods are employed in treatment, including closed reduction, overhead traction, and open reduction with internal fixation. The choice of treatment depends on the degree of displacement, the severity of associated swelling and soft tissue injury, and the preference of the surgeon in charge. Following reduction, supracondylar fractures may require 3 to 6 weeks of immobilization. During the early phases of healing, displacement may occur, and close follow-up is necessary.

The chief complication of malunion of supracondylar elbow fractures is change in the so-called carrying angle of the elbow. Ordinarily about 5 degrees of apex medial angulation exists at the elbow, producing a mild valgus angulation. Girls have a slightly greater carrying angle. Rotational and angular malalignment may increase or decrease this angle (Fig 2–20). With growth, the deformity may become more obvious. Although function is ordinarily not affected, the cosmetic results are often unpleasant. Osteotomy of the distal humerus may be required at the completion of growth to restore alignment.

Lateral Condylar and Epicondylar Fractures

The lateral condyle of the distal humerus or capitulum articulates with the radial head and forms the lateral half of the elbow joint (Fig 2–21,A). Fractures of the lateral condyle may be either type III or type IV physeal injuries (Fig 2–21,B). The small metaphyseal fragment in type IV injuries is an important diagnostic clue in minimally displaced fractures. Fat-pad signs and displacement of the secondary ossification center of the injured capitulum relative to the opposite normal elbow may be the only signs of type III injury. In some cases an arthrogram may be necessary to fully evaluate the injury.

Lateral condyle fractures are almost always intra-articular injuries. Anatomical

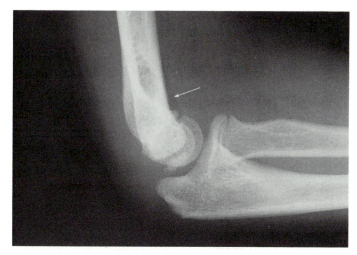

FIG 2–18.
The elusive fat-pad sign *(arrow)*. Although often a subtle sign of elbow injury, it may also occur as in incidental finding in children with no history of elbow injury. An anterior fat-pad sign is less significant than a posterior fat-pad sign; it is sometimes found in normal elbow films taken for comparison.

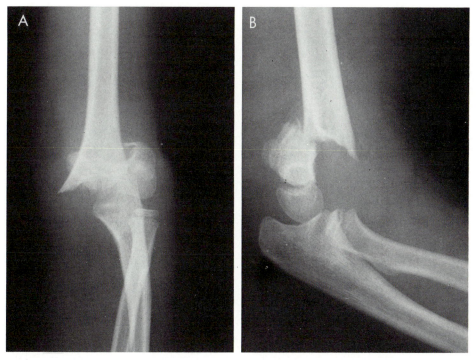

FIG 2–19.
A, supracondylar fracture of the humerus, anteroposterior view. **B,** lateral view, supracondylar fracture.

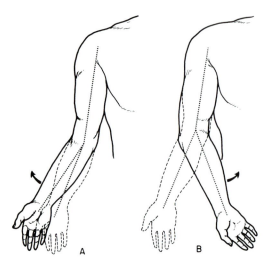

FIG 2–20.
A, valgus deformity of the elbow. **B,** varus deformity of the elbow. Permanent alterations of the normal carrying angle of the elbow may result from improper alignment of elbow fractures. (From Enneking WF, (ed): *Manual of Orthopedic Surgery,* ed 4. Chicago, American Orthopedic Association, 1972, p 138. Reproduced by permission.)

reduction is essential. Even slight displacement is unacceptable. Malunion and nonunion lead to progressive valgus angulation at the elbow joint with significant late deformity. Ulnar nerve palsy from traction across the medial side of the elbow is a common late finding. Open reduction and internal fixation are often employed to ensure prompt union and prevent late complications in lateral condyle fractures.

The lateral epicondyle is a small secondary ossification center on the lateral aspect of the distal humeral metaphysis that gives rise to the common extensor tendon of the forearm. Minor avulsions are occasionally seen as a result of pull on the extensor tendon (Fig 2–22). Epicondylar fractures do not involve the articular surface and are often of little consequence. Immobilization for 3 to 4 weeks to permit soft tissue healing to occur is usually sufficient treatment.

Medial Condylar and Epicondylar Fractures

The medial condyle, or trochlea, articulates with the proximal ulna and forms the medial half of the elbow joint. Isolated medial condylar fractures are uncommon. Medial condylar fractures may occur as part of a comminuted distal humeral fracture, however. As with other articular fractures, anatomical restoration of joint surfaces is necessary for proper function. Internal fixation is usually necessary.

The medial epicondyle is a secondary ossification center on the medial aspect of the distal humerus that gives rise to the common flexor tendon of the forearm. Like the lateral epicondyle, the medial epicondyle is extra-articular. Avulsion of the medial epicondyle may result from forced lateral rotation of the forearm or medially directed loading of the extended elbow. Medial epicondylar fracture often complicates dislocation of the elbow in adolescents (Fig 2–23).

Minimally displaced medial epicondylar fractures are usually treated by simple immobilization. Open reduction may be required in more widely displaced fractures. Internal fixation is sometimes employed to reduce the chances of painful nonunion or late elbow instability. Open reduction is necessary if the medial epicondyle was trapped in the elbow joint at the time of dislocation.

Dislocation of the Elbow Joint

Dislocation of the elbow joint may occur with or without fracture of the bones that comprise it. Dislocation without fracture is more common in older adolescents. Dislocation with fracture of the medial epicondyle or proximal ulna is more common in younger children.

The radial head should articulate with the capitulum in all views of the elbow

FIG 2–21.

Lateral condyle fracture. **A₁,** anteroposterior view of a normal elbow in a 4-year-old boy. **A₂,** lateral view. A line drawn down the anterior aspect of the humeral shaft normally intersects the secondary ossification center of the capitellum. **B₁,** lateral condyle fracture in a 4-year-old boy. This example is a type IV growth plate fracture. The fracture line extends from the metaphysis of the lateral aspect of the humerus across the growth plate and through to the articular surface of the distal humerus. **B₂,** lateral view. Forward displacement is not severe in this example. Although an attempt at management by nonoperative methods is acceptable in minimally displaced fractures of the lateral condyle, most are best treated by open reduction and internal fixation.

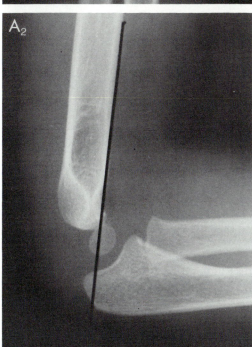

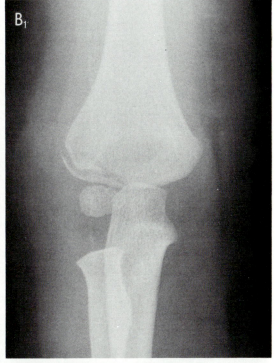

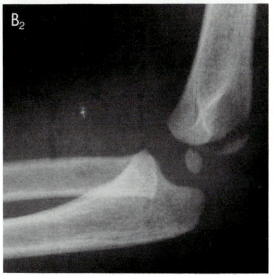

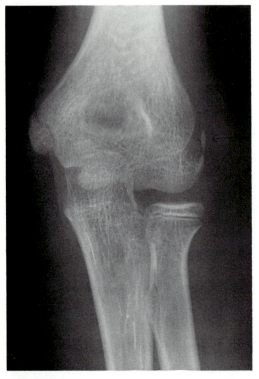

FIG 2–22.
Lateral epicondyle fracture. Avulsions often arise from the pull of the common extensor tendon origin.

(Fig 2–24). Displacement in any projection indicates dislocation. Radial head dislocation associated with proximal ulnar fracture is an often missed combination (Fig 2–25).

Elbow dislocations can usually be treated by closed reduction. If the medial epicondyle has been displaced into the joint, however, open reduction is advisable to remove the fragment from the joint prior to reduction. After closed or open reduction, a long arm cast or splint is usually employed for 3 to 4 weeks to permit soft tissue healing to occur.

Proximal Radial Injuries

The radial shaft tapers slightly before flaring out to form the proximal radial metaphysis. The radial head caps the metaphysis and articulates both with the proximal ulna and with the capitulum. During pronation and supination, the radial head rotates in the radial notch of the ulna. During flexion and extension, it glides anteriorly and posteriorly against the capitulum. The radial head is held in

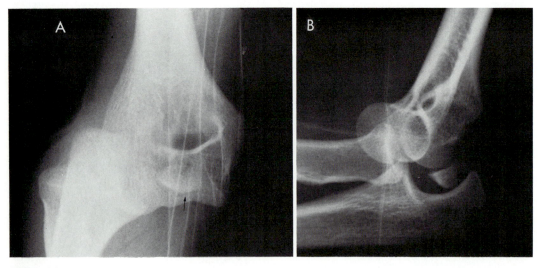

FIG 2–23.
A, anterior view of dislocation of elbow, with displacement of medial epicondyle into the elbow joint. **B,** lateral view shows epicondyle within the elbow joint.

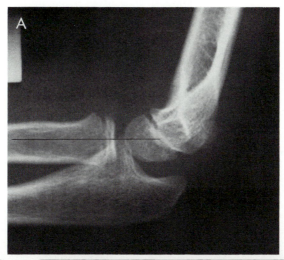

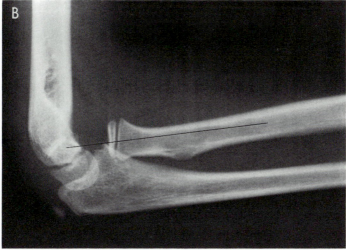

FIG 2–24.
Lateral views of the elbow, aged 10 years. **A,** a line drawn down the shaft of the radius should always intersect the capitulum. **B,** anterior dislocation of the proximal radius.

position by a fibrous cuff composed of the radial collateral ligament and the annular ligament, a transverse band of fibrous tissue that surrounds the head and proximal metaphysis of the radius. Irregularities in the contour of the radial head or malalignment of the head on the shaft after fracture may block the smooth motion necessary for full elbow function.

Pulled elbow, or nursemaid's elbow, is one of the most common musculoskeletal injuries of childhood. It is seen most often between ages 1 and 5 years, with peak incidence between ages 2 and 3 years. The injury is usually the result of a combination of traction and pronation forces, commonly generated by lifting a recalcitrant child by the forearm (Fig 2–26). Pathologic studies indicate that a transverse tear occurs at the attachment of the annular ligament to the neck of the radius and that a portion of the annular ligament may become trapped in the joint (Fig 2–27).

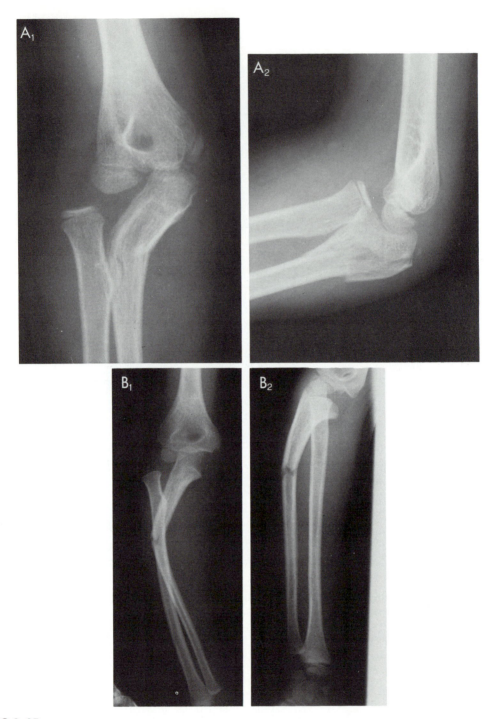

FIG 2–25.
Two examples of fracture of the ulnar shaft with dislocation of the radius from the capitulum. This injury is referred to as the Monteggia's fracture. Closed reduction of the ulnar fracture and radial head dislocation is usually possible in children; open reduction and internal fixation are sometimes required in adolescents and adults. **A₁,** in the anteroposterior view, the radial head is laterally displaced. A fracture line passes through the proximal ulna. **A₂,** in the lateral view, the radial head is superiorly displaced, and proximal ulnar fracture is obvious. **B₁, B₂,** in this example, the ulnar fracture is more distal, and radial head dislocation might be missed unless the elbow joint is included in the film.

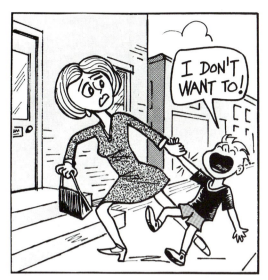

FIG 2–26.
Nursemaid's elbow—a common mechanism of injury. (From Rang M: *Children's Fractures.* Philadelphia, JB Lippincott, Co, 1974, p 121. Reproduced by permission.)

Affected children usually present with a history of sudden onset of elbow pain following a traction injury, although parents are sometimes reluctant to discuss the accident. The arm is held in slight flexion and mild pronation. Limited active motion is present, and passive motion is vigorously resisted. A point of maximal tenderness to palpation is usually present over the proximal radial metaphysis. Roentgenograms of the elbow are usually normal.

Treatment is simple. Quick and firm supination of the forearm unlocks the annular ligament and permits interposed tissues to escape the joint. A click may often be felt or heard as the radial head is reduced. Relief of pain is usually dramatic in children treated shortly after injury. Children with more long-standing symptoms may not experience such rapid relief. Following reduction, immobilization in a splint or sling for 7 to 10 days permits healing of soft tissues to occur. Parents should be cautioned against lifting the child by one hand since recurrence is common up to age 4 or 5 years.

Fractures of the proximal radius are occasionally seen following a fall on the outstretched arm. Most often such fractures are either type II injuries of the proximal radial physis or compression fractures of the proximal radial metaphysis (Fig 2–28). Pain, tenderness, and discoloration over the proximal metaphysis are consistent findings.

Displacement of proximal radial frac-

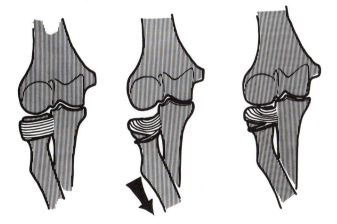

FIG 2–27.
The pathology of pulled elbow. The annular ligament is torn when the arm is pulled *(arrow).* The radial head moves distally and when traction is discontinued, the ligament is carried into the joint. (From Rang M: *Children's Fractures.* Philadelphia, JB Lippincott, Co, 1974, p 121. Reproduced by permission.)

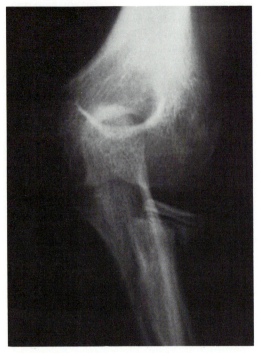

FIG 2–28.
Type II fracture of the proximal radius. A triangular fragment of metaphysis is attached to the proximal fracture fragment.

tures is usually measured by the degree of deviation of the articular surface of the proximal radius from horizontal. Treatment depends on the degree of displacement. Minimally displaced fractures, those with less than 20 to 30 degrees of tilt, usually require only a brief period of splintage for comfort. Little or no functional impairment follows minimally displaced radial head and neck fractures.

More severely displaced fractures require reduction and should be referred for treatment since limitation of rotation and flexion will follow if healing occurs in this unsatisfactory position. In most cases, a trial of closed reduction under adequate sedation is employed. Open reduction and internal fixation are necessary if an acceptable and stable closed reduction cannot be obtained.

Forearm Fractures

Forearm fractures follow a wide variety of trauma. The location and nature of the fracture are determined both by the characteristics of the deforming force and by the mechanical properties of the involved bones. Failure may occur in any segment of the radius or ulna, and fractures of both bones are common. Incomplete greenstick and buckle fractures occur frequently in young children; complete fractures are more common in older children and adolescents.

Fractures that result from large-magnitude or rapidly applied forces may be associated with muscle, nerve, and arterial damage. Careful assessment of neurovascular function must precede fracture management and continue after reduction. Swelling within the closed fascial spaces of the forearm may irreversibly damage deep musculature. Persistent pain after splintage, paresthesia, and pain on attempted motion of the fingers indicate impending ischemia and are urgent danger signals. Prompt removal of compressive dressings is vital. At times surgical decompression may be necessary to salvage limb function.

Radial and ulnar shaft fractures commonly follow falls from trees, gymnastic sets, and picnic tables. Most fractures in children younger than age 10 years are incomplete, with failure of bone on one side and bending on the other (Fig 2–29). Complete fractures occur more commonly in adolescence as cortical bone assumes more adult characteristics. In some cases, displacement is minimal, and no reduction is necessary. Most often, however, angular deformity is present, and reduction is required. These injuries should be referred to an orthopedist for treatment.

Diaphyseal fractures of the radius and ulna are usually easily reduced in young children. The thick surrounding perios-

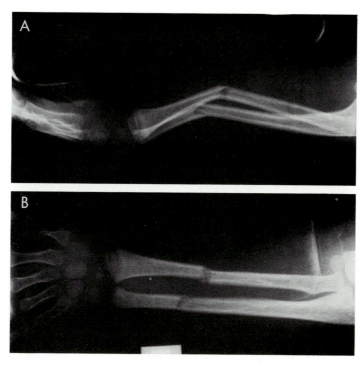

FIG 2–29.
A, lateral view of incomplete fractures of radial and ulnar midshafts. The elbow joint was mistakenly not included on the initial roentgenogram. **B,** anterior view of the forearm. Note associated dislocation of the elbow. The joints above and below a fracture should always be included on the initial x-ray examination.

teum serves as a hinge on which reduction can be based. Side-to-side apposition of fracture fragments and mild residual angulation in the plane of motion of the wrist and elbow are acceptable. Rotary malalignment and radial or ulnar deviation will not remodel and should not be accepted. Discrepancy in width of proximal and distal fragments at the fracture site after reduction may be the only indication of mild rotational malalignment (Fig 2–30).

In most cases reduction can be obtained in the outpatient department using intravenous or intramuscular sedation and local anesthesia at the fracture site. Union usually occurs within 6 weeks in a long arm cast or splint. An additional 2 to 4 weeks' protection in a short arm splint may be necessary in older children and

adolescents or children in whom satisfactory alignment cannot be achieved by closed methods. Following final cast removal, patients should refrain from contact sports for 1 to 2 additional months.

Buckle (or torus) fractures of the distal radial and ulnar metaphyses are incomplete compression fractures common in childhood (Fig 2–31). They frequently result from minor trauma and usually cause little deformity. Many are probably not recognized. They are stable injuries and heal rapidly. A brief period of cast immobilization for comfort and protection is sufficient treatment.

Types I and II distal radial and ulnar physeal fractures are common during adolescence (Fig 2–32). In most cases, the distal radial and ulnar fracture fragments are displaced dorsally, with resultant apex

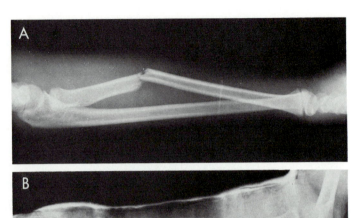

FIG 2–30.
A and **B,** rotational malalignment of
forearm fracture. Note discrepancy in
width of proximal and distal
fragments at fracture site.

volar angulation. Compression of the median nerve may complicate fractures with
extreme displacement or severe swelling.
The presence of a puncture wound or lac-
eration over the apex of the fracture usually indicates that the fracture is open and
that surgical debridement will be required, no matter how small the wound.

Closed reduction is usually successful
in closed fractures after intravenous sedation or regional block. General anesthesia
may be necessary to obtain sufficient relaxation in difficult fractures. Mild angulation in the plane of wrist motion will remodel, especially in younger children.
Postreduction immobilization in a bi-
valved long arm cast or long arm splint is
appropriate to prevent neurovascular
compromise from postreduction swelling.

In most cases, 3 to 4 weeks' immobilization is sufficient. A short arm cast or
splint is often used for an additional 3 to
4 weeks for protection in older children.

Since these fractures involve the
physis, damage to the growth plate at the
time of injury may result in premature
closure. Parents must be forewarned, and
patients must be followed carefully for 6
to 12 months after injury.

WRIST AND HAND INJURIES

Ossification centers in the bones of
the wrist and hand appear in a regular
and well-documented sequence throughout childhood. The radiologic appearance
of the epiphysis may be used as an index
of skeletal age and is useful in estimating
overall growth potential. The secondary
ossification centers of the metacarpals and
phalanges are sometimes confusing.
When necessary, comparison views of the
normal hand should be made.

Carpal Fractures

Fractures and fracture dislocations of
the carpus are usually adult injuries. Fractures of the navicular bone are occasionally seen in adolescents, however. Pain
and tenderness on the radial side of the
wrist following a fall on the outstretched
hand should raise the suspicion of navicular fracture. These fractures are often difficult to identify on roentgenograms made
immediately after injury. Special navicular
views of the wrist are often necessary to
confirm the diagnosis of navicular frac-

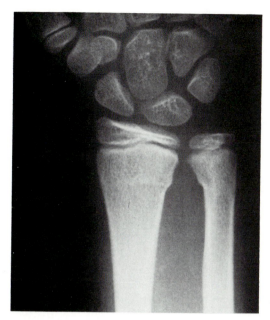

FIG 2–31.
Stable compression fracture of the distal radius. No reduction is necessary. Splintage for comfort is appropriate; a short arm cast provides adequate immobilization.

ture. As bone resorption occurs after fracture, the fracture site becomes more obvious (Fig 2–33). Patients with suspected navicular fractures should have follow-up roentgenograms made 7 to 10 days after injury for positive diagnosis. Protective splinting should be used in the interval between examinations.

Navicular fractures heal slowly, and prolonged cast immobilization may be necessary. The nonunion rate is high, and surgical treatment is sometimes required. Because of the possibility of delayed union or nonunion, patients with suspected navicular fractures should be referred for treatment.

Fractures of the bones of the hand in children and adolescents are usually the result of a direct blow. Children frequently trap the hand or fingers in closing doors or beneath falling objects. Football, baseball, basketball, and fistfights are responsible for most metacarpal and phalangeal fractures in teenagers.

Fractures and dislocations in the hand often appear deceptively uncomplicated to the physician who treats these injuries only occasionally. Many of the radiologic

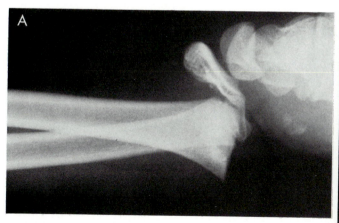
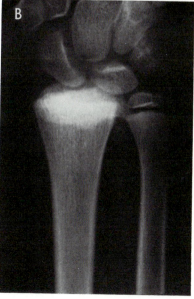

FIG 2–32.
A and **B,** anterior and lateral views of the distal radius and ulna in a type II fracture of the growth plate.

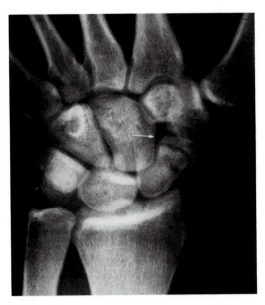

FIG 2–33.
Fracture through the distal one third of the carpal navicular bone in an adolescent boy. This roentgenogram was made 10 days after injury.

features of hand injuries are quite subtle
and easily overlooked. Unfortunately, the
hand is much less forgiving of errors in
diagnosis and treatment than are other
parts of the upper extremity. Shortening
and rotational malalignment may not be
apparent on standard anteroposterior and
lateral roentgenograms, but will result in
malunion and permanent impairment of
function unless corrected. Small chip fractures off the base of the middle or distal
phalanx may be associated with avulsions
of flexor or extensor tendons that may require operative repair. Most hand injuries
should be referred for treatment.

Metacarpal and Phalangeal Fractures

Fractures of the metacarpals of the index through small finger rays usually occur after direct blows or through a combination of a direct blow and a twisting
injury. The boxer's fracture of the neck of
the small finger metacarpal is a familiar
example. Other metacarpals are occasion-

ally involved (Fig 2–34). Longitudinally
directed forces tend to produce fractures
of the neck of the involved metacarpal;
spiral and oblique shaft fractures result
from torsional loads. Examination usually
shows depression of the knuckle of the
involved ray and asymmetric shortening
in comparison with the metacarpals of the
opposite hand. Rotary malalignment is
less obvious. Normally, the fingernails lie
in the same plane when the hand is
cupped. Tilting of one nail indicates rotational deformity of the proximal segments
of the ray. Unless this is reduced, the affected finger will overlap the other digits
when the hand is clenched.

Fractures of the small- and ring-finger
metacarpals angulated less than 25 or 30
degrees in the posterior direction without
rotational malalignment may be treated
by immobilization in a plaster gutter
splint (Fig 2–35). Fractures with greater
angulation or rotational malalignment require reduction and should be referred for
treatment. Closed reduction under local
anesthetic block almost always is successful in metacarpal neck fractures that do
not involve a split of the articular surface
of the metacarpal. The remodeling potential of such fractures is high, and 50 degrees or more of residual angulation after
closed reduction is acceptable. Fractures
of the shaft of the fifth metacarpal can
usually be treated by closed reduction and
immobilization in a plaster splint. Fractures of the shafts of other metacarpals
may be more difficult to treat, especially if
shortening or rotational malalignment
persists after closed reduction. Open reduction or percutaneous pin fixation after
closed reduction may be necessary to
maintain alignment (Fig 2–36).

Fractures through the growth plates
of the phalanges are common childhood
injuries. Most are type II injuries caused
by abduction or rotation.

Type III injuries result from avulsion
of a portion of the articular surface by at-

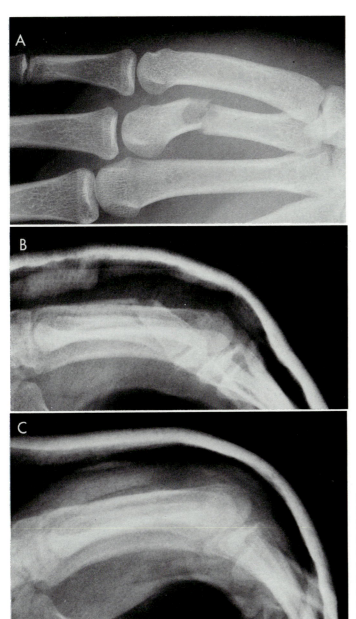

FIG 2–34.
Fracture of the shaft of the ring finger metacarpal. **A,** anteroposterior roentgenogram showing slight shortening and rotational malalignment. **B,** unacceptable angular malalignment after attempted reduction. **C,** acceptable alignment after repeat reduction.

tached tendon or ligament. Type II fractures can usually can be treated by closed reduction after infiltration or digital block with local anesthesia (Figs 2–37 and 2–38). Epinephrine-anesthetic combinations must not be used since they may cause irreversible vascular spasm. Reduction may be attempted by placing the thumb at the apex of deformity and using the distal digit as a lever. These fractures are usually stable once reduced and can be immobilized on a padded curved splint. Remodeling of residual angulation can be expected, especially in the proximal phalanx. Remodeling is less predictable in the distal and middle phalanx. Rotational malalignment

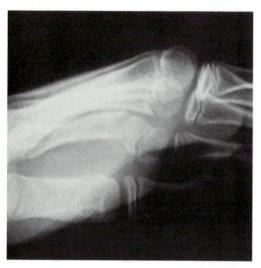

FIG 2–35.
Fracture of the distal portion of the small-finger metacarpal, commonly called a boxer's fracture. Little or no functional impairment will occur if this fracture is treated without reduction, but a slight depression of the knuckle will be noticeable.

sports injuries. Many can be successfully reduced with local anesthesia or mild parenteral sedation. At times, however, dislocations may be locked by intra-articular displacement of ligaments or tendons. This is especially true of metacarpal-phalangeal dislocations. Open reduction may be necessary if gentle attempts at closed reduction are unsuccessful.

Roentgenograms are essential before and after reduction to permit accurate diagnosis and assess adequacy of reduction. Dislocations associated with intra-articular fractures may require internal fixation after reduction to restore joint congruity

is not acceptable since it will not remodel and will result in permanent deformity. Consultation should be obtained if any difficulty is experienced in obtaining or maintaining reduction.

Displaced phalangeal shaft fractures with rotational and angular malalignment can be difficult to treat by closed methods. The pull of flexor and extensor tendons spanning the phalanx is difficult to overcome. Operative fixation is often necessary.

Type III fractures that involve a significant portion of the articular surface of the phalanx are often best treated by operative reduction and internal fixation. Accurate realignment of fractures that involve the joint surfaces is essential. Small avulsion fractures can sometimes be treated nonoperatively, but displaced intra-articular phalangeal fractures require operative realignment.

Dislocations of the metacarpal phalangeal and interphalangeal joints (Fig 2–39) are common consequences of adolescent

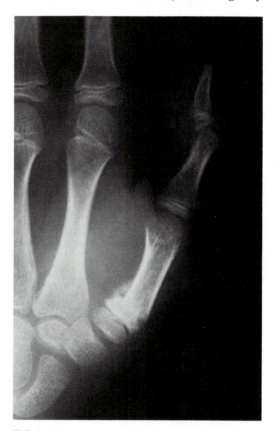

FIG 2–36.
Healing fracture through the proximal shaft of the thumb metacarpal. The alignment of this fracture is acceptable; often, however, the pull of tendons attached to the thumb distal to the fracture makes closed reduction impossible to maintain, and pin fixation may be necessary.

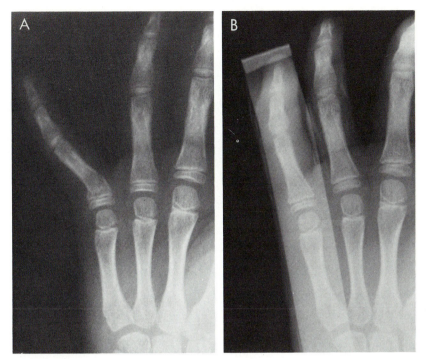

FIG 2–37.
Type II fracture of the base of the proximal phalanx of the small finger. **A,** although slight angulation in the plane of joint motion is acceptable, angulation in other planes must usually be corrected. **B,** anteroposterior roentgenogram after closed reduction and immobilization with a curved aluminum splint.

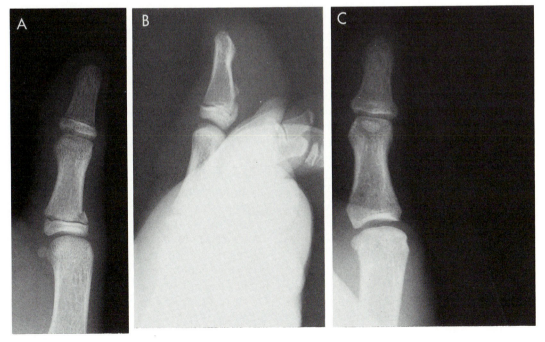

FIG 2–38.
Mild angular malalignment after treatment of a type II fracture of the proximal thumb phalanx by immobilization alone, without reduction. **A** and **B,** roentgenograms made at the time of fracture. **C,** radiologic appearance at maturity.

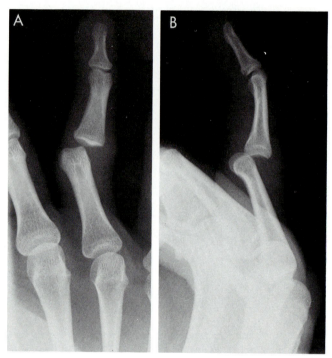

FIG 2–39.
Anteroposterior **(A)** and lateral **(B)** roentgenograms of a dislocation of the ring finger proximal interphalangeal joint.

and stability. Following reduction, injured joints must be protected to permit healing of damaged soft tissues. A period of 2 to 3 weeks is recommended. Buddy-taping to an adjacent normal finger during sports activities for an additional 1 to 2 months provides extra protection. Dislocations that significantly damage articular supporting structures may result in acute instability after initial reduction. Repair of soft tissues has been advocated by some surgeons if instability is present after successful closed reduction.

A direct blow to the tip of a finger that forces the distal joint into flexion may rupture the extensor tendon insertion into the dorsal aspect of the distal phalanx. The resulting flexion deformity is termed mallet finger. At times, it may be associated with avulsion of a fragment of underlying bone. Although such injuries usually result in little disability if untreated, splintage of the joint in extension may restore full function. Splinting such

avulsions is often technically difficult, and referral is appropriate. Avulsions associated with fractures should be referred for treatment.

Acute longitudinal compression of the interphalangeal joints may result in the "jammed finger" common in football, baseball, and basketball. Although the precise pathology of these injuries is unclear, they may represent grade I sprains or strains of the ligaments or tendons around the involved joint or result from compression injury of the articular surfaces. If a full range of active motion is present, no instability is noted on medial or lateral stress, and no fractures are apparent on x-ray examination, such injuries may be safely treated by immobilization on a gently curved padded aluminum splint. Straight splints and tongue blades should not be used since they may cause permanent extension contractures. After a week to 10 days of immobilization, the involved finger may be buddy-taped to its neighbor, and motion is started. The joint should be protected by buddy-taping during sports for 4 to 6 weeks after injury; swelling and soreness in the area may persist for several months.

Nail avulsions after crush injuries are often associated with fractures of the underlying distal phalanx. The fracture fragments frequently penetrate the nail bed, and contamination of the fracture is probable. Meticulous debridement and thorough irrigation of the fracture surfaces are essential prior to reduction. The fingernail should be removed if nearly detached. If the nail bed is lacerated, it should be meticulously repaired with 6-0 or 7-0 absorbable suture. The finger should be protected with a padded curved splint following reduction, and broad-spectrum oral antibiotics should be given for 2 weeks. Partial nail regeneration can be expected, although scarring is likely. Parents must be informed of this at the time of the initial treatment.

Fingertip Amputations

Fingertip amputations are common in childhood. Depending on the level of amputation and the age of the patient, regeneration of the amputated fingertips may be expected. Amputations distal to the proximal one third of the lunula of the nail can be expected to regenerate nearly completely in children younger than age 10 years. Some regeneration will occur in older children and in children with amputations between the nail base and the distal interphalangeal joint. Regeneration will not occur in amputations through or proximal to the distal interphalangeal joint. Amputation wounds should be treated by thorough cleansing and debridement. Sterile paper adhesive strips can be used to approximate wound edges before a bulky dressing is applied. The wound should be redressed at 4- to 5-day intervals during healing.

FRACTURES OF THE PELVIS

Like spine fractures, pelvic fractures in children are usually the result of significant violence. Automobile accidents are the most frequent cause. Although overall morbidity and mortality after pelvic fractures in children are lower than in adults, the potential complications in individual cases are equally serious. Forces sufficient to produce pelvic fractures often damage abdominal viscera and great vessels; in many cases, musculoskeletal damage is less significant than associated soft tissue damage.

Contusions on the lower trunk suggest the possibility of pelvic fracture, especially when tenderness over the symphysis pubis, iliac crests, or sacroiliac joints is present. Pain on bimanual compression of the iliac wings is another sign of fracture of the pelvic ring. Abdominal tenderness, guarding, and rigidity suggest associated visceral injury. Blood loss from ruptured organs, lacerated pelvic vessels, and cancellous fracture surfaces can be extensive, and hypovolemic shock may develop rapidly. Thorough, repeated examinations and appropriate blood replacement are essential.

Genitourinary tract injury is the most common complication of pelvic fracture (Fig 2–40). Renal parenchymal damage, ureteral avulsion, bladder rupture, and urethral lacerations all may result from the intrapelvic compression and shearing forces generated at the time of injury. Hematuria, either microscopic or gross, is a danger sign that indicates the need for urologic evaluation. Intravenous pyelograms and voiding cystourethrograms are mandatory when hematuria is present. If a child cannot void spontaneously, careful catheterization should be performed. This must be done gently; traumatic catheterization may cause further damage to a torn urethra or contaminate a previously sterile hematoma. In the male, scrotal he-

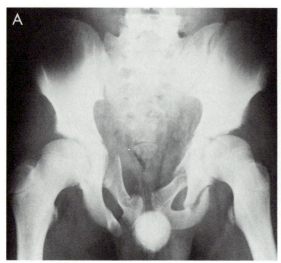
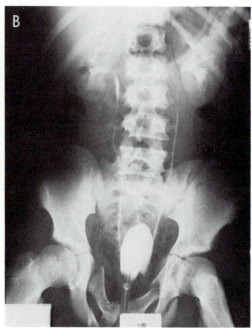

FIG 2–40.
A, fractures of the pelvis result from significant injuring forces. The combination of bilateral superior and inferior pubic ramus fractures has a high incidence of associated visceral injury. **B,** intrapelvic bleeding is manifested by displacement of the bladder.

matoma or blood at the urethral meatus are signs of urethral injury. Retrograde urethrography should be performed before catheterization is attempted. Urologic consultation should be obtained if there is any evidence of genitourinary injury.

Immobilization is the first step in the orthopedic management of pelvic fractures. Further displacement of fracture fragments and possible further damage to pelvic vessels can be avoided by splinting the trunk with sandbags or pillows while more urgent problems are cared for. After the patient's condition has stabilized, attention can be directed to fracture care.

Stable pelvic fractures require little treatment in children. In many cases, only a brief period of bed rest is necessary. Walking may be started when the child is comfortable. Unstable or displaced fractures may require skeletal traction or open reduction to achieve alignment. Fractures

that involve the acetabulum in particular must be restored as nearly as possible to anatomical alignment; internal fixation is at times required.

LOWER EXTREMITY FRACTURES

Fractures and Dislocations of the Hip

Fractures and dislocations of the femoral head and neck occur much less often in children than adults and, like fractures of the pelvis, are most often the result of automobile accidents. As with other fractures that occur after violent injury, careful evaluation and treatment of airway injury, cardiovascular damage, head and neck injury, and abdominal trauma take precedence over orthopedic problems. Splintage on a backboard will suffice until the child is stable.

Proximal femoral fracture may occur

through the proximal growth plate, the femoral neck, the intertrochanteric region, or the subtrochanteric region. Hip pain, limitation of active motion, and resistance to passive motion are consistent findings in the conscious child with such a fracture. Lateral rotation and apparent shortening of the affected limb are usually present in displaced fractures. The diagnosis can be confirmed with anteroposterior and cross-leg lateral roentgenograms of the hip; it is not necessary to move the injured extremity to obtain these views. Attempts to move the injured hip to obtain frog-leg lateral views are painful and unnecessary.

Accurate reduction and immobilization of fracture fragments must be obtained in proximal femoral fractures. The prognosis for uncomplicated healing depends to a large extent on the fracture level. Physeal and neck fractures are often associated with damage to the vessels that supply the proximal epiphysis, and the potential for avascular necrosis and malunion is high with these fractures. Intertrochanteric and subtrochanteric fractures, on the other hand, are rarely complicated by avascular necrosis. Nondisplaced fractures can be treated by immobilization in a body cast, but displaced fractures are best treated by reduction and internal fixation.

Traumatic dislocation of the hip is rare in children. The mechanism of injury varies with age. In young children, dislocation may result from a minor fall. In older children and adolescents, motor vehicle accidents are the most common cause, and hip dislocation may be associated with other fractures or visceral damage. In most cases, the femoral head dislocates posteriorly (Fig 2–41). The affected limb then lies in a position of hip and knee flexion, adduction, and medial rotation. The femoral head may be palpable beneath the gluteal muscles in the buttock. Sciatic nerve damage, a rare compli-

cation, is manifested by paresis of the muscles of the lower leg.

Avascular necrosis of the proximal femoral epiphysis is the principal musculoskeletal complication of traumatic hip dislocation. Interruption of the blood supply to the femoral head may occur through rupture of the intracapsular vessels at the time of dislocation or by tamponade resulting from intracapsular swelling. Prompt reduction decreases the risk of avascular necrosis; delay of more than 24 hours is associated with poor outcome. In most cases closed reduction under anesthesia is possible. Open reduction may be necessary if closed reduction is unsuccessful or if acetabular fractures accompanied dislocation.

Following reduction, the hip must be protected until soft tissue healing occurs. Bed rest for 3 to 6 weeks followed by a variable period of partial weight bearing is usually employed. Spica cast immobilization may be used. Prolonged follow-up is necessary since avascular necrosis may not be manifested for up to 3 years after dislocation.

Femoral Shaft Fractures

Most femoral shaft fractures before walking age are the result of accidental falls from dressing tables or parents' arms. Direct blows or twisting forces may produce femoral fractures in unfortunate victims of child abuse. Later in childhood, pedestrian, bicycle, and motor vehicle accidents become the most common causes. During adolescence, football accidents are occasionally responsible for femoral fractures.

The amount of damage sustained by the soft tissues of the thigh at the time of fracture depends on the magnitude of the injuring force. As a child grows, the femur increases in size and strength, and more force is required to produce a fracture. Damage to the muscles of the thigh

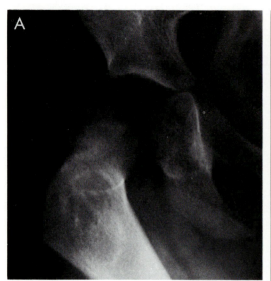

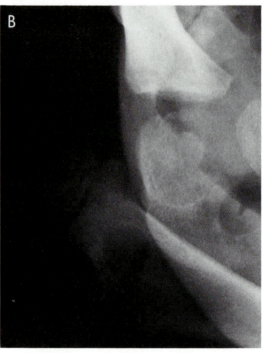

FIG 2–41.
A, anteroposterior view of a posterior dislocation of the hip. **B,** oblique view shows the dislocation more clearly.

consequently is usually greater in older children. The morphology of the fracture surfaces often provides information about the characteristics of the injuring force. Transverse fractures are usually the result of direct loads applied perpendicularly to the femur; car bumpers are frequently culprits. Spiral fractures follow torsional loading, which might occur in a football tackle or when the leg is caught beneath a falling bicycle. Comminution of a fracture implies rapid, high-magnitude loading with release of large quantities of stored energy at the time of fracture.

Blood loss after femoral fracture is significant. Even patients with minimally displaced fractures will lose one to two units at the fracture site during the first 48 hours after fracture. Patients with comminuted or open fractures may lose much more blood, especially if damage to major vessels has occurred at the time of fracture. Hypovolemic shock may develop rapidly in patients with other fractures or abdominal or chest injury.

Almost all children's femoral shaft fractures can be treated nonoperatively (Fig 2–42). In many cases, a short period of traction is employed to restore fracture alignment and to permit preliminary healing to occur. A spica cast is used until healing is complete. Skin traction with adhesive strips applied carefully to the legs is often used in infants less than 1 year old who weigh less than 10 kg. Meticulous attention is required to prevent circulatory impairment in the legs. Older children are often better treated with skeletal traction before cast application since the traction forces required may be greater than those that can safely be achieved with skin traction.

In some instances, femoral fractures can be treated by closed reduction and immediate spica cast application. This technique is particularly useful in children less than 10 years old with oblique or spiral distal fractures and without other injury. Immediate cast techniques avoid the prolonged period of hospitalization nec-

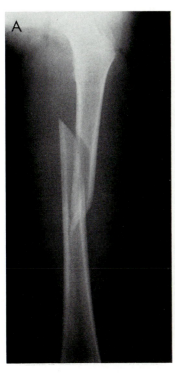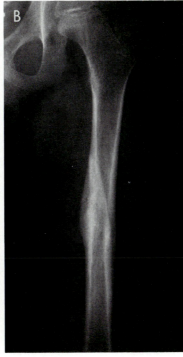

FIG 2–42.
A, long oblique femoral shaft fracture treated by traction and subsequent cast immobilization. **B,** roentgenographic appearance 12 weeks after injury.

essary for traction treatment but do not shorten the overall period required for fracture healing. Careful follow-up is necessary throughout treatment to guard against unacceptable displacement during healing.

Open reduction and internal fixation are rarely necessary in uncomplicated femoral shaft fractures in children. In special circumstances, however, internal fixation of femoral shaft fractures may be a necessary part of overall management of a multiply injured older child. Comatose and combative patients who cannot be controlled in traction and badly burned patients for whom bed rest is impossible may be best treated operatively. Some trauma specialists believe that children with multiple extremity and visceral injuries recover faster with less risk of systemic complication if fractures are internally fixed and patients rapidly mobilized. Fortunately, such circumstances are uncommon.

Femoral shaft fractures stimulate growth of the affected side in immature patients. One to 2 centimeters of overgrowth of the fractured femur often occurs if anatomical reduction of the fracture is obtained during treatment. The potential for overgrowth appears to be less in children less than 2 years of age, probably because they are in a period of overall rapid growth. For the same reason, femoral shaft fractures in adolescents have been said to be less likely to stimulate growth. Children between ages 2 and 12 are most prone to overgrowth. In these patients, slight override of fragments is desirable if it can be obtained without accompanying angulation. Overdistraction of the fracture should be avoided if possible. Some residual angular deformity is acceptable, especially if the apex of the angulation is anteriorly directed. Rotational malalignment must be avoided to prevent permanent deformity.

Fractures of the distal femoral growth

plate, like fractures of the proximal femur, are usually the result of significant trauma. In juvenile patients, auto accidents and falls from windows are frequent causes; in adolescents, football and soccer accidents are common causes as well. As with proximal femoral fractures, the prognosis after fracture through the distal femoral physis is not uniformly as good or as predictable as in physeal injuries of the upper limb. The forces required to produce distal femoral fracture are great, and damage to the germinal layers of the physis may occur even in minimally displaced injuries. Bridging of the physis with resultant partial or complete growth arrest is unfortunately common; in some series, this occurred in more than 50% of cases. In younger patients, premature growth plate closure is especially damaging since it consistently causes significant angular deformity and/or leg-length inequality. Adolescents approaching the age of growth plate closure are less likely to develop leg-length inequality requiring treatment, but measurable discrepancy is a common sequela of such fractures. Anatomic reduction is the best insurance against premature arrest, and open reduction may be necessary to obtain alignment. Even under the best of circumstances, however, physeal arrest may occur, and the prognosis for normal growth of the distal femur is guarded. Careful follow-up after initial reduction is necessary to identify premature closure or partial bridging; resection of the bridge is sometimes possible when the area involved is not great and significant angular deformity has not yet developed.

Fractures through the distal femoral growth plate may mimic knee ligament injuries in their clinical appearance. Instability of the knee may be present on physical examination. Stress roentgenograms are necessary to distinguish between the two injuries. Anatomical realignment of the fracture fragments is essential, and

open reduction and internal fixation may be necessary. Even with anatomical reduction, however, the chance of angular deformity secondary to growth plate injury is high.

Tibial Fractures

Because of its unique configuration, the growth plate separating the secondary ossification center of the proximal tibial epiphysis from the tibial metaphysis is often confused with a fracture line. The proximal tibial growth plate is capped by an epiphysis that forms the tibial portion of the knee joint. A tongue-like projection of the epiphysis extends downward along the anterior crest of the tibia and serves as the site of attachment for the patellar tendon. Separate ossification centers within this extension are often mistaken for fracture fragments. Comparison views of the opposite knee are helpful in making the distinction (Figs 2–43 and 2–44).

Abnormal forces applied to the knee may result in failure through ligamentous structures or through underlying bone. In young children, failure usually occurs through bone, producing typical growth plate fractures. In older children and adolescents, failure may occur through either soft tissues or through bone. The clinical signs of ligamentous injury and tibial fractures are quite similar. Fractures that involve the growth plate or epiphysis usually produce a prompt bloody effusion, as do significant ligament injuries. Active motion is restricted, and passive motion is painful. Point tenderness will be present both at the site of fracture and over the site of ligamentous injury. Joint instability may be present in either case.

Careful evaluation of vascular and neurologic function is imperative. The major vessels and nerves to the lower leg lie in close proximity to the growth plate and may be damaged by sharp fracture fragments or compromised by fracture

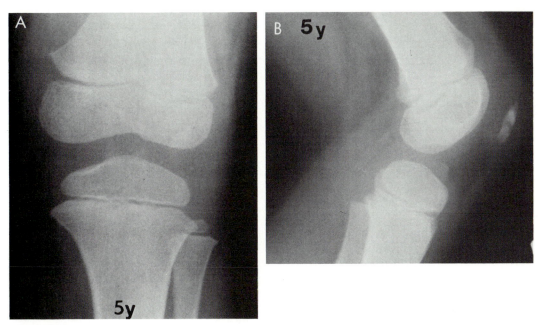

FIG 2–43.
A, anterior view of ossification centers around the knee in a 5-year-old child. Secondary centers are visible in the distal femur, proximal tibia, and proximal fibula. **B,** lateral view, aged 5 years. The ossification center for the patella is present.

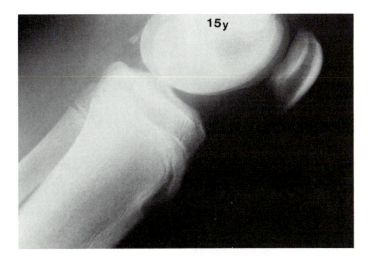

FIG 2–44.
Lateral view of the knee—15-year-old male. The growth plates at the distal femur, proximal tibia, and proximal fibula have nearly closed. Union between the tibial tubercle and proximal tibial metaphysis is not yet complete. A small normal accessory ossicle, the fabella, is present posterior to the femoral condyles in this patient.

displacement. The signs of ischemia in the lower leg are identical to those in the forearm. Pain in the leg despite immobilization, pain on passive dorsiflexion of the toes, pallor in the distal limb, paresthesia in the foot, lack of active dorsiflexion or plantar flexion of the foot or toes, and absence of posterior tibial or dorsalis pedis pulses are cardinal signs of vascular compromise. Impending ischemia is an absolute surgical emergency.

Initial radiographic evaluation of patients with suspected fractures around the knee should consist of anteroposterior and lateral roentgenograms made through temporary radiolucent splints. Tunnel views made through the flexed knee may be necessary if preliminary films suggest intra-articular fractures. Stress views of the knee may be needed to separate instability secondary to fracture from instability caused by ligament injury (Fig 2–45).

Avulsion fractures of the tibial tubercle occur occasionally in adolescence after athletic, bicycle, or motor vehicle accidents (Fig 2–46). The injuries are probably the result of violent quadriceps contraction against a flexed knee; after the pull of the patellar tendon initiates failure at the distal pole to the proximal tibial physis, the fracture propagates proximally through the zone of hypertrophic cartilage. In some cases, the fracture stops short of the articular surface; in others the fracture line may extend into the joint. Pain, tenderness, and knee effusion are consistent findings. Active knee extension against gravity may be difficult or impossible. Lateral roentgenograms confirm the diagnosis. Minimally displaced incomplete avulsion fractures are usually treated by cast immobilization; fractures with wide separation or joint incongruity are best treated operatively.

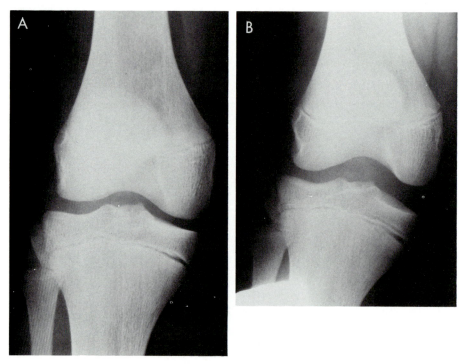

FIG 2–45.
Stress views of the knee in a 13-year-old boy with instability after injury. **A,** unstressed view. **B,** stressed view demonstrating medial ligamentous instability.

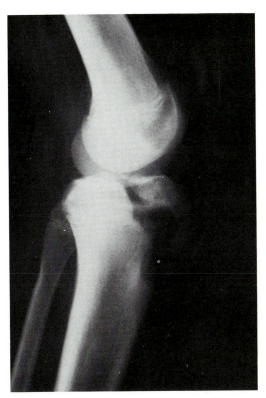

FIG 2–46.
Proximal tibial growth plate fracture through the tibial tubercle.

Fractures through the anterior or posterior tibial spine may occur if loads applied through the cruciate ligaments exceed the failure limits of underlying bone. Posterior spine fractures are much less common than anterior spine fractures. Both result in anteroposterior instability on manual testing. Operative fixation is usually required (Fig 2–47).

Proximal tibial physeal fractures are rare injuries and are usually the result of motorcycle or athletic accidents. The risk of vascular compromise is high because of the proximity of the popliteal vessels to the posterior border of the proximal tibia. In addition, damage to the peroneal nerve may occur at the time of injury or as a result of subsequent swelling. Careful assessment of neurologic and vascular function is the first step in the management of these fractures. If adequate circulatory function is not present, arteriography and surgical exploration may be necessary to restore blood flow. Fasciotomy of the closed muscular compartments of the lower leg may be required to prevent severe muscle damage.

Type I and II fractures of the proximal tibial growth plate can usually be treated nonoperatively when vascular compromise is not present. The incidence of late complications, such as premature growth plate closure with leg-length inequality or angular deformity, is higher than that of similar fractures in other parts of the body, and patients must be carefully followed until completion of growth. Type III and IV fractures with joint incongruity often require open reduction and internal fixation (Fig 2–48). The incidence of premature plate closure is high, and late joint incongruity may result in deformity and premature degenerative disease.

Tibial shaft fractures may result from perpendicular loads, torsional forces, or combinations of both. As with femoral fractures, the configuration of the fracture surfaces indicates the nature of the deforming force and the severity of the injury to surrounding soft tissue (Figs 2–49 and 2–50). Tibial shaft fractures in adults are often difficult to reduce and heal slowly; open reduction and internal fixation may be necessary to maintain reduction. Most children's fractures are much simpler to treat. Closed reduction and cast immobilization are usually successful. A small amount of override can be accepted if rotary and angular malalignment are avoided. Comminution of a tibial fracture indicates greater damage to surrounding soft tissues (Fig 2–51). Fracture fragments may be stripped of blood supply, and delayed healing can be expected. Open comminuted fractures of the tibial shaft are among the most difficult frac-

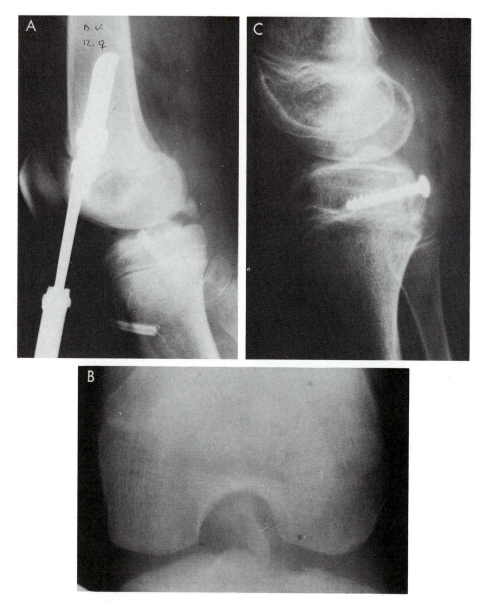

FIG 2–47.
Preoperative **(A** and **B)** and postoperative **(C)** roentgenograms of posterior tibial spine fracture.

tures to treat successfully. Surgical debridement is mandatory, and external fixation devices may be required to maintain
alignment. Bone and skin grafting are often necessary during the course of treatment.

Ankle Injuries

Sprains, strains, and fractures around
the ankle joint are usually the result of a
combination of twisting and bending
forces. Often the foot is caught and fixed

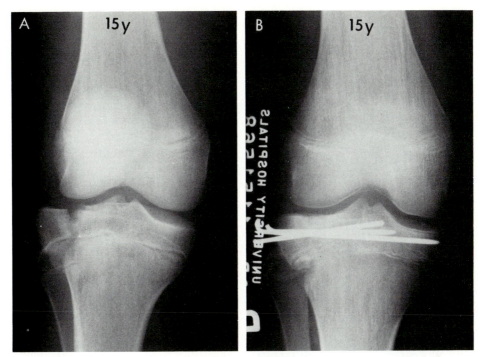

FIG 2–48.
A, type IV proximal tibial fracture. **B,** roentgenogram made after open reduction and internal fixation.

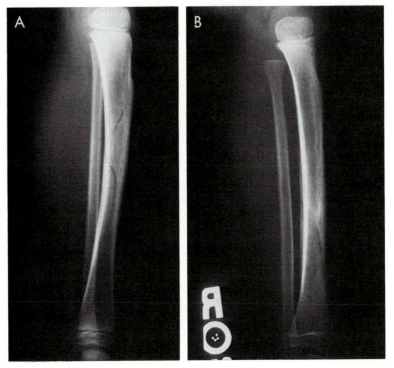

FIG 2–49.
A, minimally displaced spiral tibial shaft fracture resulting from a twisting force in a child abuse victim. **B,** 4 weeks after injury. Note periosteal elevation along the shaft.

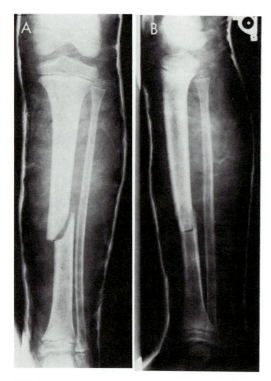

FIG 2–50.
Short oblique tibial fracture in a child who was trapped beneath a falling bicycle. **A,** anteroposterior view. **B,** lateral view.

while the body rotates around it. If the foot is forced into an inverted position, injuries of the lateral ligaments or the lateral malleolus occur first. When the foot is forcibly everted, medial injuries occur first. As in other parts of the body, fractures are more common than ligament injuries in young children; sprains become more common in older children and adolescents.

Many of the clinical findings of ankle injury are common to both bone and soft tissue lesions. Pain, localized tenderness, and restriction of motion are the rule. Joint swelling, manifested by obliteration of the slight depression normally found anterior to the lateral malleolus, may follow intra-articular fractures of severe ligament injuries. Gross deformity usually indicates underlying fracture, but fractures

may also be present in the absence of obvious deformities.

Careful radiologic evaluation of patients with suspected ankle injuries is essential. Anteroposterior, lateral, and oblique views should always be obtained. The extremity should be splinted before the patient is moved to the x-ray department to minimize pain and prevent further damage. Air splints must be used with care since they may further compromise limited circulation.

The radiologic appearance of the growth plates of the distal tibia and fibula is not complex (Fig 2–52). The secondary ossification center for the distal tibial epiphysis usually appears during the first year. Between ages 7 and 8 years, a comma-shaped prolongation of ossification within the medial malleolus occurs.

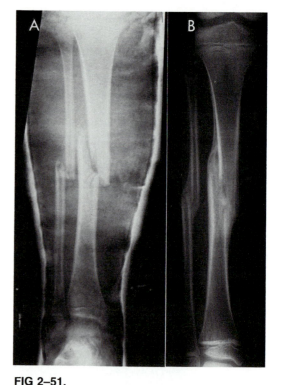

FIG 2–51.
A, comminuted, oblique tibial shaft fracture in a young skier. **B,** roentgenographic appearance 20 weeks after injury. Growth stimulation will compensate for the slight override of the fracture fragments.

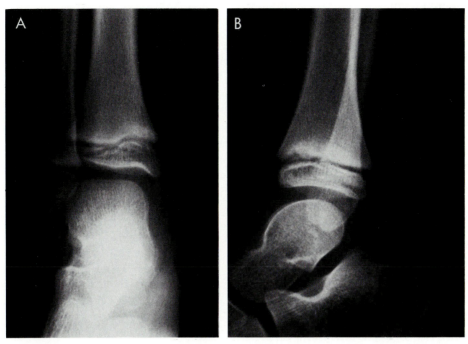

FIG 2–52.
A, Anteroposterior view of ankle, aged 6 years. **B,** lateral view of ankle, aged 6 years.

Closure of the growth plate usually occurs between ages 14 and 17 years. The secondary ossification center of the distal fibula appears by age 2 years, and the physis closes at about the same time as the distal tibial growth plate. Comparison views of the opposite extremity should be obtained when a question exists.

In the absence of roentgenographic evidence of bone injury, pain, tenderness, and limitation of motion should be taken as signs of ligament sprain. Tenderness around the medial malleolus indicates deltoid ligament damage; tenderness around the distal fibula indicates injury to lateral supporting ligaments. Of these, the anterior talofibular ligament running from the anterior portion of the fibula to the anterolateral portion of the talus is the most commonly injured ligament. At times, careful inspection of the roentgenograms will show a small fleck of bone at the site of ligament avulsion.

Ankle sprains not associated with joint instability or fracture can be treated acutely in a soft compression dressing. Ice and elevation in the immediate postinjury period are useful to minimize swelling. Active range of motion exercises can be started as soon as acute symptoms subside, and progressive weight bearing may be started 2 to 3 days post injury. Full return to function can be expected in 7 to 10 days. More serious ankle sprains may require a period of immobilization to permit ligamentous healing to occur before motion can be resumed. At times operative repair of complete ruptures is necessary, although this is very uncommon in patients with open growth plates.

Fractures around the ankle require careful orthopedic treatment. The ankle is one of the major weight-bearing joints; residual angular deformity and joint incongruity are tolerated poorly. Type I fractures of the distal fibula and tibia usually heal without complication if anatomical reduction is obtained. The prognosis in type II fractures of the distal tibia is more guarded. In some cases, distraction of the medial portion of the physis may be accompanied by crush injury of the lateral portion. Premature closure of a portion of the growth plate will follow, and angular deformity will occur with growth. Accurate reduction of type II injuries is required, but even if anatomical alignment is obtained, the outcome is unpredictable.

Open reduction of ankle fractures that involve the articular surface is frequently necessary to secure anatomical alignment (Figs 2–53 and 2–54). The risks of partial growth plate closure are high in these injuries, and parents must be advised of the possibility of late deformity at the start of treatment. Crush injuries of the distal growth plate have an especially poor prognosis. Shortening and angular deformity may develop with growth.

Fractures in the Foot

Tarsal fractures are uncommon in children. Calcaneal fractures sometimes follow a fall in the standing position. When calcaneal fractures are minimally displaced, protection with a bulky dressing and crutches for 3 to 4 weeks is adequate treatment. More significantly displaced calcaneal fractures require careful manipulative or surgical reduction to restore congruity of the calcaneotalar joint.

Fractures of the talus and fracture dislocations of the tarsometatarsal joints occur occasionally in adolescent motorcyclists. Surgical reduction is usually necessary. Talar neck fractures have a guarded prognosis; the blood supply to the talus is tenuous, and avascular necrosis with late degenerative arthritis often complicates fracture.

Minimally displaced metatarsal fractures can be adequately treated with a short leg cast and crutches for 3 to 4 weeks (Fig 2–55). Closed reduction may be necessary in displaced fractures. Phalangeal fractures can usually be treated by taping the injured toe to its neighbor for 3 weeks (Fig 2–56). A piece of cotton gauze should be interposed to prevent maceration. Weight bearing in a firm sole shoe can be permitted as tolerated.

SPINE INJURY

Spine injury in children is usually the result of extraordinary trauma. Automobile accidents, falls, diving mishaps, football, and trampoline accidents account for most vertebral column injuries. The mobile and unprotected cervical spine is most often involved; thoracic and lumbar spine fractures and dislocations occur less

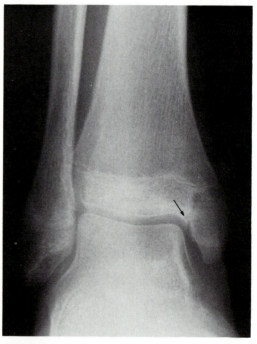

FIG 2–53.
Minimally displaced type III fracture of the medial malleolus *(arrow).*

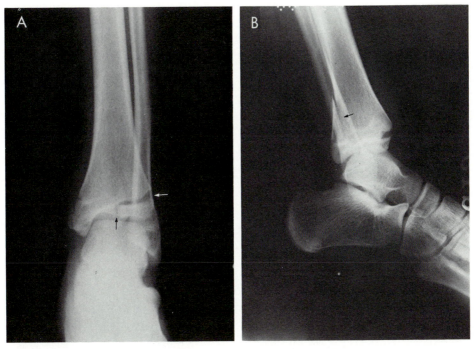

FIG 2–54.
Type IV fracture of the distal tibia—the so-called triplane fracture. **A,** anterior view demonstrates sagittal *(black arrow)* and horizontal *(white arrow)* fracture planes in the distal tibial epiphysis. **B,** lateral view demonstrates a frontally oriented metaphyseal fragment *(arrow).*

often. The upper cervical segments are most often involved in young children; lower cervical spine levels are more often involved in adolescents.

Vertebral column injury may occur without spinal cord damage or may be associated with neurologic deficit ranging from weakness and paresthesia to complete paralysis. Spinal cord damage often is sustained at the time of injury; unfortunately, neurologic damage may also occur during transportation or initial clinical or radiologic examination. This late damage is almost always preventable.

Evaluation of the child with suspected spinal injury can be quite difficult. Young patients cannot relate details of accidents well and may describe symptoms poorly. Careful neurologic examination may be impossible because of pain and apprehen-sion. Fortunately, clues to the nature and extent of damage are often present.

The combination of neck or back pain and soft tissue injury in a conscious patient strongly suggests spine injury. When the vertebral column is injured by direct blows from flying missiles, falling objects, or blunt weapons, overlying soft tissue damage may localize the site of spinal injury. Contusions on the forehead or occiput after an automobile accident or a fall, when associated with neck pain, may indicate acute hyperflexion or hyperextension of the neck. Eccentric contusions imply rotational forces during injury.

In most cases, the severity of symptoms correlates well with the degree of spine injury in conscious children. Patients with little pain or tenderness in the

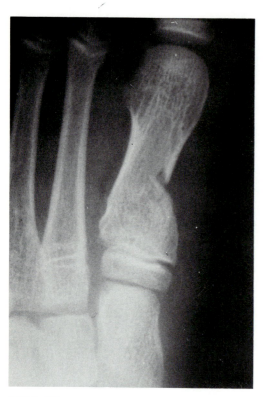

FIG 2–55.
Minimally angulated fracture of the great toe metatarsal. Reduction is not necessary in this case.

neck, minimal muscle spasm, and no neurologic compromise usually do not have significant spine injury. Pain, tenderness, muscle spasm, and guarding, with or without neurologic abnormalities, imply more serious injury in the conscious patient. The unconscious patient with suggestive soft tissue injury or appropriate history should be considered to have spinal column injury until proved otherwise.

Any patient with suspected spinal injury must be handled with care. The patient should be splinted on a backboard and his head held in neutral position with sandbags or blocks. Extreme caution is essential while positioning the backboard. Once immobilized, the patient should not be moved again until a diagnosis is established and appropriate treatment begun.

Radiology of Spine Injury

High-quality roentgenograms are essential for evaluation of the potentially injured spine. Anteroposterior and lateral views should be obtained without moving the child from the backboard. Flexion, extension, and oblique views should be made only after careful review of films for which no motion of the spine is required. Tomography and computed tomography are often necessary to precisely define suspected injury.

Roentgenograms of the immature spine are difficult to interpret. Normal os-

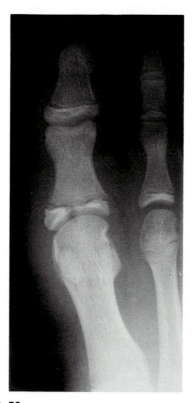

FIG 2–56.
Type III fracture of the proximal phalanx of the great toe. No reduction is necessary.

sification centers may be mistaken for fracture fragments, and the junctions of incompletely ossified vertebral elements may resemble fracture lines. The normal hypermobility of the child's spine may be mistaken for subluxation. At times, damage to vertebrae is obvious on initial roentgenograms. In other cases, vertebral fractures, subluxations, and dislocations may not be immediately evident. In these instances, alterations in the normal contour of spinal segments and displacement of normal soft tissue shadows may suggest more serious spinal injury.

Spasm in the supporting muscles of the spine after injury alters spinal configuration. As a result, the normal lordotic and kyphotic curves of the vertebral column may appear flattened on lateral views. Scoliosis may be present on anteroposterior views. Bleeding into the soft tissues around the spinal column may be manifested by displacement of the tracheal air shadow in the cervical spine or by obliteration of the psoas muscle shadows or renal outlines in the thoracolumbar spine. Ileus may be a manifestation of sympathetic and parasympathetic trunk irritation.

Radiologic signs of cervical spine injury in the child (Figs 2–57 through 2–61) include:

1. Loss of height, angular deformity, or fragmentation of a vertebral body.
2. Soft tissue swelling in the prevertebral area, manifested by anterior displacement of the tracheal air shadow.
3. Loss of normal cervical lordosis in older children and adolescents. (This may be normal in young children.)
4. Displacement of more than 3 mm of one vertebral body onto another in the lateral projection.
5. Posterior displacement of the odontoid process more than 5 mm from

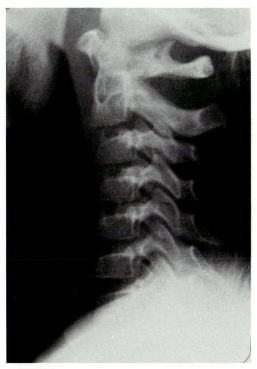

FIG 2–57.
Normal lateral roentgenogram of the cervical spine in a 10-year-old patient. Absence of normal adult cervical lordosis may be normal in children but may also indicate soft tissue injury. The anterior and posterior borders of vertebral bodies usually are in line. Up to 3 mm of forward displacement of one vertebral body on another may be normal in young children. Note relationship of tracheal air shadow to the anterior aspect of the vertebral column.

the posterior edge of the first cervical vertebral body.

Signs of injury in the thoracic and lumbar spine include:

1. Vertebral fragmentation, wedging, or loss of weight.
2. Displacement of one vertebral body onto another in either the anteroposterior or lateral direction.
3. Loss of thoracic kyphosis or lumbar lordosis, or acute scoliosis.
4. Ileus resulting from sympathetic

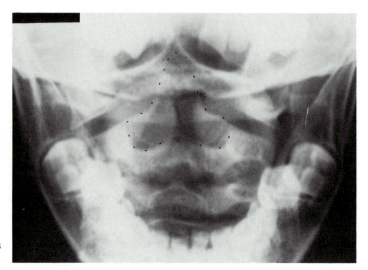

FIG 2–58.
Open-mouth view of the odontoid
process. The odontoid fits like a
bottle stopper into the lateral arches
of C-2.

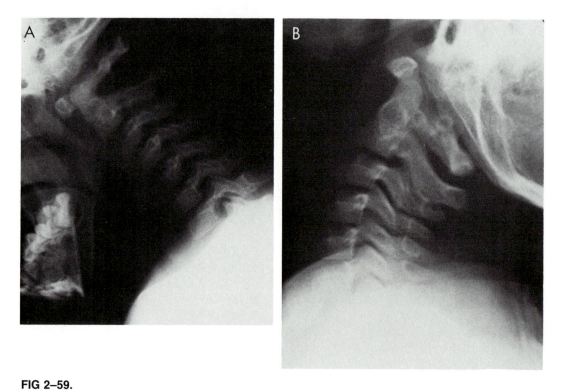

FIG 2–59.
Flexion **(A)** and extension **(B)** views of the normal cervical spine. More than 5 mm of anterior displacement of the
arch of C-1 from the odontoid process indicates cervical instability. Forward or backward displacement of individual vertebral bodies should normally not exceed 3 mm.

and parasympathetic nerve trunk damage.

Small triangular secondary ossification centers are often seen at the superior and inferior corners of the anterior portion of normal vertebral bodies in adolescents. These should not be mistaken for fracture fragments in asymptomatic patients. Symptomatic patients with suggestive radiologic findings require immediate orthopedic or neurosurgical consultation. The costs of underdiagnosis of spine injury are high.

Management

Children with suspected spinal injuries should be immobilized immediately. A rapid search for respiratory and cardiovascular injury should be conducted next. Extreme caution must be used in maintaining an airway. Neck hyperextension must be avoided. Usually the airway can be opened by lifting the mandible forward. Oral airways may induce vomiting and should be avoided. Intubation may

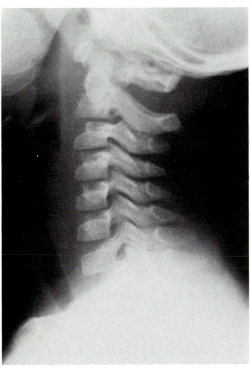

FIG 2–60.
Anterior displacement of the tracheal air shadow in a child who sustained a hyperextension injury of the cervical spine with no neurologic or vertebral damage (see Fig 2–57).

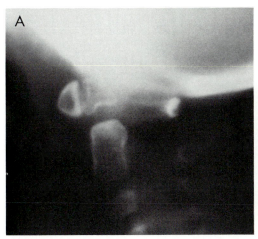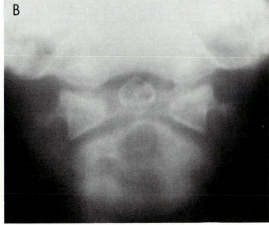

FIG 2–61.
Lateral **(A)** and anterior **(B)** tomograms of the upper cervical spine in a 6-year-old child with nonunion of a presumed fracture through the odontoid process. The radiolucent area between the fracture fragments is well above the usual synchondrosis of the odontoid and the lateral masses of C-2 (see Fig 2–58). This has led some authors to conclude that this lesion may be developmental rather than traumatic.

be necessary but should be performed only by experienced personnel; inept attempts at orotracheal or nasotracheal intubation may result in permanent neurologic damage.

The initial neurologic examination of a child with spinal trauma is critical in determining treatment and prognosis. Without moving the patient from the backboard, motor function in the major flexor and extensor muscle groups of the extremities should be determined. Deep tendon reflexes at the elbows, wrists, knees, and ankles should be recorded. Sensory deficits in the upper and lower extremities must be noted. Perianal sensation and rectal sphincter tone are critical indicators of the degree of spinal cord injury. Sensory sparing in the perianal region suggests an incomplete spinal cord lesion, despite apparent quadriparesis.

Treatment of the neurologic damage resulting from spine injury depends on the nature of the lesion. Patients with immediate and complete paralysis in most cases do not benefit from decompressive laminectomy; in fact, laminectomy may render the spine even more unstable. Patients with incomplete and progressive neurologic damage require prompt spinal cord decompression. The role of spinal cord decompression for patients with incomplete and unchanging or improving neurologic signs is not firmly established.

The orthopedic management of spine injury is based on the probability of either acute or chronic vertebral column instability. Injuries such as vertebral compression fractures without neurologic damage are stable and require only symptomatic care. Other injuries may be either acutely or chronically unstable and may lead to further neurologic damage or severe spine deformity unless adequately immobilized or surgically stabilized.

SUGGESTED READINGS

Hollinshead WH: *The Back and Lower Limbs: Anatomy for Surgeons*, ed 2. New York, Harper & Row, 1969, vol 3.

Ozonoff MB: *Pediatric Orthopedic Radiology*. Philadelphia, WB Saunders Co, 1979.

Rang M: *Children's Fractures*. Philadelphia, JB Lippincott, Co, 1974.

Rubin P: *Dynamic Classification of Bone Dysplasias*. Chicago, Year Book Medical Publishers, 1972.

Salter RB, Harris WR: Injuries involving the epiphyseal plate. *J Bone Joint Surg Am* 1963; 45:587.

Surgical Staff, Hospital for Sick Children, Toronto, Canada: *Care for the Injured Child*. Baltimore, Williams & Wilkins Co, 1975.

Child Abuse
Akbarnia B, et al: Manifestations of the battered child syndrome. *J Bone Joint Surg Am* 1974; 56:1159.

Helfer RE, Kempe CH (eds): *The Battered Child*, ed 2. Chicago, University of Chicago Press, 1974.

McNeese MC, Hebeler JR: The abused child: A clinical approach to identification and management. *Clin Symp* 1977; 29(5).

O'Neill JA, et al: Patterns of injury in the battered child syndrome. *J Trauma* 1973; 13:332.

Injuries Around the Shoulder
Campbell J, Almond HGA: Fracture-separation of the proximal humeral epiphysis: A case report. *J Bone Joint Surg Am* 1977; 59:262.

Rowe CR, Pierce DS, Clark JG: Voluntary dislocation of the shoulder. *J Bone Joint Surg Am* 1973; 55:445.

Injuries of the Elbow
Conwell HE: Injuries to the Elbow. *Clin Symp* 1969; 21(2):35.

Jakob R, et al: Observations concerning fractures of the lateral condyle in children. *J Bone Joint Surg Br* 1975; 57:430.

Salter RB, Zaltz C: Anatomic investigations of the mechanism of injury and pathologic anatomy of pulled elbow in young children. *Clin Orthop* 1971; 77:134.

Smith L: Deformity following supracondylar fracture of the humerus. *J Bone Joint Surg Am* 1960; 42:235.

Fractures of the Forearm and Wrist
Davis DR, Green DP: Forearm fractures in children. *Clin Orthop* 1976; 120:172.

Mikic Z: Galeazzi fracture-dislocation. *J Bone Joint Surg Am* 1975; 57:1071.

Piero A, Andres F, Fernandez-Esteve F: Acute Monteggia lesions in children. *J Bone Joint Surg Am* 1977; 59:92.

Hand Injuries
Dickson GL, Moon NF: Rotational supracondylar fractures of the proximal phalanx in children. *Clin Orthop*; 1972; 83:151.

Engber WD, Clancy WG: Traumatic avulsion of the fingernail associated with injury to the phalangeal epiphysis plate. *J Bone Joint Surg Am* 1978; 60:713.

Illingworth CM: Trapped fingers and amputated fingertips in children. *J Pediatr Surg* 1974; 9:853.

Leonard MH, Dubravcik P: Management of fractured fingers in the child. *Clin Orthop* 1970; 73:160.

Rosenthal LJ, Reiner MA, Bleicher MA: Nonoperative management of distal fingertip amputations in children. *Pediatrics* 1979; 64:1.

Injuries Around the Pelvis
Cook GT, Barkin M, Schillinger JF: Urologic injuries: II. Upper and lower genito-urinary tract, in the Surgical Staff, Hospital for Sick Children, Toronto, Canada (eds): *Care for the Injured Child*. Baltimore, Williams & Wilkins Co, 1975, pp 166–169.

Kay SP, Hall JE: Fracture of the femoral neck in children and its complications. *Clin Orthop* 1971; 80:53.

Miller WE: Fractures of the hip in children from birth to adolescence. *Clin Orthop* 1973; 92:155.

Pearson DE, Mann RJ: Traumatic hip dislocation in children. *Clin Orthop* 1973; 92:189.

Pennsylvania Orthopedic Society: Traumatic dislocation of the hip joint in children. *J Bone Joint Surg Am* 1968; 50:79.

Fractures of the Leg and Lower Leg
Cooperman DR, Spiegel PG, Laros G: Tibial fractures involving the ankle in children: The so-called triplane epiphyseal fracture. *J Bone Joint Surg Am* 1978; 60:1040.

Griffin P, et al: Fractures of the shaft of the femur in children: Treatment and results. *Orthop Clin North Am* 1972; 3:213.

Irani R, Nicholson J, Chung S: Long term results in the treatment of femoral shaft fractures in young children by immediate spica immobilization. *J Bone Joint Surg Am* 1976; 58:945.

Jackson DW, Cozen L: Genu valgum as a complication of proximal tibial metaphyseal fractures in children. *J Bone Joint Surg Am* 1971 53:1571.

Ogden JA, Tross RB, Murphy MJ: Fractures of the tibial tuberosity in adolescents. *J Bone Joint Surg Am* 1980; 62:205.

Spiegel PG, Cooperman DR, Laros GS: Epiphyseal fracture of the distal ends of the tibia and fibula. *J Bone Joint Surg Am* 1978; 60:1046.

Spine Injury
Cattell HS, Filtzer DL: Pseudosubluxation and other normal variations of the cervical spine in children. *J Bone Joint Surg Am* 1965; 47:1295.

Dawson EG, Smith L: Atlanto-axial subluxation in children due to vertebral anomalies. *J Bone Joint Surg Am* 1979; 61:582.

Fielding JW: Selected observations on the cervical spine in childhood, in Ashstrom JP (ed): *Current Practices in Orthopaedic Surgery*. St Louis, CW Mosby Co, 1973, pp 31–55.

Hubbard DD: Injuries of the spine in children and adolescents. *Clin Orthop* 1974; 100:56.

Sherk HH, Nicholson JT, Chung SM: Fractures of the odontoid in young children. *J Bone Joint Surg Am* 1978; 60:921.

3

Lower Extremity Development

The child is neither an anatomical nor a functional model of the adult. A toddler's progress to mature form and function is punctuated by stumbling, tripping, and falling. The wide range of acceptability in lower limb configuration and gait development is often poorly understood by new parents, and unexpected idiosyncrasies can be the source of great concern. Friendly advice is readily available but often results in prolonged, expensive, and unnecessary treatment. This chapter examines early gait development and variations in lower extremity configuration.

DEVELOPMENT OF GAIT

Normal Gait

Children ordinarily take their first tentative steps with external support between ages 9 and 14 months. The interval between this assisted ambulation and independent walking varies greatly, but most children are free of external support by age 18 months. The angular and rotational movements of adult gait develop slowly in toddlers, and their absence accounts for many of the peculiarities of early walking.

In mature gait, walking on smooth, level ground entails a repetitive cycle of identical events in each limb (Fig 3–1). Each limb sequentially contacts the ground, bears the weight of the body, and then leaves the ground as the other limb makes contact. The gait cycle is defined as the interval between foot contacts of the same limb and is divided into stance and swing phases. Each phase is composed of a number of distinct events. Foot contact is the initial event of stance phase; this occurs by heel strike in normal gait. Contact response occurs next; in normal mature individuals, contact response is plantar flexion of the ankle. At midstance the foot is flat on the ground, and the hip and knee are extended. Midstance

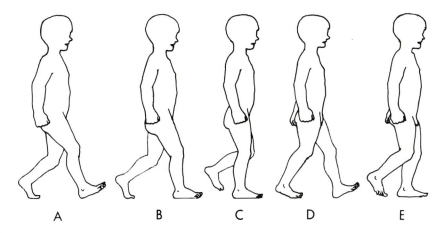

FIG 3–1.

Phases of gait in a 4-year-old child. Reciprocal arm motion is not as pronounced in a child of this age as in an adult. **A,** heel strike of the right foot occurs before the left foot leaves the ground, giving a period of double stance that is characteristic of walking. In this child, the right hip is flexed and the right knee nearly fully extended at heel strike. **B,** dorsiflexion of the foot follows, to achieve a foot-flat position as the left foot toes off. The knee is slightly more flexed and the hip less flexed as the body moves forward. **C,** at midstance the foot is flat on the ground, and the knee and hip are very slightly flexed. The left leg is in midswing phase. **D,** terminal stance phase begins as the right heel leaves the ground. Hip and knee extension are present on the right side. Heel strike has occurred on the left. **E,** toe-off of the right foot ends right stance phase. Hip and knee flexion occurs to advance the right leg.

ends as the center of gravity passes over the ankle and the heel leaves the ground. Stance phase ends as the foot pushes off the ground.

Swing phase begins as the foot leaves the ground and the limb accelerates forward. By convention, swing phase is divided into three periods: initial swing, which immediately follows toe off and ends as the ankle passes forward of the opposite tibia; midswing, which ends as the tibia of the swing limb passes the other limb and becomes vertically aligned; and terminal swing, during which the limb slows in preparation for foot contact. Swing phase ends at foot contact, the initial event of stance phase of another cycle.

In normal adult gait, stance phase occupies about 60% of the gait cycle and swing phase about 40%. The resultant period of double stance, in which one limb has made foot contact and the other is preparing to push off, is characteristic of walking. There is no period of double

stance in running, jogging, or hopping. The duration of the double stance phase of gait is longer in toddlers than in adults; with increasing maturity, swing phase occupies a greater proportion of the gait cycle.

A number of mechanisms are employed to make walking smooth and efficient. Coordinated movement of the pelvis, knee, and foot minimizes the vertical translation of the body's center of gravity and flattens its path to a sinusoidal curve. This reduces the energy expenditure in walking and lessens the impact force across the joint surfaces of the lower limb that occurs each time the foot makes contact with the ground. Stability in stance phase and foot clearance in swing phase are provided through coordinated action of flexor and extensor muscle groups around the ankle, knee, and hip.

Reciprocal ankle plantar flexion and dorsiflexion are characteristic of normal mature gait. The ankle is dorsiflexed at the start of stance phase, and foot contact is made with heel strike in mature gait. Plantar flexion of the ankle immediately follows; this is controlled by the muscles of the anterior compartment of the calf. Controlled relaxation of these muscles decelerates the limb and prevents the foot from slapping on the ground. As the body moves forward, dorsiflexion of the ankle again occurs, so that at midstance the ankle is in neutral position, and the foot is flat on the ground. Plantar flexion follows midstance, and at toe off, contraction of the posterior muscles of the calf occurs to accelerate the limb forward. Dorsiflexion of the ankle occurs during swing phase to provide clearance for the foot and to prepare the limb for heel strike at the start of stance phase. Toddlers may start stance phase with toe touch or foot flat instead of heel strike. A tiptoe posture may be maintained throughout stance phase in normal children for several months after walking begins. By age 18 months to 2 years, the adult pattern of heel strike, ankle plantar flexion, foot flat, and toe off are present at least part of the time in most normal infants. Persistent plantar flexion at the start of stance phase may be a sign of underlying neurologic abnormality.

Cyclic knee flexion and extension are characteristic of mature gait. In adults, the knee is in nearly full extension at the start of stance phase and flexes immediately as the body moves forward (Fig 3–2). At midstance the knee is slightly flexed and then extends prior to toe off. Knee flexion occurs at toe off, and during swing phase the knee passes from flexion to extension in preparation for heel strike at the start of stance phase. The smooth knee flexion-extension wave characteristic of adult gait is absent in immature gait. Toddlers often start stance phase with the knee in flexion; knee extension may follow heel strike, or the knee may be held in the same degree of flexion throughout stance

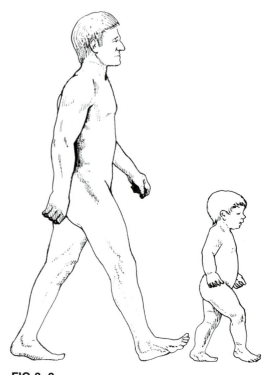

FIG 3–2
Early stance phase, right side, in adult and toddler. The adult starts stance with heel strike, dorsiflexed ankle, and a nearly fully extended knee. A toddler may begin stance with toe touch and a flexed knee.

phase. This pattern of knee motion in stance phase in young children causes an increased vertical translation of the center of gravity and contributes to the bobbing appearance of the toddler's gait.

At the start of stance phase, the adult hip is flexed and slightly laterally rotated. Extension and medial rotation occur during stance phase as the center of gravity of the body passes forward of the hip joint. At toe off, the hip is maximally extended and medially rotated. During swing phase, rapid extension and lateral rotation occur as the hip flexors and adductor muscles pull the limb forward. The normal range of flexion and extension in the adult is from approximately 40 degrees flexion at the start of stance to 20 degrees flexion at the time of toe off. This arc is much less in the toddler; although hip flexion at the start of stance phase may approach the adult angle, extension of the hip during stance is limited, and in early walking, full hip extension may not occur. This results in a disproportionately shorter stride length, and a longer period of double stance in the toddler. In addition, lateral rotation is often greater, especially when walking first begins, most probably as a result of posterior hip capsular and muscular contractures that have persisted since birth.

Other more subtle differences exist between early and mature gait. Toddlers' gait tends to be wide based; the feet are often placed outside the lateral margins of the trunk. Synchronous reciprocal arm motion is absent. The arms may be widely abducted and are often held forward of the body (Fig 3–3). Cadence is high, but overall velocity of gait is low because of the short stride length. Increases in velocity must be achieved by increases in cadence rather than by increases in stride length or decreases in the period of double limb stance. All of the idiosyncrasies of early gait are accentuated when the child begins to run.

As the child matures, rhythmicity and reproducibility improve. By age 2 years, stance phase is initiated by heel strike, and the foot is flat at midstance. The knee flexion-extension wave has begun to develop; the knee flexes after foot strike and extends prior to toe off. The base of stance is decreased as the feet fall within the margins of the trunk when viewed from the front. Reciprocal arm swing has begun to develop. By age 3 years, most of the characteristics of adult gait are present at least part of the time in normal children, although stride length is still short, and velocity is low. With further maturation and growth, stride length and velocity increase, and cadence decreases. Although wide variations exist in otherwise normal children, the synchronous patterns of adult gait are usually present by age 3 years, and consistent by age 7 years. Delay in gait development or obligate repetition of an immature gait pattern such as tiptoeing or wide arm abduction may indicate underlying neuromuscular disease.

Limping

Abnormalities of development, trauma, neurologic disorders, and muscle diseases that produce alterations in the expected patterns of gait are manifest as limping. When a child limps, he attempts to shorten single stance phase on the affected limb as much as possible to decrease pain and minimize instability. Stride length decreases, and the period of double stance increases. Alterations in the normal angular motions of lower limb joints are present. Evaluation of the limping child often is confusing, but thorough observation and correlation with normal walking patterns usually permits accurate primary diagnosis (see Fig 1–16).

Careful review of the patient's history is the first step in the evaluation of limp. Delay in onset of walking or abnormal gait patterns in a child whose neonatal

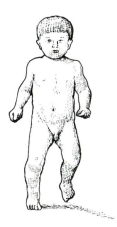

FIG 3–3.
Abduction and forward flexion of both arms are characteristic of early gait. The feet are placed outside the lateral margins of the trunk.

period was stormy strongly suggest underlying neurologic disorders. Asymmetry of right and left gait cycles in a child whose motor milestones are otherwise normal more likely is the result of unilateral structural abnormalities such as congenital hip dysplasia. The acute onset of a painful limp in a previously normal child suggests inflammatory or traumatic processes. The gradual onset of limping with intermittent or mild discomfort in an older child may be a sign of either one of the developmental disorders of the lower limbs, such as Legg-Calvé-Perthes disease or slipped capital femoral epiphysis, or may indicate the presence of a previously unsuspected spinal dysraphism or myopathic or neuropathic disease.

Visual evaluation of gait requires patience and practice. The first step in examining a child with a perceived limp is to classify the limp as asymmetric or symmetric. In asymmetric limping, the gait cycle on the uninvolved side is normal. In symmetric limping, the gait cycle on both sides is abnormal. Identification of the involved limb is simple in the child with asymmetric limp; it is the limb with the shortest period of single stance. Evaluation of symmetric limp is more difficult; comparison of observed patterns of motion to expected patterns for a normal child at the same stage of development is necessary. Relative duration of stance and swing phase and the duration of the period of double stance provide clues. Prolongation of double stance, shortened swing, decreased stride length, and decreased velocity are characteristic of symmetric limp.

After initial characterization of a limp, an attempt should be made to identify its cause and localize if possible the affected limb segment. Sequential comparison of angular motions at the hip, knee, and ankle to either the opposite unaffected side in a patient with asymmetric limp or to expected values in a child with symmetric limp often discloses the source of the limp. Decreased angular excursion of a joint may result from reflex guarding to diminish pain or may be the result of attempts to minimize instability when weakness is present. In other instances, decreased motion may be the result of muscular or ligamentous contracture. Palpation, determination of active and passive ranges of motion, and evaluation of strength in the limb usually permit primary identification of the problem.

Idiopathic Toe Walking

Tiptoe gait is normal during the first months after independent walking begins. By age 2 years, most normal children have established a pattern of heel-toe gait at least part of the time. Persistent tiptoe gait after age 2 years is abnormal and requires evaluation. Although some normal children continue to toe walk past age 2 years, persistent toe walking may be an early sign of underlying neuromuscular disease. Children with mild spastic cerebral palsy often toe walk; in these patients, a suggestive neonatal history, delay in achieving milestones in gross motor development, and the finding of exaggerated deep tendon reflexes or of clonus at the ankle indicates a central neurologic lesion. Unilateral tiptoe gait with wide abduction of the ipsilateral arm is characteristic of hemiplegia; bilateral tiptoe gait with increased hip and knee flexion, exaggerated trunk motion, and abduction of both arms is a sign of diplegic involvement.

The insidious development of tiptoe gait in a previously normal child is especially ominous. Toe walking is one of the early signs of myopathic diseases such as Duchenne type muscular dystrophy. A family history of myopathy and trunk weakness suggests that generalized muscle disease is present. Toe walking may also be the result of occult spinal cord lesions. Abnormal tethering of the spinal cord by fibrous bands or bony spurs often affects lower limb function and may present as increasing foot and ankle deformity. A number of benign spinal cord tumors may present in a similar fashion. Clinical and radiographic examination of the spine should be part of evaluation of persistent tiptoe gait.

A group of children exists who persist in toe walking past the expected time of resolution and in whom no neurologic or myopathic cause for toe walking can be identified. The diagnosis of idiopathic toe walking is justified only when other possible causes of toe walking have been excluded. Sometimes these patients are capable of heel-toe gait on command but prefer to walk on tiptoe. Others are incapable of heel-toe gait. Mild knee hyperextension may be present at midstance in these children. In normal children, passive dorsiflexion of the ankle past 15 degrees is possible. Restriction of passive dorsiflexion in the absence of other musculoskeletal or neurologic abnormalities implies that a short gastrocnemius-soleus muscle group may be responsible for tiptoe gait. The etiology of contracture is controversial. It was originally thought to be congenital but may also be the result of adaptation to the habit of toe walking. Electromyographic studies of tiptoe walkers have to date been inconclusive.

Treatment of idiopathic toe walking depends on the severity and duration of contracture. In patients less than 3 years old in whom normal passive dorsiflexion of the ankle is possible, a period of observation is warranted. Older children or children with fixed contracture are best treated by passive stretching and cast applications for a period of 1 or 2 months. Persistence or recurrence of contracture may require surgical heel cord lengthening.

TORSIONAL DEFORMITIES OF THE LEGS

Wide variation in lower extremity configuration occurs in normal children. The rotational and angular alignment of the legs change during growth and development until skeletal maturity is reached late in adolescence. Toe-in and toe-out postures, bowlegs, and knock-knee occur in many children and may be the source of great concern. Concern about lower limb alignment is probably the single greatest reason that parents seek orthopedic referral. Fortunately, most rotational and angular alignment problems correct spontaneously; active treatment is rarely necessary. Careful examination, explanation, and reassurance usually suffice.

The description of lower limb alignment is confusing, and until recently, there has been no uniform system of terminology. The Subcommittee on Torsional Deformity of the Pediatric Orthopaedic Society recommended a classification system that takes into account many of the variables of limb rotation and provides a standardized vocabulary for those who deal with limb alignment in children. The primary references in this system are the transverse and sagittal planes of the body (Fig 3–4). Angular and rotational alignment are described in relation to these planes. Normal limb alignment and joint range of motion are defined as those which occur within two standard deviations of the mean. Rotational problems with values within this range are termed *rotational variations*, and those outside the normal range are termed *torsional deformities*.

Rotational and angular alignment have been intensively investigated radiographically and clinically over the past four decades. Roentgenographic methods of determining limb alignment using con-

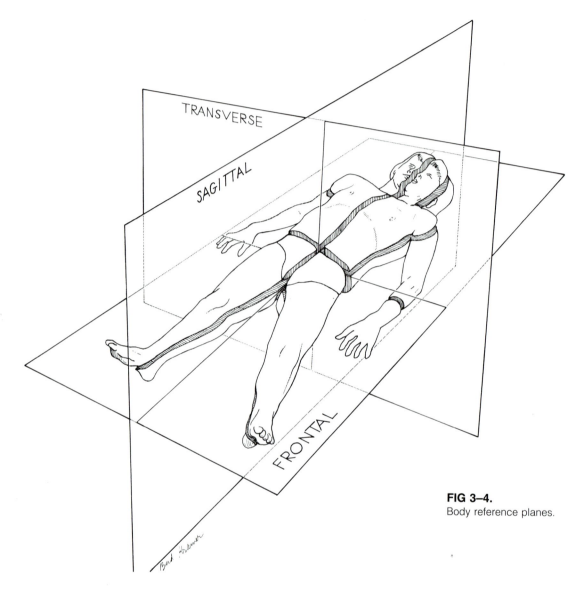

FIG 3–4.
Body reference planes.

ventional radiographic techniques and complex geometric conversions were developed by Dunlop and Shands, Ryder and Crane, and others. More recently, computed tomography has been employed to study torsional alignment. Such techniques are expensive and sometimes involve considerable radiation exposure. Fortunately, in most cases clinical examination alone is sufficient. Many of the pa-

rameters of normal have been established by Staheli and co-workers in large studies of children and adolescents with no evidence of musculoskeletal abnormalities. Using these guidelines, most rotational and angular alignment problems can be accurately documented and appropriately treated without extensive radiographic evaluation.

The terminology system recommended by the Pediatric Orthopaedic Society is as follows:

The terms *adduction, abduction,* and *rotation* are used to describe position, alignment, or direction of motion of an extremity segment (Fig 3–5):

1. *Adduction* is motion toward the sagittal plane.
2. *Abduction* is motion away from the sagittal plane.
3. *Rotation* is motion parallel to the transverse plane. The terms medial and lateral are preferable to internal and external in describing rotational alignment since the latter terms are most often used to describe that which is inside or outside the body wall, as in external fixation of a fracture or an internal derangement of the knee.

Version is the normal angular difference between the transverse axis of each end of a long bone (Fig 3–6). In the tibia, version is the angular difference between the transcondylar axis of the knee and the transmalleolar axis of the ankle. In the femur, version is the angular difference between the transcondylar axis of the knee and the head-neck axis of the femur at the hip joint. Version can also be defined for flat bones. Acetabular version is the normal inclination of the acetabulum in reference to the sagittal plane.

The rotational alignment of the lower limbs present at birth is the result of intrauterine molding. During fetal development, the hips are flexed and laterally rotated, while the limbs distal to the hips are medially rotated. At birth, lateral rotation of the hips exceeds medial rotation, but the overall alignment of the limbs beneath the hips is medially deviated. Realignment of the bones along their long axes takes place during growth and development. Arrested remodeling of version at one or more segments alters the align-

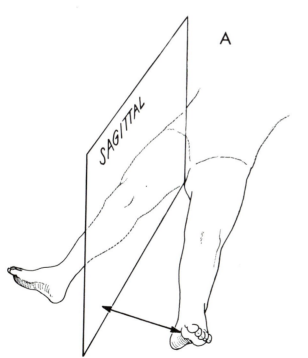

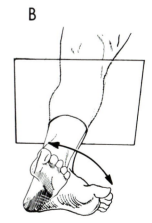

FIG 3–5.
A, abduction and adduction of the leg. Abduction is motion away from the sagittal plane; adduction is motion toward the sagittal plane. **B,** medial and lateral rotation.

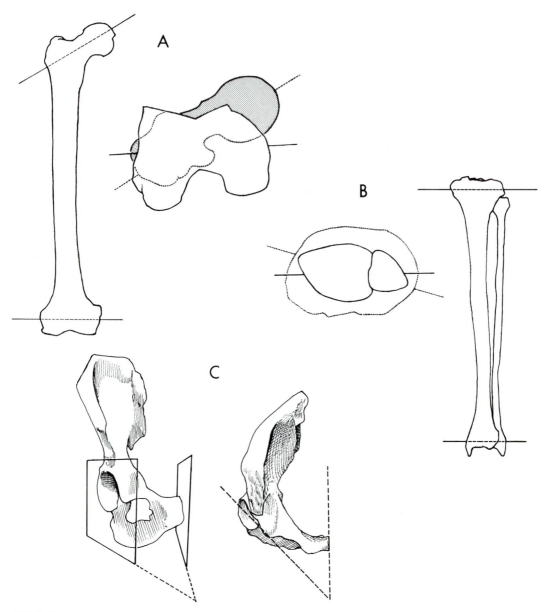

FIG 3–6.
Lower extremity version. **A,** superimposition of the transcondylar and femoral head-neck angles defines the angle of femoral version. **B,** superimposition of the transcondylar axis of the knee and the transmalleolar axis of the ankle defines the angle of tibial version. **C,** the angle of acetabular version is defined by the intersection of the sagittal plane of the body and a plane parallel to the acetabular edges.

ment of the entire limb, producing a rotational or angular deformity.

The terms *torsion, varus,* and *valgus* are used to define deformity:

1. Tibial and femoral torsion are said to be present when abnormal version is present in either bone at a given age. Acetabular torsion is abnormal acetabular inclination.

2. Varus angulation of a limb segment is present when the extremity distal to the segment in question is deviated toward the midline of the body (Fig 3–7,A).

3. Valgus angulation exists when the extremity distal to the segment in question deviates away from the midline (Fig 3–7,B).

When walking, jogging, or running, the body moves forward along a path called the *line of progression.* The *foot axis* is a line that runs from the midpoint of the foot at the heel to the midpoint of the foot at the metatarsal heads. The intersection of the foot axis with the line of progression of the body is called the *foot-progression angle* (Fig 3–8). Toeing-in and toeing-out are medial and lateral deviations of the foot-progression angle beyond normal ranges.

Staheli and co-workers found the foot-progression angle to be greatest and most variable during infancy. Decreases in the foot-progression angle occur during the first years of life, and by adolescence, the mean foot-progression angle is approximately +10 degrees (see Fig 3–8,D). The normal range of the foot-progression angle is quite wide, and a considerable number of otherwise normal infants and children have a negative foot-progression angle and are perceived to toe-in. The normal range at skeletal maturity is con-

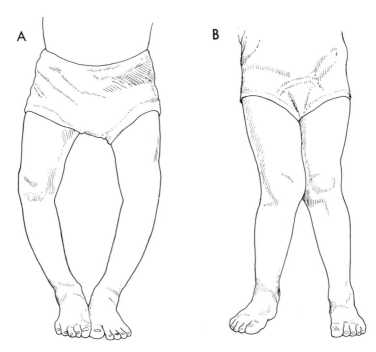

FIG 3–7.
A, bowleg deformity. Bowlegs are referred to as varus angulation because the legs distal to the knees are tilted toward the midline of the body. **B,** knock-knee or valgus deformity of the knees. The extremity distal to the knee is tilted away from the midline.

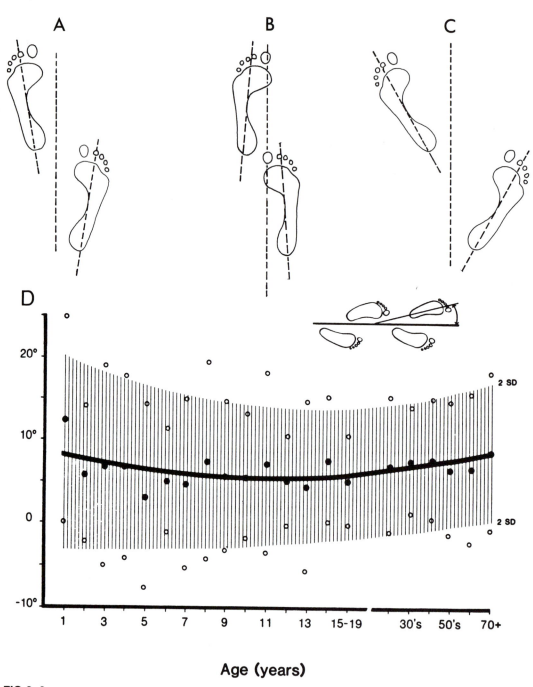

FIG 3–8.
The foot-progression angle is the intersection of the long axis of the foot and the line of progression of the body. **A,** usual foot-progression angle. **B,** toeing-in. **C,** toeing-out. **D,** changes in the foot-progression angle with increasing age. The *solid line* shows the mean change with age; the *shaded area,* different age groups; and the *open circles,* plus or minus 2 SD for the same mean measurements. (From Staheli LT, Corbett M, Wyss C, et al: Lower extremity rotational problems in children. *J Bone Joint Surg Am* 1985; 67:39–47. Reproduced by permission.)

sidered to be between -3 and $+20$ degrees.

The foot-progression angle is the net result of structural and dynamic influences at several segments. Bone configuration, muscle balance, and joint capsule contracture all may contribute to the final alignment of the lower limb. Toeing-in or toeing-out may be the result of torsion, imbalance, or contracture at one or several segments. Compensation for medial torsion of one segment may occur through lateral torsion or increased lateral rotation at another. The net foot-progression angle may be normal, even though torsional malalignment of individual segments of the limb may be present.

Femoral Version

Superimposition of the transcondylar and head-neck axes of the femur produces the angle of femoral version (Fig 3–9). Anatomical and radiologic studies have indicated that the normal angle of femoral version at birth is approximately 30 degrees and that spontaneous correction occurs at the rate of about 1 degree per year until skeletal maturation. *Anteversion* is the term applied to normal angular difference between the transcondylar plane of the knee and the head-neck plane of the proximal femur. Abnormal increases in femoral anteversion at a given age are termed *medial femoral torsion*. *Lateral femoral torsion*, or *femoral retrover-*

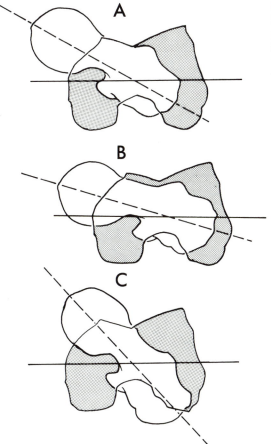

FIG 3–9.
Normal and abnormal femoral version. **A,** the normal angle of femoral version in the neonate is 25 to 30 degrees. **B,** the normal angle of adult femoral version is 15 degrees. **C,** an angle of 45 degrees is abnormal and constitutes a torsional deformity.

sion, is abnormally decreased femoral version.

Uncompensated femoral anteversion and medial femoral torsion are often found in children who toe-in. If the femoral head is held in a constant relationship to the acetabulum, medial femoral torsion is associated with inward rotation of lower extremity segments distal to the hip (Fig 3–10). Lateral femoral torsion will produce external rotation of the distal segments.

Clinical estimation of the effect of femoral anteversion or medial femoral torsion on lower limb alignment can be made by placing the child in the prone position with the hip extended and the knee flexed (Fig 3–11,A). Medial and lateral rotation of the hip is then measured, allowing gravity to determine the end point. The amount of rotation possible at the hip joint in each direction varies with the age of the child being tested.

In infants, medial rotation of the hips is ordinarily quite limited, even though the angle of femoral anteversion is greatest at this time. This is probably the result of contractures of the capsule of the hip joint resulting from the fetal position. As the infant begins to walk, capsular contractures stretch out, and medial rotation increases. Staheli found that medial rotation in males exceeds medial rotation in females; from the middle of childhood on the mean medial rotation of the hip possible in male subjects is about 50 degrees, with a range of 25 to 65 degrees (Fig 3–11,B). In females, the mean is approximately 40 degrees, with a range of 15 to 60 degrees (Fig 3–11,C).

Lateral rotation of the hips is greatest in infancy and decreases throughout childhood. There appears to be no difference between sexes. From middle childhood on, mean lateral rotation is about 45 degrees, with a normal range between 25 and 65 degrees (Fig 3–11,D). Older children who present for evaluation of toeing-in often have decreased lateral rotation at the hip. In some instances it may be impossible to laterally rotate the hip even to the neutral position. Femoral torsion is usually present in these children.

A number of radiographic techniques

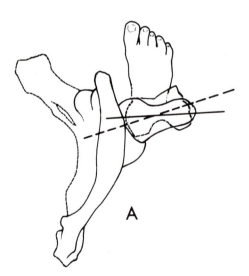
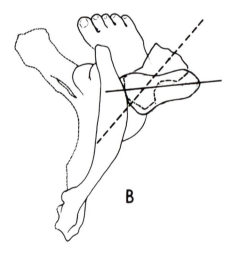

FIG 3–10.
Relationship of femoral version to toe-in. **A,** with normal femoral version, the lower extremity below the hip aligns parallel to the sagittal plane. **B,** with medial femoral torsional deformity, the lower leg rotates toward the sagittal plane. A toed-in gait may result.

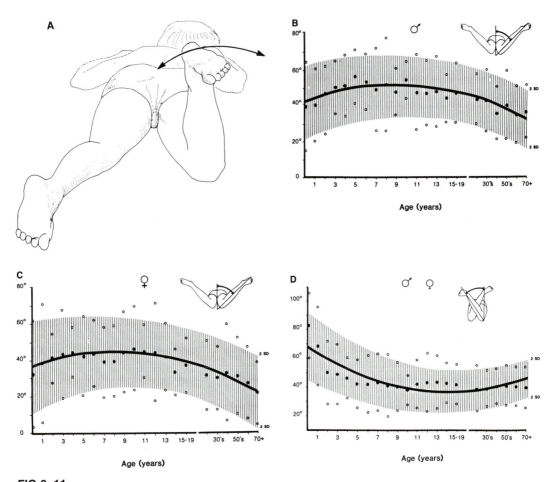

FIG 3–11.
A, position for clinical estimation of femoral version. The child is placed prone to hold the hips in extension. The knee is flexed and the lower leg used as lever to rotate the femur in the hip joint. Medial rotation of the flexed lower leg rotates the femur laterally. Lateral rotation of the lower leg rotates the femur medially. The arc of medial and lateral rotation in children over age 5 is usually symmetric. Infants may have more lateral rotation than medial rotation because of tight posterior hip capsular ligaments and short external rotator muscles. In patients with medial femoral torsional deformities, lateral rotation of the femur is restricted, and medial rotation appears increased. **B,** medial rotation of the hip in males. **C,** medial rotation of the hip in females. **D,** lateral rotation of the hip in children of both sexes. See Figure 3–8D for key to B, C, and D. (**B, C,** and **D** from Staheli LT, Corbett M, Wyss C, et al: Lower-extremity rotational problems in children. *J Bone Joint Surg Am* 1985; 67:39–47. Reproduced by permission.)

are available to measure femoral torsion more accurately. Biplanar radiography, fluoroscopy, and computed axial tomography have been used successfully. Radiation exposure and expense can be excessive, however, and routine radiographic examination of children with suspected femoral torsion is not necessary.

Toe-in gait due to femoral anteversion or medial femoral torsion usually corrects spontaneously. Derotation of the proximal femur occurs with normal growth and development in most children. In others, compensation for medial femoral torsion occurs through development of lateral tibial torsion or dynamic external rotation at the hip joint. Exercise programs, physical therapy, orthotics, and modifications of sitting and sleeping habits are not necessary. Spontaneous correction occurs at the same rate in treated and untreated children. There is little evidence that the medial femoral torsion that persists in these children is of functional significance or that it predisposes to premature degenerative joint disease.

Tibial Version

The tibia, like the femur, is medially rotated on its long axis at birth. Spontaneous derotation takes place during normal childhood growth and development. Persistent medial tibial version, often referred to as internal tibial torsion, can contribute to toe-in gait.

It is more difficult to measure tibial version than femoral version. An estimate may be obtained by flexing the knee to 90 degrees and palpating the medial and lateral malleoli with thumb and index finger. In the adult, the medial malleolus ordinarily lies about one finger breadth forward of the lateral malleolus. In the neonate, the malleoli may be parallel, or the medial malleolus may lie behind the lateral malleolus. Staheli and Engel have proposed a caliper method for measuring tibial version (Fig 3–12,A). The child is seated over the edge of a table with the heel resting against a firm surface. The medial and lateral malleoli are marked, and the distance between the malleoli and the surface measured. The intermalleolar distance is then measured with a caliper, and the angle of tibial version is calculated geometrically (Fig 3–12,B).

The *thigh-foot angle* may also be used to estimate tibial version. In this test the child is placed prone, and the knee is flexed. The angle between the foot axis and the long axis of the thigh is then estimated. In normal individuals, there is a close correlation between the thigh-foot

axis and the transmalleolar axis of the tibia. The normal thigh-foot angle present at birth is approximately −15 degrees, with a normal range between −30 and +20 degrees. By age 3, the thigh-foot angle is approximately +5 degrees, with a normal range between −10 and +20 degrees. From the middle of childhood until skeletal maturity, the normal mean thigh-foot angle is about +10 degrees, with a normal range between −5 and +30 degrees (Fig 3–12,C).

The thigh-foot angle is a composite measurement of both tibial version and hindfoot version, and as such, abnormalities of the talus or midfoot may interfere with this measurement. For practical purposes, differentiation between tibial and hindfoot version is clinically unimportant.

Persistent tibial version or medial tibial torsion frequently contributes to toeing-in in young children. Spontaneous correction of tibial torsion occurs in almost all cases. The rate of change is greatest during the first year, before the child has begun to walk, but further correction will occur for at least 2 or 3 more years.

A wide variety of orthotic devices have been employed for treatment of the child with persistent medial femoral and/or tibial version or torsion. Beneficial results have been reported with twister cables, external rotation shoe bars, shoe wedges, torque heels, and derotation casts. Controlled studies are lacking, however, and critical biomechanical analysis of many of the orthoses has not yet been performed. It seems likely that many devices may exert their external rotation effect on the soft tissues of the lower extremity rather than on the bones of the lower limb. Besides being awkward and uncomfortable, brace treatment may cause iatrogenic angular knee and ankle deformity. Shoe modifications are expensive, uncomfortable, and usually unnecessary. There is very little evidence that "corrective" shoes accelerate the rate of

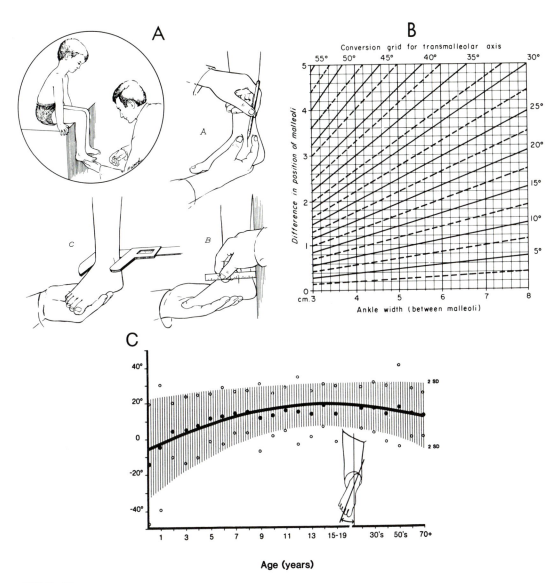

FIG 3–12.
A, estimation of tibial version. The child is seated with knee flexed to 90 degrees against a firm surface. The medial and lateral malleoli are marked *(A)*. An estimate of the degree of tibial version can be made by measuring the distance from the malleoli to the posterior surface *(B)*. The medial malleolus ordinarily lies farther forward than the lateral malleolus. A more accurate measurement of torsional deformity can be obtained by measuring the width of the ankle at the malleoli *(C)* and using the conversion grid in Figure 3–12,**B** to determine the transmalleolar axis. (From Staheli LT, Engel GM: Tibial torsion: A method of assessment and a survey of normal children. *Clin Orthop* 1972; 86:183. Reproduced by permission.) **C,** changes in the thigh-foot angle with increasing age. See Figure 3–8,D for key. (From Staheli LT, Corbett M, Wyss C, et al: Lower extremity rotational problems in children. *J Bone Joint Surg Am* 1985; 67:39–47. Reproduced by permission.)

spontaneous correction of medial tibial torsion.

There is little evidence that persistent femoral or tibial torsional deformity predisposes to limitation of function or premature degenerative joint disease in adult life. Structural or dynamic compensation for persistent malalignment usually occurs with growth and development. In very rare instances, however, extreme torsional deformities may present unacceptable cosmetic or functional problems. In these instances, surgical correction may be considered. Although effective, surgery is a last resort since the possible operative risks often outweigh the benefits of realignment.

VARUS AND VALGUS DEFORMITIES OF THE LEGS

The angular alignment of the lower extremities varies normally with age. Most neonates appear bowlegged if supported in the standing position. This varus angulation, often referred to as physiologic bowing, reverses with growth, and by age 3 to 4 years, most children are slightly knock-kneed. By age 5 to 7 years, the mild valgus angulation corrects, and adult lower limb alignment is evident.

Prospective radiologic studies indicate that the angle between the long axis of the femur and the long axis of the tibia is about 15 degrees varus at birth in normal children (Fig 3–13). The angle decreases to 0 degrees between ages 18 and 24 months. By age 3 or 4 years, 10 degrees of valgus angulation may be present. By age 5 to 7 years, the tibiofemoral angle usually has decreased again to the normal adult range of 7 to 9 degrees valgus in girls and 4 to 6 degrees valgus in boys.

When correction fails to occur on schedule or when the magnitude of varus or valgus exceeds that expected at a given age, angular deformity exists. Bowlegs

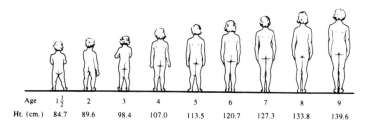

Age	1½	2	3	4	5	6	7	8	9
Ht. (cm.)	84.7	89.6	98.4	107.0	113.5	120.7	127.3	133.8	139.6

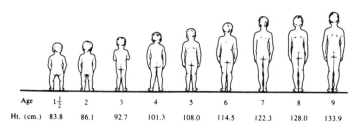

Age	1½	2	3	4	5	6	7	8	9
Ht. (cm.)	83.8	86.1	92.7	101.3	108.0	114.5	122.3	128.0	133.9

FIG 3–13.
Angular development. Children usually are slightly bowlegged when they start to walk. Knock-knee develops between ages 3 and 5 years. Normal limb alignment is usually present by age 9 years. (From Smart MS, Smart RC: *Children: Development and Relationships.* New York, Macmillian Publishing Co, 1972. Reproduced by permission.)

and knock-knees are not specific diseases but rather the common clinical manifestations of a number of normal or abnormal physiologic processes. Often, perceived deformity is only an exaggeration of normal alignment and will correct spontaneously. At times, however, varus or valgus alignment of the knees may be caused by more serious underlying bone dysplasia.

Bowlegs

The terminology used to refer to bowleg deformity is confusing. Clinical course and radiologic appearance have been used to divide genu varum in otherwise healthy children into several categories. Conflicting reports of incidence and behavior and the lack of convincing pathophysiologic data have made this separation at times confusing, but several general patterns have been identified. The varus angulation found in normal infants is usually termed *physiologic bowing*. Varus angulation greater than 20 degrees in toddlers is considered *severe physiologic bowing*. Severe varus bowing associated with radiologic changes in the proximal tibial epiphysis is known as tibia vara, Blount's disease, or osteochondrosis deformans tibiae.

The physiologic bowing and medial tibial version of infancy usually begin to correct by age 18 months. This is manifest clinically by gradually decreasing distance between the knees when the ankles are held together and the patellae point straight ahead. The thigh-foot angle becomes gradually more positive as lateral rotation of the tibia occurs. Such correction occurs with or without the benefit of specially designed children's shoes, and no braces or therapy programs are necessary.

Spontaneous correction occasionally does not occur on schedule, however, and the distance between the knees may remain static or increase. In the absence of other abnormalities or a family history of metabolic or dysplastic bone disease, such children may be followed clinically until age 18 months to 2 years. If correction has not begun by then, further investigation is justified. Laboratory studies of calcium and phosphorus metabolism may be necessary, and standing roentgenograms of the lower extremities should be obtained. In children over age 2 years, these roentgenograms permit both measurement of the tibiofemoral angle and analysis of the growth centers around the knee. In younger children, however, there is often insufficient ossification for definitive interpretation, and diagnosis may be difficult.

Medial metaphyseal beaking of both the proximal tibial and the distal femur, medial cortical thickening in both the tibia and the femur, and varus angulation of greater than 20 degrees are characteristic findings in severe physiologic bowing (Fig 3–14). No pathologic changes are present in the proximal tibial epiphysis.

Spontaneous correction can be expected to occur in most children with moderate or severe physiologic bowing in the absence of underlying metabolic bone disease and in whom no radiographic signs of Blount's disease are present. Improvement usually begins before the second birthday, and correction to neutral by age 6 or 7 years is the rule. Occasionally mild varus angulation may persist throughout the juvenile period into adolescence and may be cosmetically unacceptable. Functional problems caused by residual varus angulation are uncommon in teenagers, but premature degenerative arthritis may develop in early adult life if significant varus deformity is present at skeletal maturity.

A number of orthotic devices and shoe modifications have been proposed for treatment of severe bowing. These have included long leg braces, night

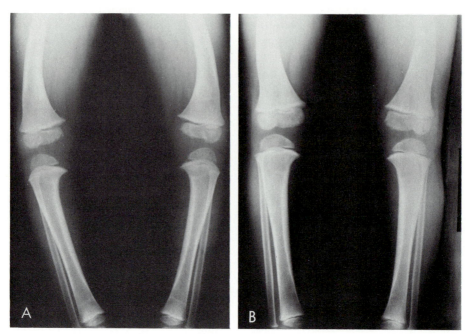

FIG 3–14.
Physiologic bowleg deformity. **A,** at age 18 months. Bilateral bowleg deformity is present; beaking of the medial metaphysis is present at both the distal femur and proximal tibia. **B,** at age 30 months. Spontaneous correction has occurred without treatment.

splints, shoe bars, shoe wedges, and arch supports. Biomechanical studies of most such devices are lacking, and their efficacy is questionable. Bracing is recommended for treatment of severe physiologic bowing only when there is clinical and radiologic evidence of worsening deformity. If braces are chosen for treatment, they must be carefully fitted and monitored. A lateral upright long leg brace with no knee joint that applies medially directed force to the lateral aspect of the proximal tibial metaphysis is usually employed. Results are most satisfactory if the brace is applied before age 2 years and is used at least during waking hours until correction has been obtained.

Tibia Vara (Blount's Disease)

Erlacher in 1922 is credited with reporting the first case of tibia vara. Blount in 1937 reviewed 15 reported cases of tibia

vara and presented 13 additional cases of what subsequently has become known as Blount's disease. True Blount's disease is uncommon but not rare. Smith noted in 1982 that approximately 500 cases had been reported, and several large series have been reported since Smith's review. The disorder is far less common than severe physiologic tibial bowing, however. It occurs in both infantile and adolescent forms and can be associated with extreme tibia vara.

The etiology of tibia vara is unclear and may differ in the infantile and adolescent forms of Blount's disease. It was originally thought to represent osteochondrosis or avascular necrosis of the medial corner of the proximal tibial epiphysis. Histologic support for this contention is lacking, however. More recently, it has been proposed that tibia vara is a manifestation of altered endochondral bone formation in response to abnormal loading of the medial tibial epiphysis in a child with severe physiologic tibial bowing. It is well known that compression across an active growth plate will retard growth (the Heuter-Volkman law) and that distraction across a growth plate will accelerate growth (Delpeck's law). Experimental models indicate that compressive stress across the medial tibial physis is greatly increased when abnormal varus angulation exists. It has been estimated that loads across the medial aspect of the tibial physis are as much as seven times normal when varus angulation of 30 degrees is present. Obesity results in even greater loads. Such forces could well be responsible for altered physeal growth.

The infantile form of tibia vara develops in children between ages 1 and 3 years. A strong family history has been reported in some series, and the disease is often bilateral. Affected children are often heavy and often walk early. Laxity of the collateral ligaments of the knees has been noted in some reports and if present may contribute to varus angulation. The disorder has been reported to be more frequent in blacks but occurs in other races as well.

Infants with Blount's disease are initially indistinguishable from children with severe physiologic bowing. After age 18 to 24 months, roentgenograms of affected children begin to show angulation beneath the posteromedial proximal epiphysis, metaphyseal irregularity and beaking in the proximal tibia, and wedging of the proximal epiphysis (Fig 3–15). In untreated cases, premature closure of the medial epiphysis and underlying metaphyseal change result in severe varus angulation.

Spontaneous correction has been reported in a few cases of early onset infantile tibia vara. In such cases, resolution of deformity occurred between ages 2 and 5 years without treatment, even though radiographic evidence of potential or early Blount's disease was present. Because of

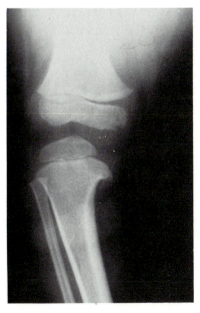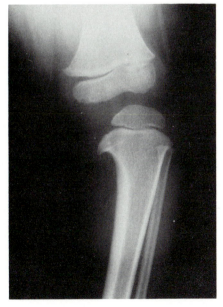

FIG 3–15.
Blount's disease. Bowleg deformity is pronounced. There is prominent beaking of the proximal tibial medial metaphysis only.

the potential for some cases of tibia vara to correct spontaneously, reports of correction with bracing must be viewed with caution, and surgical treatment should be reserved for those patients in whom progression has been documented.

Orthotic treatment may be successful in some children with Blount's disease. To be effective, bracing must be started between ages 18 and 24 months and continued at least during waking hours for an average of 2 years. If progression occurs in spite of brace treatment, or if patients are older at the time of diagnosis, surgical treatment will be necessary. Realignment osteotomy is most effective when performed before age 5 years, probably because the growth plate has not yet undergone permanent damage in young patients. Results are less predictable in patients with the infantile form of tibia vara in whom treatment is delayed.

The adolescent form of Blount's disease develops in previously normal children after age 8 years. The disease is more often unilateral and has been reported much more commonly in blacks than in other races. Most affected patients have been markedly obese. Some appear to have had incompletely resolved physiologic tibial bowing. Radiographs often show paradoxical widening of the most medial portion of the proximal tibial physis, with physeal narrowing and frequent bridging of the physis just lateral to the widened portion. The few biopsy specimens available show disorganization of the usual orderly process of endochondral bone formation similar to that seen in patients with slipped capital femoral epiphysis. Although the initiating event in affected patients is most often unclear, it appears that the loads applied to the medial aspect of the joint in obese adolescents with severe varus deformity may cause growth arrest and medial bridging.

Surgical correction is necessary, and recurrent deformity has been reported after surgery. Brace treatment is not effective in adolescent onset tibia vara.

Knock-knee

Knock-knee, or genu valgum, is a less common problem than bowlegs. Most normal children are slightly knock-kneed between ages 3 and 5 years; excessive knock-knee develops later in childhood or early in adolescence when normal knock-knee fails to remodel. Defective development of the lateral femoral condyle, laxity of the medial collateral ligaments of the knee, flatfoot, and obesity all have been implicated as causes of knock-knee; in most cases, however, the exact cause is unknown. Like severe physiologic bowing or Blount's disease, knock-knee may represent accentuation of normal angulation caused by abnormal forces across the knee.

Knock-knee usually presents as a cosmetic problem often associated with flatfeet and an awkward gait. Pain is almost never present. Running accentuates the awkward appearance. A clinical estimate of the amount of valgus can be made by measuring the distance between the medial malleoli of the ankles when the child stands with patellae pointing forward and the knees just touching. Standing roentgenograms provide a more accurate measurement. Girls usually have slightly more valgus than boys; angulation of greater than 9 degrees in girls and 6 degrees in boys is perceived as knock-knee.

Although knock-knee is usually of cosmetic importance only, in rare cases, exaggerated knock-knee may predispose to late degenerative arthritis of the lateral compartment of the knee. Although some correction can be expected to occur spontaneously in young children, older children with knock-knee usually do not improve without treatment. Shoes and shoe modifications have not been reliably demonstrated to change the natural course of knock-knee. Long leg bracing has been advocated for treatment of children with excess valgus at the knees, but as in bow-leg deformity, mechanical analysis of the effects of bracing is not available. Bracing may be effective in younger children, but adolescents with cosmetically unacceptable knock-knee are best treated by medial femoral epiphyseal arrest or osteotomy.

DISORDERS OF THE FEET

Variations in the configuration of the foot at birth and during childhood are quite common and are often the cause of considerable parental anxiety. In many instances no treatment at all is necessary, but in other cases, prompt therapy may prevent significant later deformity and disability.

The Normal Foot

A review of the anatomy and development of the normal foot is necessary before considering variations and anomalies. There are a number of important surface landmarks that aid in examination of the child's foot.

Surface Anatomy

The skin of the dorsal surface of the foot, like the skin of the dorsal surface of the hand, is thin and freely movable. There is little subcutaneous tissue between it and the underlying deep structures. The dorsalis pedis artery, a continuation of the anterior tibial artery, is palpable on the dorsal surface midway between the medial and lateral malleoli (Fig 3–16,A). The deep peroneal nerve lies just lateral to it. Superficial veins are often prominent, and the extensor tendons of the toes can be easily traced to their insertions. The anterior tibial tendon is palpable just forward of the medial malleolus

on the medial aspect of the dorsum of the foot.

Behind the medial malleolus, the pulse of the posterior tibial artery can be felt (Fig 3–16,B). The tendons of the tibialis posterior, flexor digitorum, and flexor hallucis muscles run behind the medial malleolus. The tibialis posterior tendon is palpable over the medial border of the navicular bone when the foot is actively inverted. The prominence of the sustentaculum tali, a bony ridge on the calcaneus that supports the talus, can be palpated slightly below and forward of the medial malleolus.

The lateral malleolar prominence of the distal fibula is palpable on the outer border of the ankle. It lies slightly behind the medial malleolus in older children but may be forward of the medial malleolus in normal infants with internal tibial torsion. The tendons of the peroneal muscles run behind the lateral malleolus.

Bones of the Foot

The bones of the foot are analogous to the bones of the hand and wrist (Fig 3–17). The tarsal bones comprise the talus, calcaneus, navicular, cuboid, and the three cuneiforms. There are five metatarsal bones. The phalanges of the toes correspond in number to those of the hand. Numerous accessory and sesamoid bones have been described in the foot and ankle; they are sometimes confused with fractures.

At birth, ossification centers are present in only three of the seven tarsal bones: the calcaneus, the cuboid, and the talus. Initially the ossification centers are oval and bear little likeness to the shape of the surrounding cartilage model of the tarsal bone. Ossification centers for the navicular and cuneiform bones appear between ages 1 and 4 years.

Secondary ossification centers for the metatarsals appear around age 3 years. The secondary center for the first metatar-

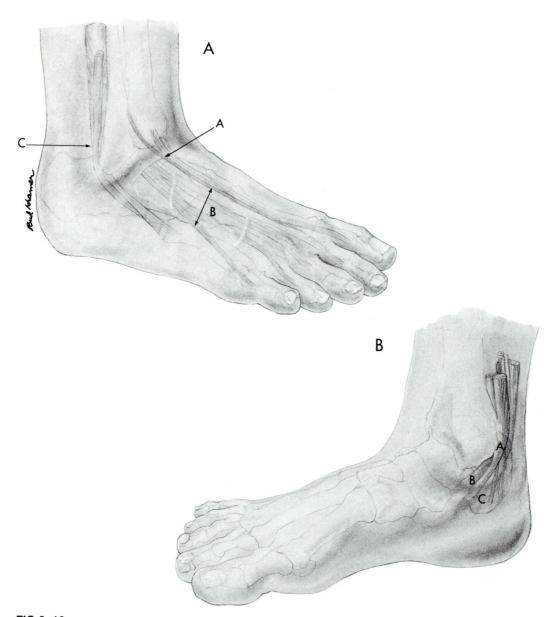

FIG 3–16.
A, dorsolateral surface of the foot. The dorsalis pedis artery *(A)* is palpable on the dorsal surface of the foot, midway between the medial and lateral malleoli. The tendons of the toe extensor muscles *(B)* and the peroneal tendons *(C)* are readily palpable. **B,** dorsomedial surface of the foot. The pulse of the posterior tibial artery is palpable *(A)* behind the medial malleolus. *B* indicates the navicular bone and insertion of the tibialis posterior tendon. *C* indicates bony prominence of the sustentaculum tali process of the calcaneus.

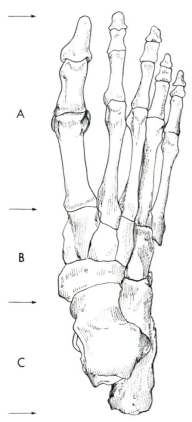

FIG 3–17.
Bones of the foot. The metatarsal bones and phalanges comprise the forefoot *(A)*. The three cuneiforms, cuboid, and navicular bones are located in the midfoot *(B)*. The hindfoot is composed of the talus and calcaneus *(C)*.

sal is located at the proximal end of the bone; the centers for metatarsals two through five are located at the distal end of the bone. The secondary ossification centers for the phalangeal epiphyses appear at about the same time.

Longitudinal and transverse arches are present in the normal foot. The medial side of the longitudinal arch is higher than the lateral side (Fig 3–18). The medial border of the normal foot is in contact with the ground at the heel and at the first metatarsal head; the lateral border of the foot rests on the ground along its entire length (Fig 3–19). The bony longitu-

dinal arch passes through the anterior part of the calcaneus and the head of the talus to the navicular and cuneiform bones, and then down through the medial metatarsals to the metatarsal heads. The lateral longitudinal arch passes through the calcaneus to the cuboid and then through the lateral metatarsals.

The transverse arch of the foot is more difficult to define. The bones of the midfoot are arranged so that the plantar surface of the foot is concave and the dorsal surface is convex. The transverse arch is most distinct at the tarsometatarsal joint (Fig 3–20). Anteriorly the arch flattens rapidly, so that the heads of all metatarsals lie flat when the feet are supporting the weight of the body in a standing position.

The bones and ligaments of the foot are the primary supports of the transverse and long arches. In the normal foot, muscular forces are not required for support at rest. In quiet stance, about 50% of body weight is borne by the calcaneus. The rest is shared by the metatarsal heads, with the first metatarsal bearing more than the others. Force distribution changes rapidly with motion.

Dorsiflexion and plantar flexion of the foot involve not only tibiotalar hinged motion but also subtalar and intertarsal translation. The joints of the midfoot and hindfoot are complex and permit the foot to adapt to a wide variety of gait patterns and walking surfaces.

At all phases of growth, the foot is relatively larger than the rest of the lower limb. The foot reaches 50% of its eventual length by the middle of the second year of life. The remainder of the leg does not reach 50% of growth until age 3 to 4 years. The growth rate remains fairly constant at approximately 0.9 cm/year until age 12 years in girls and age 14 years in boys and then declines rapidly. Full length is usually present by age 14 years in girls and 16 years in boys.

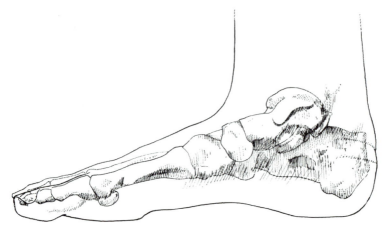

FIG 3–18.
Medial long arch of the foot. The medial border of the foot ordinarily contacts the ground at the metatarsal heads and at the heel.

Deformities of the Foot

Deformities of the feet are among the most often noticed orthopedic problems of the infant and child. Some foot deformities are flexible and mild and correct spontaneously with growth. Others persist into adult life but cause little or no functional handicap. Some foot deformities are quite rigid and, unless treated early in life, will result in significant adult disability. In most instances, early recog-

nition and prompt treatment improve the final result.

Talipes Equinovarus

Talipes equinovarus, or clubfoot, is a common congenital deformity. It was described by Hippocrates and has been the subject of many classic orthopedic tracts. The clubfoot is obvious at birth (Fig 3–21). The principal components of the deformity are plantar flexion or equinus of the ankle, inversion or varus of the heel, and

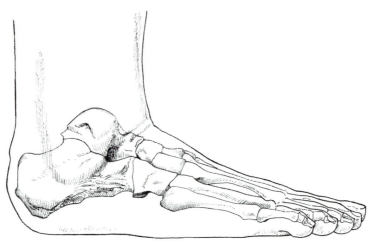

FIG 3–19.
Lateral border of the foot. The lateral aspect of the foot rests on the ground along its entire length.

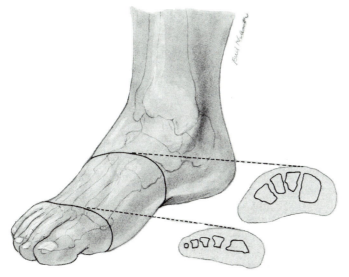

FIG 3–20.
Transverse arches of the foot.

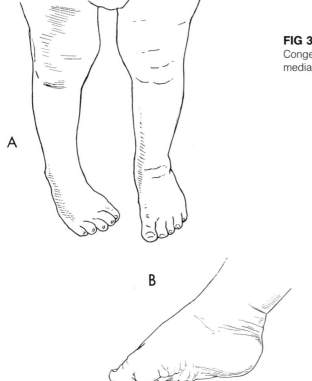

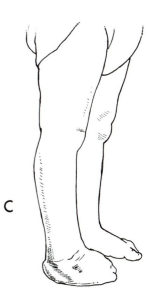

FIG 3–21.
Congenital right clubfoot. **A,** anterior view. **B,** medial view. **C,** lateral view.

adduction of the forefoot. In some children, clubfoot is the result of more generalized musculoskeletal or neuromuscular disease. It is frequently seen in myelomeningocele and arthrogryposis. In most cases, however, the etiology is less clear.

Typical clubfoot occurs in about 1 in 1,000 live births. Boys are affected about twice as often as girls. The incidence of clubfoot in a family with one affected first-degree relative is much greater, probably about 1% to 2%. The risk to subsequent children is increased about 20 times. Male relatives of a female patient appear to be particularly at risk. In nonidentical twins, the deformity is shared in about 3% of cases. This risk is approximately the same as for nontwin siblings. Identical twins share the deformity in about one case in three. These incidence studies indicate an underlying genetic factor in the production of talipes equinovarus.

Abnormal intrauterine pressures probably contribute to the development of clubfoot as well. The clubfoot frequently looks as though it had been abnormally molded in utero. Clubfoot has been associated with a small uterus, abnormal fetal position, and multiple births, but the associations are not invariable. Many such pregnancies terminate without clubfoot.

Typical congenital clubfoot is probably neither purely genetic nor purely environmental. According to Wynne-Davies, the more alike the parental genetic constitutions, the greater the risk to the child. It is likely that abnormal intrauterine pressures at a critical time in fetal development produce clubfoot in a genetically predispositioned patient.

There has been a great deal of dispute over the primary pathology in talipes equinovarus. Anatomical studies of the bones of the foot in stillborns with clubfoot have repeatedly demonstrated osseous abnormality. Most often there is distortion of the talus, with shortening, medial deviation, and plantar flexion of the talar neck. The navicular bone may be wedge shaped, displaced medially, and articulate with the medial malleolus. Abnormalities of the subtalar joints between the talus and calcaneus are often present. Abnormal coalitions between the tarsal bones have been reported both at autopsy and at surgery. Even though such osseous alterations have been consistently found in clubfoot specimens, they may represent the effect of intrauterine molding rather than primary malformation of the foot.

It has been suggested that genetically induced shortening of muscle tendon units with subsequent muscular fibrosis and contracture may cause clubfoot deformity by pulling the cartilaginous anlage of the developing foot into an abnormal intrauterine position. In disorders such as arthrogryposis multiplex congenita, the generalized muscle fibrosis and atrophy secondary to a presumed anterior horn cell lesion can produce a very rigid and severe equinovarus contracture. Histologic studies of the neuromuscular junction in patients with isolated clubfoot deformity have not been consistently abnormal, however. In some cases, muscle atrophy may be a secondary development. It is probably most likely that the clubfoot position is the common end result of a number of pathologic processes that may affect the osseous, neurologic, and muscular components of the lower limb.

In patients with clubfoot deformity, the foot is plantar flexed, inverted, and medially deviated. The calcaneus is small and often difficult to palpate. Marked calcaneal varus is often present. The skin overlying the lateral malleolus is often thin and taut, while the skin overlying the medial side of the foot may appear redundant. The normal posterior creases at the ankle and subtalar joint may be obliterated. Plantar fascial contractures are often present and result in an exaggerated medial arch with a prominent transverse crease at the midfoot. Flexion contractures of the toes may be present. The foot is often smaller in size than the opposite normal foot, and atrophy of calf musculature is usually noticeable in older infants and children with clubfoot. In some cases, the deformity is supple and yields to gentle passive manipulation. In others, however, the equinovarus contractures are quite rigid.

Successful treatment of clubfoot requires reduction of the displaced navicular on the head of the talus, mobilization of tight joint capsules in the ankle and foot, and elongation of the tendons of the posteromedial aspect of the foot and ankle. In some cases, this can be achieved by serial manipulation and casting. In other instances, surgical treatment is necessary.

During the first few weeks of life, the ligaments of the foot are elastic and often yield to gentle manipulation. Primary nonoperative treatment usually involves a combination of manipulation and casting to reduce the talonavicular displacement and stretch the tight posteromedial structures. Serial manipulation and casting are employed to avoid excessive pressure on soft tissues.

Nonoperative treatment is most successful if started in the newborn nursery and repeated at 2- to 4-day intervals during the first few weeks. If the clubfoot responds to treatment, the interval between cast changes can be increased. Three months or more of casting may be required to attain full correction. Modified shoes and/or night splints may be employed at the end of cast treatment to maintain correction.

Many children with clubfoot do not respond completely to manipulative treatment. As many as 50% may require some form of surgical treatment. A number of surgical procedures are employed, depending on the nature and severity of residual deformity. In the past, it was common to perform a series of limited releases throughout childhood for the patient with resistant clubfoot. More recently, a trend toward early surgical treatment has developed. Complete one-stage release of contracted tissues and realignment of the foot appear to be highly successful in the child between ages 9 months and 2 years. In selected cases, it can be performed in younger infants and older children with excellent results. Appearance and function are markedly improved in most cases, although calf atrophy and a smaller than normal foot may persist into adult life regardless of treatment.

Clubfoot is a complex problem. A successful outcome requires prompt diagnosis and early referral. A trial of night splints or special shoes is never indicated for primary care of talipes equinovarus. In many cases, manipulation and serial casting are successful. In most others, carefully chosen and skillfully performed surgical releases will yield good results. A trial period of observation before referral for treatment is never warranted.

Metatarsus Adductus

Many infants have feet that appear to curve inward at the midfoot. In some, the toe-in position is due to physiologic tibial version. In others, the posture is caused by overpull of the abductor hallucis muscle, causing a dynamic hallux varus deformity, or by medial deviation of the first metatarsal ray without medial deviation of the rest of the foot (metatarsus primus varus). In many, however, the medial deviation of the foot results from medial deviation of the forefoot on the hindfoot, commonly called metatarsus adductus. Simple metatarsus adductus and its more complex variants are among the most common orthopedic problems of infancy and childhood. In many cases, the deformity is mild and supple. Spontaneous correction occurs in these children with growth. In others, however, the foot is more rigid, and spontaneous correction does not occur. Unless treated early in infancy, deformity of the foot will persist into adult life. Although persistent metatarsus adductus is rarely associated with alterations in foot function, it may be disfiguring and may interfere with shoe wear.

A number of terms have been used to refer to incurving of the forefoot. Besides metatarsus adductus, these include metatarsus varus, metatarsus internus, skewfoot, hooked foot, and one-third clubfoot. Because of the conflicting terminology applied to the deformity and the paucity of data that permits comparison of studies of affected patients, it is difficult to correlate existing studies. As advocated by Berg, it appears reasonable to consider metatarsus adductus a collection of closely related foot deformities that produce incurving of the forefoot. In simple metatarsus adductus, adduction of the forefoot on the hindfoot occurs in the plane of the sole of the foot as a single disorder. In metatarsus varus, the forefoot is inverted with respect to the hindfoot; if the hindfoot is

held in the neutral position in such patients, the forefoot appears to be twisted medially rather than adducted. Skewfoot is a combination of forefoot adduction and hindfoot valgus deformity. If the adducted foot is placed in the weight-bearing position, the heel appears everted. "Complex skewfoot" is the term applied by Berg to the combination of forefoot adduction, hindfoot eversion, and lateral translation of the forefoot with respect to the hindfoot.

In normal patients, the medial border of the sole of the foot is straight, and the lateral border is straight to slightly concave. In patients with metatarsus adductus, the sole of the foot is convex laterally and concave medially (Fig 3–22,A). A prominence is present along the lateral border of the foot at the base of the fifth metatarsal and cuboid bones. A high arch may be present, and the great toe may be widely separated from the others. When the child is placed in a standing position, the heel may roll into a valgus position (Fig 3–22,B). Bleck has stated that a line bisecting the long axis of the heel in normal patients passes through the interspace between the second and third toes. In patients with metatarsus adductus, the line falls lateral to the second-third inter-

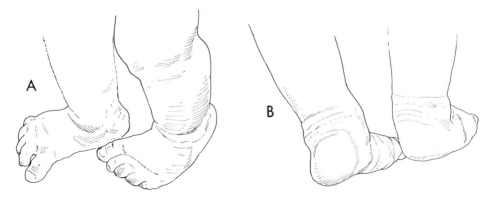

FIG 3–22.
Bilateral metatarsus adductus. **A,** dorsomedial and dorsolateral views. The medial border of the foot is concave; the lateral border of the foot is convex. The medial arch may be accentuated. **B,** posterior view. Slight valgus of the hindfoot may be present in the standing position.

space. The relationship of the heel bisector to the forefoot may be used to grade the clinical severity of deformity but may not be useful in categorizing more precisely the nature of the underlying deformity (Fig 3–23). Differentiation of the varieties of metatarsus adductus by physical examination can be quite difficult, and in some cases, radiographs may be necessary before treatment is begun (Fig 3–24).

The etiology of metatarsus adductus is unclear. Like many orthopedic problems in children, it appears to be a multifactorial condition. Both genetic and intrauterine mechanical factors seem to be involved. The overall incidence is about 1 in 1,000 live births, but the incidence in siblings is about 1 in 20. Male children are affected slightly more often than females, and male children of women with metatarsus adductus are particularly at risk. There is an increased incidence in twin births and breech births. It appears that abnormal intrauterine pressures in a genetically susceptible patient combine to produce the deformity. Congenital hip dysplasia has been found by some workers to occur more frequently in patients with metatarsus adductus and may be another manifestation of increased intrauterine pressure.

Treatment of metatarsus adductus during infancy is usually recommended for cosmetic reasons. As previously noted, persistent metatarsus adductus in adult life rarely causes functional problems, although it may lead to abnormal shoe wear and secondary local callus formation. The relationship of persistent metatarsus adductus to bunions in adult life is at best unclear. Many authorities frankly doubt an etiologic role of metatarsus adductus in hallux valgus.

It is often difficult to decide which children with apparent metatarsus adductus require treatment. Children with mild adductus will often actively overcorrect the deformity if the lateral border of the foot is gently stroked. Passive overcorrection is easily obtained if gentle pressure is applied over the base of the fifth metatarsal and behind the first metatarsal head. Many pediatric orthopedists, this author included, believe that infants with mild

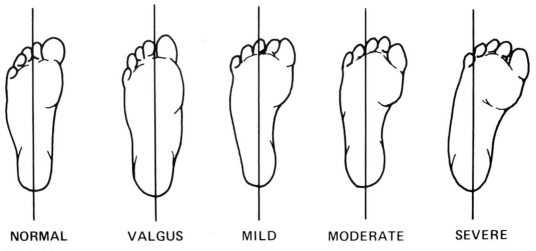

NORMAL   VALGUS   MILD   MODERATE   SEVERE

FIG 3–23.
A line bisecting the heel can be used to clinically grade the severity of metatarsus adductus. Normally this line bisects the second and third toes. It falls progressively more lateral in patients with metatarsus adductus. (From Bleck EE: Metatarsus adductus: Classification and relationship to outcomes of treatment. *J Pediatr Orthop* 1983; 3:2. Reproduced by permission.)

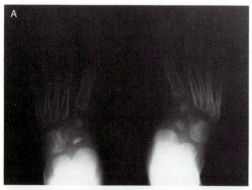

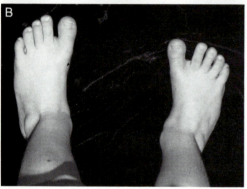

FIG 3–24.
A, roentgenograms of a patient with bilateral metatarsus adductus. **B,** the deformity is much more severe on the right. Note the lateral shift of the metatarsals with respect to the hindfoot on the right side.

and supple deformities require no treatment.

The chief hallmark of severe metatarsus adductus is rigidity (Fig 3–25). Active correction is absent, and passive correction is difficult or impossible in children with severe metatarsus adductus. Often the prominence of the fifth metatarsal base is quite pronounced, and heel valgus may be marked. Spontaneous correction will not occur in these cases, and early treatment is recommended. Gentle manipulation and serial plaster immobilization are the treatment methods of choice. Shoe modifications and stretching exercises are of little or no value in severe adductus and are not necessary in mild,

spontaneously resolving adductus. Abduction night bars do not affect the primary deformity in severe adductus and may cause a severe flatfoot (Figs 3–26,A and B).

Treatment of metatarsus adductus is most effective if started early in life. If begun before age 5 or 6 months, correction can often be obtained with 6 to 8 weeks of casting. Longer periods may be necessary if treatment is delayed. After age 1 year, cast treatment is difficult, and after age 2 years, it is of little value. Older children with metatarsus adductus can be treated surgically if the deformity is severe. A variety of procedures have been described, including release of soft tissue contractures of the midfoot in younger children and osteotomy of the midfoot in older children. The results of surgery are never as gratifying as those obtained with early cast treatment.

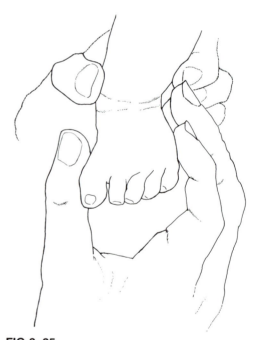

FIG 3–25.
Metatarsus adductus. Rigidity is the chief characteristic of severe metatarsus adductus; passive correction of the deformity is not possible.

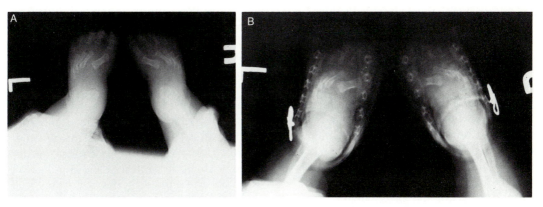

FIG 3–26.
Outflare shoes are not effective treatment for metatarsus adductus. **A,** roentgenograms of the feet of a child with metatarsus adductus. **B,** roentgenograms made with shoes on; there is no effect on the alignment of the foot even though the shoes appear to be flaring outward.

Flatfoot

Flatfoot, or pes planus, is the descriptive term applied to a number of conditions in which the medial longitudinal arch of the foot is depressed or absent. Few other areas of musculoskeletal development cause so much parental concern.

There are numerous types of flatfoot. In many cases, the deformity is quite flexible, and no serious structural abnormalities are present. These children are rarely symptomatic. In other cases, however, alterations in the anatomy of the midfoot and hindfoot may lead to severe, painful deformity in adolescent and adult life.

Flexible Flatfoot

Children with flexible flatfoot appear to have normal foot contour when seated. The longitudinal arch flattens or disappears when the child stands (Fig 3–27). This is the most common type of flatfoot. The clinical diagnostic criteria are quite subjective. Frequently the toddler is brought for evaluation shortly after he begins to stand. At this age, the combination of normal ligamentous laxity and persistent baby fat can make evaluation of a low arch very confusing. Later in child-

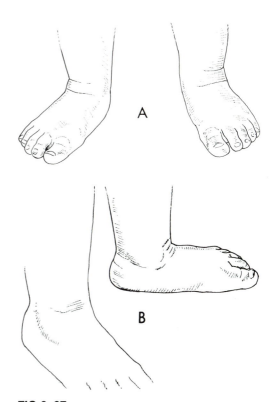

FIG 3–27.
Anterior **(A)** and medial **(B)** views of flexible flatfoot.

hood when the foot is larger, flexible flat-foot is more obvious.

There been a great deal of controversy regarding the etiology of flexible flatfoot. Skeletal malformation, incompetent intrinsic and extrinsic musculature, and ligamentous laxity have all been incriminated, but no single factor has been uniformly implicated. Radiologic and anatomical studies have shown little or no deformity of tarsal bones in common flexible flatfoot, suggesting that osseous malformation is not the cause of deformity. Electromyographic studies have indicated that little or no muscular activity is present in the muscles of the normal foot during quiet stance. Weakness of intrinsic muscles therefore is unlikely to be a major cause of flexible flatfoot. It seems likely that most cases of flexible flatfoot are caused by excessive laxity of the joint capsules and ligaments of the plantar aspect of the foot. If the ligaments are lax, the tarsal arch will collapse when loaded.

Several radiologic criteria have been proposed to aid in the evaluation of flatfoot. These are based on the shift of the tarsal bones that accompanies significant collapse of the arch. In the patient with flexible flatfoot, weight bearing causes abduction of the forefoot, medial displacement and plantar flexion of the head and neck of the talus, and lateral rotation and eversion of the calcaneus. When standing and sitting x-ray films of the feet are com-

pared, depression of the arch is noted on the lateral view (Fig 3–28).

Routine radiologic evaluation of flatfoot is not necessary. If a painful or rigid deformity is present, x-ray films can be helpful in diagnosis and treatment. Since nearly complete tarsal ossification is necessary for evaluation of these roentgenograms, they are most useful in the older child with flatfoot. Appropriate studies should include anteroposterior, lateral, and oblique views of the unloaded foot and weight-bearing anteroposterior and lateral views.

Most children with flatfeet are asymptomatic at the time of initial evaluation and will remain so throughout life. The low arch ordinarily is much less troublesome than an excessively high arch, or cavus deformity. Flexibility is perhaps the most important characteristic of benign flatfoot. If normal foot contour is present when seated, and if the ankle, midfoot, and hindfoot are freely movable, the flatfoot present on standing will rarely be troublesome. Rigidity of deformity, restriction of motion, or pain at the time of initial evaluation implies more serious problems and indicates the need for further evaluation.

In most cases, no treatment is necessary for children with mild to moderate flexible flatfoot deformities. Although many nonoperative treatment programs have been advocated, there is no convinc-

FIG 3–28.
Lateral radiograph of flexible flatfoot. The long arch of the foot is flattened

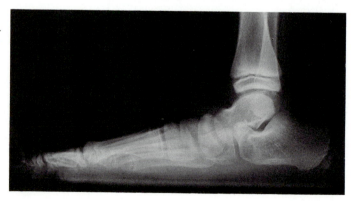

ing evidence that special shoes or shoe modifications will alter foot development or lessen the low possibility of foot pain in adult life. Exercise programs designed to strengthen foot musculature seem to be of little theoretical or practical value. Some children with flexible flatfeet rapidly wear out the medial border of standard shoes. In these cases a more sturdy shoe, such as an orthopedic oxford, may be more durable. In some cases, a scaphoid pad or medial heel wedge may prolong shoe life. These modifications are by no means a medical necessity.

Flexible flatfoot may on occasion become quite severe. This is especially true in some cerebral palsy patients or children with neuromuscular developmental delay. These patients present a difficult management problem. In children who are vigorous walkers, severe flatfoot may lead to pressure sores on the medial border of the foot and predispose to early degenerative arthritis. A number of operative and nonoperative methods have been proposed for management of this problem, but no protocol is universally successful or accepted. It seems reasonable to attempt to provide comfortable, supportive shoe wear in most cases of severe flatfoot and to reserve surgical intervention for very active children with severe deformity.

Tarsal Coalitions

Abnormal union between tarsal bones may be associated with rigid, painful flatfeet in late childhood and early adolescence. Tarsal coalitions have been demonstrated in fetal specimens and probably represent incomplete segmentation during embryonic development. Calcaneonavicular and talocalcaneal coalitions are most common. Talonavicular and calcaneocuboid coalitions have been described as well.

Tarsal coalition is a rare condition. The incidence in the general population is unknown, but it is probably significantly less than 1 per 1,000.

The etiology of tarsal coalition is unclear. Genetic factors appear to be important, and talocalcaneal coalition has been reported to be an autosomal dominant trait.

Tarsal coalitions are initially fibrous or cartilaginous and flexible. Ossification occurs later in childhood, with resultant restriction of hindfoot motion. Disruption of synchronous, smooth motion is presumed to be the reason for the aching foot pain frequently found in these patients. Spasm of the peroneal muscles occurs on occasion, with accompanying calf pain and tenderness. Degenerative arthritis may develop in patients with untreated coalitions and may cause continued foot pain in later life.

A careful radiologic search for signs of tarsal coalition should be made in older children and teenagers with symptomatic flatfoot. Calcaneonavicular bridging is easily demonstrated with oblique views of the foot (Fig 3–29). Talar beaking and loss of talocalcaneal joint space seen on lateral views suggest talocalcaneal coalition. Axial views of the calcaneus and lateral tomograms of the talocalcaneal joint will demonstrate underlying talocalcaneal coalition. Talonavicular and calcaneocuboid coalitions can be seen on anteroposterior views of the foot.

Treatment of tarsal coalitions depends on the severity of symptoms, the location of the bridge, and the presence of associated degenerative joint disease. If symptoms are not severe, a trial of firm shoes with medial arch supports is justified. Anti-inflammatory medications and a period of cast immobilization are appropriate in more severe cases. Surgical treatment is necessary in many cases. Excision of the coalition and interposition of soft tissue is useful in treatment of calcaneonavicular coalitions without advanced degenerative disease. More extensive surgi-

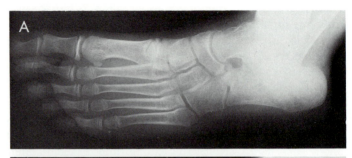

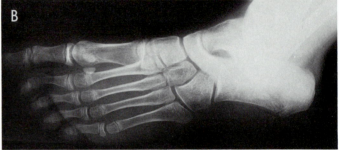

FIG 3–29.
Calcaneonavicular tarsal coalitions.
A, fibrous bar with incomplete ossification. **B,** complete bony bridge
between talus and calcaneus.

cal treatment is required in older children
with other types of coalition or associated
degenerative changes.

Congenital Vertical Talus

Congenital vertical talus, or convex
pes valgus, is a rare condition in which
the talus is vertically oriented and the navicular is displaced onto the dorsal surface of the talus. The structural abnormalities produce a characteristic rigid rocker-
bottom deformity at birth (Fig 3–30). The
etiology is unclear, but in many cases, it
appears to be related to abnormal muscular or neurologic development. It is often
associated with arthrogryposis multiplex
or spinal dysraphism.

Congenital vertical talus is sometimes

FIG 3–30.
Medial views of bilateral congenital vertical
talus deformities and severe flatfeet.

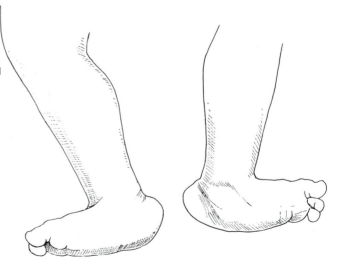

confused with more common congenital calcaneovalgus deformity. Rigidity is the principal differential feature. Achilles tendon and posterior tibiotalar and subtalar contractures are present in congenital vertical talus. Even though the foot may appear to be in a neutral or mild calcaneus position, the calcaneus itself is plantar flexed. Forced dorsiflexion bends the foot at the midtarsal joint and accentuates the rocker-bottom deformity.

Roentgenograms confirm the vertical alignment of the talus with regard to the long axis of the calcaneus (Fig 3–31). In older children, the ossified navicular can be seen to be displaced onto the neck of the talus. Calcaneal deformity and calcaneocuboid subluxation are often present.

Congenital vertical talus presents a difficult management problem. In many cases, a trial of manipulation and cast treatment is partially successful if started early in infancy, but most children will require surgical intervention to achieve a painless, plantigrade foot. A variety of surgical procedures are employed, depending on the patient's age and the severity of the deformity. As in other congenital foot deformities, early diagnosis and referral make definitive treatment more successful.

Miscellaneous Foot Problems

Accessory Navicular Bones

Occasionally an extra ossicle is present at the medial border of the navicular bone (Fig 3–32). It may be fused to the bone or attached to it by fibrous tissue. The posterior tibial tendon may be partially attached to it.

Patients with accessory navicular ossicles may become symptomatic in late childhood or early adolescence. Pain and tenderness may develop over the ossicle and along the posterior tibial tendon sheath. Direct pressure from rigid footwear may cause pain, and posterior tibial muscle spasm may result from the aberrant insertion of the tendon.

Shoes cut low medially or fitted with felt heel pads may relieve local pressure symptoms. Arch supports are sometimes useful in controlling posterior tibial muscle spasm. Surgical excision of the ossicle and rerouting of the posterior tibial tendon can be performed if conservative measures fail.

Bunions

Prominence of the medial aspect of the metatarsophalangeal joint of the great toe with lateral deviation of the toe is

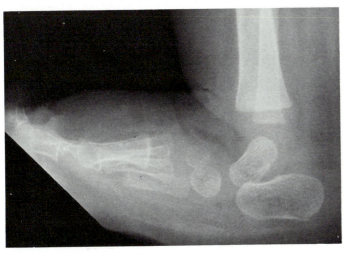

FIG 3–31.
Lateral radiograph of congenital vertical talus.

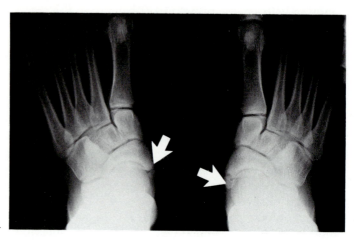

FIG 3–32.
Accessory navicular ossicles.

called *hallux valgus*, or bunion (Fig 3–33). A similar prominence at the lateral aspect of the small toe is called a bunionette, or tailor's bunion. Bunions and bunionettes are occasionally present during childhood but are rarely symptomatic until later in adult life.

Anthropological studies have shown bunions in both shod and unshod cultures. Although the precise etiology of the deformity is unclear, it probably represents a mild congenital malalignment of the first ray. Poorly fitting shoes may cause pressure symptoms over bony prominences but probably are not the cause of most bunion deformities.

Shoes with a wide toe box will prevent or relieve symptoms in most children with mild or moderate bunion deformities. Surgical treatment of severe deformities is indicated to improve appearance, relieve pain, permit the use of conventional shoes, and possibly delay the onset of late degenerative joint disease. The failure rate after surgery is high; recurrent deformity and persistent pain have been reported in 30% to 50% of cases in some series in spite of technically excellent surgical procedures. Prospective patients and their parents must be aware that even after successful realignment, narrow, pointed, high-heeled shoes may well not be permitted, and repeat surgery may be necessary in later life.

Overlapped and Undercurled Toes

Overlapped or undercurled fourth and fifth toes are occasionally seen in children (Fig 3–34,A). The deformities usually are of little cosmetic or functional importance. Symptoms may arise from impingement late in childhood or in adolescence. Surgical treatment may be required at that time if properly fitting shoes do not relieve pressure.

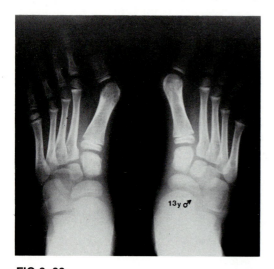

FIG 3–33.
Anteroposterior roentgenogram of a patient with severe bunion deformities.

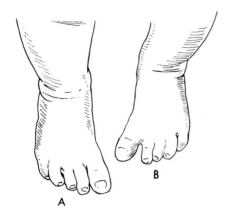

FIG 3–34.
Undercurled fourth and fifth toes **(A)** and syndactyly of the third and fourth toes **(B)**.

Syndactyly and Polydactyly

Webbing of two or more toes, or syndactyly, is a common condition (Fig 3–34,B). It is of no functional significance. Surgical correction is not required.

Accessory digits, polydactyly, are sometimes found in otherwise normal children. Surgical removal is justified for cosmetic reasons and to permit the use of standard shoes.

Ingrown Toenail

Improper trimming of the toenails may cause penetration of the surrounding soft tissue by the edge of the nail, with resultant local infection. The problem usually involves the great toe, but other toes are sometimes involved.

In many cases, the deformity can be treated successfully in the office. Warm soaks should be used for several days to reduce inflammation before definitive treatment. Systemic antibiotics should be administered if surrounding cellulitis is severe. In mild cases, elevation and excision of the offending edge of the nail under local anesthesia is sufficient.

More severe or recurrent cases may require excision of part or all of the nail, curettage of the nail bed, and excision of hypertrophic soft tissue. Such procedures are best performed with adequate regional anesthesia and under tourniquet hemostasis and should be referred for treatment.

Plantar Warts and Keratomas

Plantar warts are papillomas, probably viral, that are buried in the thick skin of the sole of the foot. They may be quite painful if present over weight-bearing areas such as the heel or metatarsal heads. The lesions are well demarcated from the surrounding skin, have a dark central area, and may occur in clusters.

Office treatment usually consists of careful applications of a salicylate solution to the central portion of the lesion. Care must be taken to avoid burning the surrounding normal skin. Electrocautery and cryotherapy of the lesions is also successful. Surgical excision is occasionally required if nonoperative measures fail. Careful dissection of the nidus from surrounding hypertrophic skin can often be done under local anesthesia in the office or in an outpatient surgery department. It should be performed only by experienced personnel, since the lesions can be quite bloody and a painful scar may result from poorly planned or executed surgery.

Plantar keratomas are areas of hypertrophic skin found over weight-bearing portions of the foot. They are the result of localized abnormal pressure points that cause local callus formation. In contrast to plantar warts, keratomas are avascular and have a clear crystalline center. The borders of a keratoma are usually not as distinct as those of plantar warts. Keratomas are painful when pressed; warts hurt more when pinched.

Keratomas are the result of focal abnormal pressure; attempts to remove the keratoma without altering underlying pressure points usually fail. Shoe modifications such as metatarsal bars and sole cutouts often are successful in relieving pressure, and spontaneous regression of the keratoma follows. Salicylate solutions should not be used for primary treatment since they do not remove the underlying cause of the keratoma and may cause severe chemical burns and secondary cellulitis.

SUGGESTED READINGS

Gait Development
Bowker JH, Hall CB: Normal human gait, in American Academy of Orthopedic Surgeons (eds): *Atlas of Orthotics.* St Louis, CV Mosby Co, 1975.

Burnett CN, Johnson EW: Development of gait in childhood: Part II. *Dev Med Child Neurol* 1971; 13:207.

Inman VT, Ralston HJ, Todd F: *Human Walking.* Baltimore, Williams & Wilkins Co, 1981.

Sutherland DH, et al: The development of mature gait. *J Bone Joint Surg Am* 1980; 62:336.

Sutherland DH: *Gait Disorders in Childhood and Adolescence.* Baltimore, Williams & Wilkins Co, 1984.

Idiopathic Toe Walking
Griffin PP, et al: Habitual toe-walkers. *J Bone Joint Surg Am* 1977; 59:97–101.

Hall JE, Salter RB, Bhalla SK: Congenital short tendocalcaneus. *J Bone Joint Surg Br* 1967; 49:695–697.

Papariello SG, Skinner SR: Dynamic electromyography analysis of habitual toe walkers. *J Pediatr Orthop* 1985; 5:171–175.

Rotational Alignment of the Legs
Staheli LT, Corbett M, Wyss C, et al: Lower extremity rotational problems in children: Normal values to guide management. *J Bone Joint Surg Am* 1985; 67:39–47.

Femoral Version
Fabry G, MacEwen GD, Shands AR: Torsion of the femur. *J Bone Joint Surg Am* 1973; 55:1726.

Staheli LT, Lippert F, DeNotter P: Femoral anteversion and physical performance in adolescent and adult life. *Clin Orthop* 1977; 129:213.

Tibial Version
Khermosh O, Lior G, Weissman SL: Tibial torsion in children. *Clin Orthop* 1971; 79:25.

Ritter MA, DeRosa GP, Babcock JL: Tibial torsion. *Clin Orthop* 1976; 120:159.

Staheli LT, Engel GM: Tibial torsion: A method of assessment and a survey of normal children. *Clin Orthop* 1972; 86:183.

Bowlegs and Knock-knees
Bateson EM: The relationship between Blount's disease and bow legs. *Br J Radiol* 1968; 41:107.

Blount WP: Tibia vara, osteochondrosis deformans tibiae, in Adams JP (ed): *Current Practice in Orthopedic Surgery.* St Louis, CV Mosby Co, 1966, vol 3, pp 141–156.

Langenskiold A, Riska EB: Tibia vara (osteochondrosis deformans tibiae). *J Bone Joint Surg Am* 1964; 46:1405.

Levine AM, Drennan JC: Physiologic bowing and tibia vara: The metaphyseal-diaphyseal angle in the measurement of bowleg deformities. *J Bone Joint Surg Am* 1982; 64:1158.

Salenius P, Vankka E: The development of the tibiofemoral angle in children. *J Bone Joint Surg Am* 1975; 57:259.

Schoenecker PL, et al: Blount's disease: A retrospective review and recommendations for treatment. *J Pediatr Orthop* 1985; 5:181.

Siffert RS, Katz JF: The intra-articular deformity in osteochondrosis deformans tibiae. *J Bone Joint Surg Am* 1970; 52:800.

Smith CF: Tibia vara (Blount's disease): Current concepts review. *J Bone Joint Surg Am* 1982; 64:630.

Thompson GH, Carter JR, Smith CW: Late onset tibia vara. *J Pediatr Orthop* 1984; 4:185.

Wenger DR, Mickelson M, Maynard JA: The evolution and histopathology of adolescent tibia vara. *J Pediatr Orthop* 1984; 4:78–88.

Talipes Equinovarus
Cowell HR, Wein BK: Genetic aspects of clubfoot. *J Bone Joint Surg Am* 1980; 62:1381–1384.

Ippolito E, Ponseti I: Congenital clubfoot in the human fetus: A histological study. *J Bone Joint Surg Am* 1980; 62:8–22.

Irani RN, Sherman MS: The pathologic anatomy of idiopathic clubfoot. *Clin Orthop* 1972; 84:14–19.

Laaveg SJ, Ponseti IV: Long-term results of treatment of congenital clubfoot. *J Bone Joint Surg Am* 1980; 62:23–30.

Turco VJ: Surgical correction of the resistant clubfoot: One stage postero-medial release with internal fixation: A preliminary report. *J Bone Joint Surg Am* 1971; 53:477–497.

Wynne-Davies R: Talipes equinovarus: A review of eighty-four cases after completion of treatment. *J Bone Joint Surg Br* 1964; 46:464–476.

Metatarsus Adductus

Berg EE: A reappraisal of metatarsus adductus and skewfoot. *J Bone Joint Surg Am* 1986; 68:1185–1196.

Bleck EE: Metatarsus adductus: Classification and relationship to outcomes of treatment. *J Pediatr Orthop* 1983; 3:2–9.

Kite JH: Congenital metatarsus varus. *J Bone Joint Surg Am* 1967; 49:388–397.

Ponseti IV, Becker JR: Congenital metatarsus adductus: The results of treatment. *J Bone Joint Surg Am* 1966; 48:702–711.

Wynne-Davies R: Family studies and the cause of congenital clubfoot: Talipes equinovarus, talipes calcaneo-valgus, and metatarsus varus. *J Bone Joint Surg Br* 1964; 46:445–476

Miscellaneous Foot Deformities

Bleck EE: Shoeing of children: Sham or science? *Dev Med Child Neurol* 1971; 13:188–195.

Harris RI: Retrospect: Peroneal spastic flatfoot. *J Bone Joint Surg Am* 1965; 47:1657–1667.

Helfet AJ, Gruebel Lee DM: *Disorders of the Foot.* Philadelphia, JB Lippincott Co, 1980.

Herndon CJ, Heyman CH: Problems in the recognition and treatment of congenital convex pes valgus. *J Bone Joint Surg Am* 1963; 45:413–429.

Inman VT: Hallux valgus: A review of etiologic factors. *Orthop Clin North Am* 1974; 5:59–66.

Scranton PE, Zuckerman JD: Bunion surgery in adolescents: Results of surgical treatment. *J Pediatr Orthop* 1984; 4:39–43.

4

The Knee

Angela D. Smith, M.D.
Peter V. Scoles, M.D.

The smooth function of the normal knee belies its complicated design. The bones of the knee do not form an intrinsically stable joint; complex arrangements of ligaments and muscles provide support and permit the three-dimensional motion required for efficient use. Although major injuries to the ligaments of the knee are not frequent in childhood, knee pain resulting from developmental variations and minor injuries is common. Assessment of the painful knee is most accurate when examination is based on careful anatomical analysis. In this chapter, knee anatomy is reviewed, including some of the common anatomical variations that cause knee pain, and childhood knee injuries and minor inflammatory conditions that affect the knee are discussed.

ANATOMY

Surface Anatomy

The major structures of the knee are close to the surface (Fig 4–1), and careful palpation can yield much information on the nature and location of underlying pathology.

The patella overlies the femoral condyles on the anterior aspect of the knee. The skin over the patella is thick and redundant. A bursal sac interposed between the skin and bone permits the skin to glide easily over the patella. The patella itself is freely movable when the knee is extended and the quadriceps muscles relaxed. Portions of the medial and lateral articular surfaces are palpable when the patella is gently displaced to the side.

The quadriceps muscles attach to the patella through a broad aponeurosis called the quadriceps tendon. The patella, in turn, is attached to the tibial tubercle

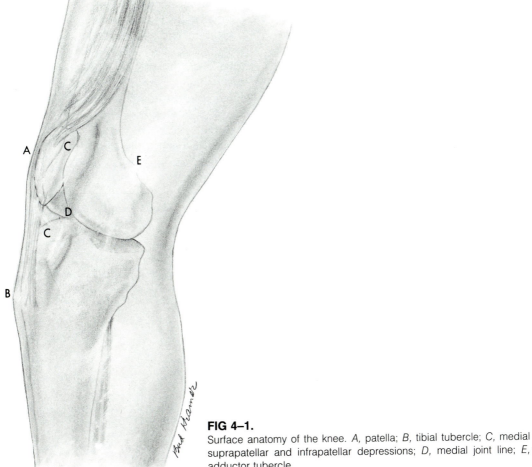

FIG 4–1.
Surface anatomy of the knee. *A*, patella; *B*, tibial tubercle; *C*, medial suprapatellar and infrapatellar depressions; *D*, medial joint line; *E*, adductor tubercle.

through the heavy patellar tendon. The tubercle is a bony prominence on the anterior aspect of the proximal tibia. In the absence of effusion within the knee joint or excessive fat around the knee, shallow depressions are present above and below the patella on either side of the quadriceps and patellar tendons. Obliteration of these depressions is an early sign of intra-articular effusion.

The notch between the distal femur and proximal tibia is easily palpable on either side of the patellar tendon when the knee is flexed. The articular faces of the distal femoral condyles are palpable above

the joint line, and the anterior surface of the tibial plateau can be felt immediately below it. The joint line can be followed medially and laterally by careful palpation. The adductor tubercle of the distal femur is palpable above the medial joint line on the medial aspect of the knee. The medial collateral ligament originates at this point and inserts several fingerbreadths below the joint line into the flare of the proximal tibial metaphysis.

The fibular head is palpable about one fingerbreadth below the joint line on the lateral aspect of the knee. The peroneal nerve runs immediately below it.

The flexion crease on the posterior aspect of the knee lies slightly above the joint line. The medial and lateral hamstring tendons mark out the popliteal fossa, and within it the popliteal pulse can be palpated.

Bones of the Knee

The knee is not a simple hinge. The shape of the distal femur and proximal tibia permits sliding, rolling, and rotational motion during flexion and extension of the knee. The femoral condyles are cam-shaped (Fig 4–2). The lateral condyle extends slightly forward of the medial condyle. A shallow groove formed by the femoral condyles is present on the anterior aspect of the knee. The patella tracks in this groove.

The proximal tibia is flared to articulate with the distal femur (Fig 4–3). The tibial plateau is composed of oval medial and lateral articular surfaces separated by the tibial spines. The cruciate ligaments arise from the tibial spines and pass upward through the intercondylar notch to insert into the distal femur. The tibial tubercle is a downward extension of the proximal tibial growth center along the anterior aspect of the tibia.

The patella is a triangular sesamoid bone interposed between the quadriceps and patellar tendons (Fig 4–4). The articular surface of the patella is covered with cartilage and is divided into medial and lateral facets. The superior-medial aspect of the medial facet is sometimes termed the *odd facet*. The patella holds the quad-

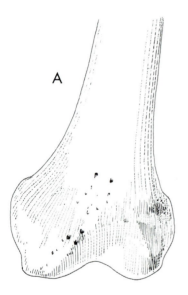

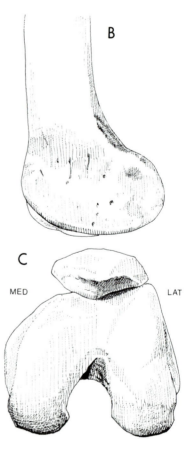

FIG 4–2.
A, anterior aspect of the distal femur. **B,** medial aspect of the distal femur. **C,** inferior aspect of the distal femur. The lateral condyle extends forward of the medial condyle; the patella articulates with the femur in the groove between the two condyles. The posterior intercondylar notch is prominent in this projection.

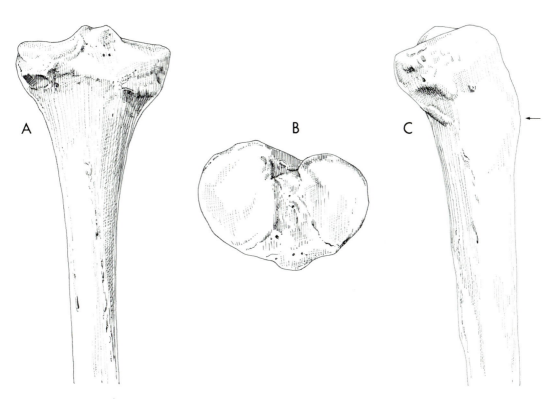

FIG 4–3.
Proximal tibia. **A,** the proximal tibia is flared for articulation with the distal femur. **B,** the tibial spines separate the tibia plateau into medial and lateral aspects. **C,** the tibial tubercle is prominent on the anterior crest of the tibia.

riceps tendon away from the femoral condyles and increases the mechanical advantage of the quadriceps muscles. There is considerable variation in patellar shape, size, and placement, as well as in depth of the groove for the patella on the ante-

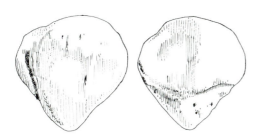

FIG 4–4.
Patella. **Left,** the inferior deep or articular surface of the patella is divided into medial and lateral (articular) facets. **Right,** the superior superficial surface of the patella is roughened to provide attachment for the quadriceps aponeurosis.

rior aspect of the femur. These variations may be important factors in patellar dislocation and subluxation.

Epiphyseal Centers

The secondary ossification center of the distal femur (Fig 4–5) is ordinarily present at birth and fuses with the femoral shaft between ages 16 and 18 years. Minor irregularities in the contour of the center are common between ages 1 and 3 years.

The secondary ossification center of the proximal tibia is also usually present at birth. The proximal growth center caps the proximal metaphysis and extends in a tongue-like projection down to the tibial tubercle. A separate secondary ossification center may appear in this extension

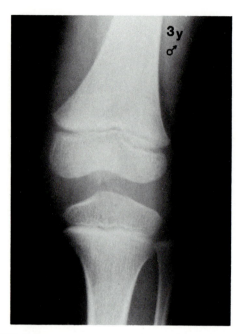

FIG 4–5.
Ossification centers around the knee in a 3-year-old boy. The distal femoral secondary ossification center is normally present at birth and normally fuses with the femoral shaft between ages 16 and 18 years. The secondary ossification center for the proximal tibia is usually present at birth and closes between ages 16 and 19 years. The secondary ossification center for the proximal fibula is barely visible in this 3-year-old child. It usually unites with the body of the fibula between ages 16 and 19 years. Ossification begins in the patella between ages 2½ and 4 years.

between ages 7 and 15 years and is often confused with a fracture. The proximal epiphysis unites with the body of the tibia between ages 16 and 19 years.

A single ossification center for the proximal fibula appears between ages 3 and 4 years and unites with the body of the fibula between ages 16 and 19 years. Ossification begins in the cartilaginous precursor of the patella around age 2½ years in girls and 4 years in boys.

The epiphyseal centers around the knee are usually said to account for 60% to 70% of the growth of the entire lower extremity. On the average, between age 4

years and maturity, the femur increases about 2 cm/year and the tibia about 1.6 cm/year.

Soft Tissues of the Knee

Ligaments

The bones of the knee are enclosed in a fibrous capsule that provides support and permits free motion (Fig 4–6). The capsule of the knee is a dense half-sleeve that surrounds the medial, posterior, and lateral aspects of the joint. It is strongly supported by extra-articular ligaments and tendons. Medial support and resistance to forces applied from the lateral direction is provided by the medial capsule

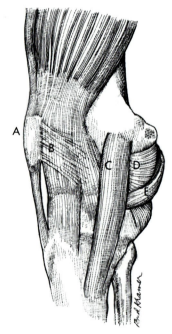

FIG 4–6.
Medial capsule of the knee. *A*, patella with superior proximal quadriceps tendon and inferior distal patellar tendon. *B*, patellar retinaculum and vastus medialis insertion reinforce the anteromedial capsule of the knee. *C*, tibial collateral ligament reinforces the midportion of the medial capsule. *D*, posterior medial corner of the knee is reinforced by *E*, the semimembranous muscle.

and its supporting ligaments and tendons. The medial capsule is thinnest in its anterior one third, where it meets the patella, and thickest in its middle one third, called the deep layer of the medial collateral ligament. The medial capsule thins out somewhat posteriorly to blend with the posterior portion of the capsule. The tibial collateral ligament (Fig 4–7), some-

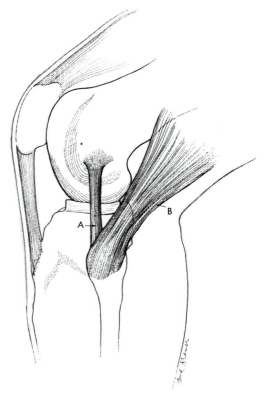

FIG 4–8.
Lateral reinforcements of the knee: *A*, lateral collateral ligament; *B*, iliotibial band. Rupture of the supporting structures is associated with lateral instability of the knee.

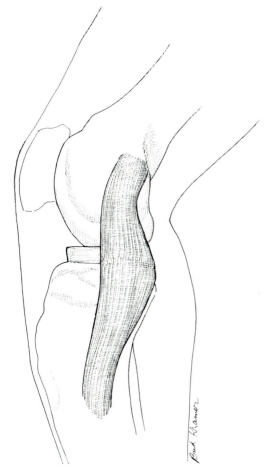

FIG 4–7.
Tibial collateral ligament. The underlying capsule of the medial aspect of the knee is not illustrated. The medial meniscus is interposed between the distal femur and the proximal tibia. The tibial collateral ligament, a discrete, strong fibrous band, originates from the adductor tubercle and inserts into the proximal tibial metaphysis. Rupture of the tibial collateral ligament is associated with medial knee instability.

times called the superficial layer of the medial collateral ligament, reinforces the medial capsule. It arises from the adductor tubercle of the femur and inserts into the medial aspect of the tibia just below the metaphyseal flare. The tendons of the semimembranous muscle and pes anserinus group provide additional support. The lateral capsule is reinforced by the lateral collateral ligaments, the iliotibial band, and the tendons of the biceps femoris and popliteus muscles (Fig 4–8).

The cruciate ligaments provide stability in the anterior and posterior directions (Fig 4–9). Although they lie within the fibrous capsule of the knee, they are out-

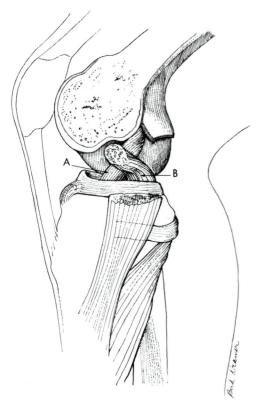

FIG 4–9.
The cruciate ligaments. The medial capsule and tibial collateral ligament have been divided, and the distal femur has been sectioned in the sagittal plane. The anterior cruciate ligament *(A)* arises from the anterior tibial spine and runs posteriorly and superiorly to insert into the posterior medial aspect of the lateral femoral condyle. The posterior cruciate ligament *(B)* arises from the posterior tibial spine and inserts into the lateral aspect of the medial femoral condyle. Cruciate ligament injuries, alone or in combination with capsular ligament injuries, render the knee unstable in the anteroposterior direction.

side the synovial lining. The anterior cruciate ligament arises from the anterior tibial spine and extends obliquely posteriorly and superiorly to insert into the posterior medial aspect of the lateral femoral condyle. The posterior cruciate ligament arises from the posterior tibial spine and crosses the anterior cruciate ligament as it passes forward and upward to insert into the lateral aspect of the posterior portion of the medial femoral condyle.

Menisci

The menisci are intra-articular fibro-cartilage crescents that lie between the tibia and the femur (Fig 4–10). They are wedge-shaped in cross section and attached at their margins to the capsule of the knee. They are firmly bound anteriorly and posteriorly to the tibia.

The menisci probably serve a number of functions in the normal knee. They provide stability under conditions of light loading and aid in joint lubrication. They may, in addition, provide a cushioning effect under heavy loads.

EVALUATION OF THE PAINFUL KNEE

Knee injuries are a common consequence of many of the activities of childhood and adolescence. Fortunately, most injuries are minor; contusions, abrasions, superficial lacerations, and minor sprains usually heal rapidly without complication. Forces sufficient to produce more serious muscle strains, ligament injuries, and fractures are generated in many popular sports, however, and at times significant articular damage does occur. Careful primary evaluation, prompt treatment, and referral when indicated in most cases will minimize disability and decrease the possibility of permanent damage.

An accurate history is essential for analysis of knee disorders. Pain and swelling that acutely follow trauma usually indicate injury to previously normal structures. Episodic pain of less well-defined onset or swelling of insidious onset and slow progression are more likely the result of developmental variations or nontraumatic inflammatory disorders. Separation of acute from chronic complaints aids greatly in establishing a diagnosis and planning subsequent treatment.

The events surrounding injury in pa-

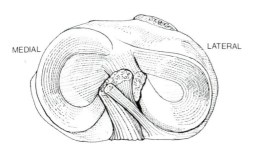

FIG 4–10.
Menisci. The medial meniscus is C-shaped and attached at its medial margin to the medial capsule of the knee. The lateral meniscus is more circular and is separate from the lateral capsule of the knee.

tients with acute knee pain of traumatic origin often give valuable clues to diagnosis. Details of the accident should be sought from both the patient and observers before they are forgotten. The position of the extremity at the time of injury and the characteristics of the deforming force should be sought. Direct anterior or posterior forces may produce cruciate ligament or posterior capsular injuries. Laterally or medially directed forces tend to produce damage to structures on the opposite side of the knee. Combinations of rotational and medial or lateral forces may injure capsular ligaments, cruciate ligaments, and menisci. Direct blows to the patella may damage articular cartilage or produce subchondral fractures on the undersurface of the patella or on the opposing femoral condyles. More oblique forces may produce patellar dislocation or subluxation; if spontaneous reduction occurs, the history of injury and findings of pain and discoloration along the medial border may be the only signs of dislocation.

The immediate response to injury often indicates the severity of damage. An individual who gets up alone and continues playing is usually, but not always, less severely injured than one who requires assistance to leave the field. The time of onset and extent of swelling are significant. Joint swelling that develops immediately after injury is usually bloody and indicates injury sufficient to tear capsular vessels or intra-articular structures. Effusion that develops 2 or 3 days later or becomes chronic may be the result of synovitis secondary to internal derangement or instability.

The patient's age frequently affects the nature of injury produced by a given force. Before closure of the growth plates, fractures through the physes or epiphyses or the distal femur or proximal tibia are more common than capsular injuries. The same injuries that may produce medial, lateral, or cruciate ligament tears late in adolescence or adult life produce avulsion fractures or type I or II physeal fractures in children. Clinical findings are often similar, but the patient's age is usually suggestive of the type of injury.

Chronic knee pain may be the result of prior incompletely treated injury or of a number of conditions that produce chronic joint irritation. The nature of the first episode of pain is significant. If it is clearly traumatic in origin, then recurrent pain may indicate internal derangement of the joint. If no definite history of trauma is present, recurrent pain or swelling may be the result of developmental variations or muscle weakness.

Patients with chronic knee pain report a number of common symptoms. True locking, usually described by the patient as inability to fully extend the knee, may be a sign of torn meniscus or an intra-articular cartilage or bone fragment that blocks motion. Instability when running on uneven ground or when turning quickly may indicate capsular or ligament damage. A sensation of "giving way" usually indicates ligamentous instability or quadriceps weakness.

Children or adolescents with nontraumatic knee or thigh pain must be carefully checked for hip disorders. Avascular necrosis of the femoral head and slipped capital femoral epiphysis often produce vague aching knee pain. Since knee examination in these patients is normal, many escape diagnosis until after permanent damage to the hip joint has occurred.

Examination of the Injured Knee

Swelling, tenderness, and discoloration, limitation of motion, and instability on stress testing are the principal signs of major knee injury. Acute effusion indicates disruption of intra-articular blood vessels. In minor degrees of injury associated with intra-articular bleeding, the normal depressions around the patella are obliterated. In more severe injuries, the knee may be tense and painful, and the patella may seem to float on the joint.

The primary site of injury can frequently be located by the point of maximum tenderness. Examination should include palpation along the medial and lateral joint lines, the medial and lateral collateral ligaments, the patella and its supporting tissues, and the prominences of the femoral condyles and tibial tubercle (Fig 4–11,A).

The usual range of motion of the knee is from about 5 degrees of hyperextension to 140 degrees of flexion. The range of comfortable active and gently assisted motion should be measured. Restriction or block may be secondary to acute pain and muscle spasm or may indicate intra-articular damage. No attempt should be made to force a full range of motion or to correct gross deformity without prior x-ray examination. Roentgenograms of the knee should be obtained before knee ligament stability is tested. The knee should be splinted with either plaster splints or commercially available prefabricated splints before x-ray studies are done. Anteroposterior and lateral views should be routinely obtained; other views may be necessary to image the patella or intracondylar area. Stress radiographs should be performed if there is tenderness to palpation along the distal femoral, proximal tibial, or proximal fibular physis. Stability of the ligaments should be tested after fractures around the knee are ruled out. To test for stability of the medial collateral ligaments of the knee, the knee is first gently flexed to approximately 15 to 30 degrees (Fig 4–11,B). The lower extremity is stabilized by holding the patient's foot against the examiner's chest. With one hand steadying the calf and thigh, the examiner uses the other hand to apply a medially directed force to the lateral aspect of the knee. Instability will be marked by a sensation of opening of the medial aspect of the joint. Ordinarily, less than 1 cm of instability is present when compared to the opposite, uninjured knee. The lateral collateral ligaments may be tested next by applying a force directed from medial to lateral to the knee. Normal knees may have slightly more lateral instability than medial instability, but in most cases, more than 1 cm of laxity is abnormal.

The stability of the anterior cruciate ligament is tested with the knee in two positions. To perform the anterior drawer test, the knee is flexed to 90 degrees, and with the patient's foot fixed on the examining table, the tibia is drawn forward (Fig 4–11,C). The anterior drawer test is repeated with the tibia in maximal medial and then lateral rotation. The Lachman test is also used to detect anterior cruciate instability. With the femur held securely and the knee flexed 15 degrees, the tibia is pulled anteriorly (Fig 4–11,D and E). The amount of displacement for each test should be compared to the patient's uninjured knee. The posterior cruciate ligament is tested similarly, except that a posterior force is applied to the tibia in the two positions.

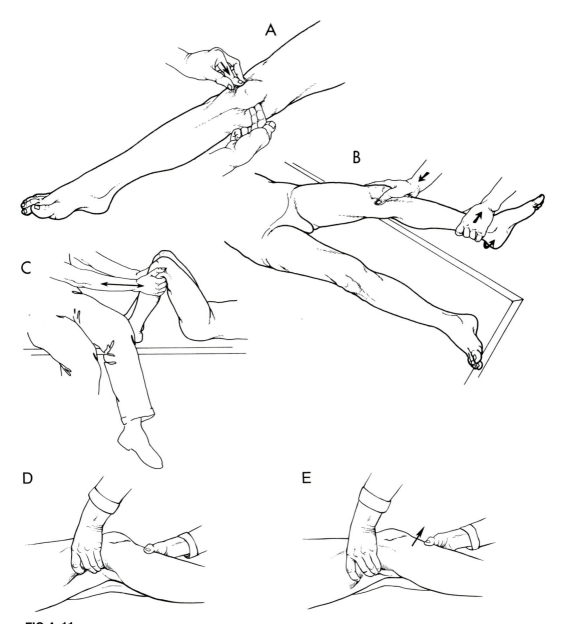

FIG 4–11.
Examination of the knee. **A,** the medial and lateral articular surfaces of the patella may be palpated by displacing the bone gently to one side while palpating its inferior surface with the other hand. **B,** stability of the medial and lateral supporting structures of the knee may be assessed by flexing the knee slightly and applying first medially and then laterally directed forces. The lower leg should be firmly held against the body or with the other hand to provide a counterpoint to forces applied at the knee. **C,** integrity of the cruciate ligaments and posterior capsule may be determined by flexing the patient's knee and fixing the foot against the table with the examiner's body. Anterior and posterior draw normally are less than 0.5 cm. By fixing the foot in a position of external rotation with respect to the rest of the patient's leg, the integrity of the posteromedial supporting structures can be assessed. The posterolateral structures may be examined by fixing the foot in internal rotation with respect to the rest of the leg. (**A–C** from Enneking WF (ed): *Manual of Orthopedic Surgery,* ed 4. Chicago, American Orthopedic Association, 1972. Reproduced by permission.) **D,** the Lachman test for anterior cruciate ligament deficiency, performed with the knee flexed 15 to 20 degrees, usually can detect laxity even in the presence of effusion. **E,** the femur is grasped firmly with one hand, while the tibia is pulled forward with the other. Displacement of more than 1 cm is abnormal.

TREATMENT OF ACUTE KNEE INJURIES

Abrasions, Lacerations, and Contusions

Most abrasions around the knee can be treated at home or in the office by careful cleansing and application of dry sterile dressings. If foreign material is deeply imbedded in the skin, debridement under anesthesia may be necessary to prevent tattooing or deep infection. Hexachlorophene or povidone-iodine soaks should be used for antibacterial effect. Nonadherent pads minimize uncomfortable sticking of the dressing to the wound and may be held in place with cotton elastic gauze loosely wrapped around the knee. Dressings should be changed daily until eschar formation is well under way. Diluted hydrogen peroxide solution may be used to help remove adherent dressings with minimal discomfort. Fresh lacerations around the knee must be carefully evaluated before closure for signs of retained foreign material or intra-articular extension. A sensation of crepitation on palpation around the patella strongly suggests the presence of intra-articular air and indicates communication of the wound with the joint cavity. Roentgenograms should be obtained to check for radiopaque foreign bodies or subtle intra-articular air shadows. Superficial lacerations that clearly do not involve the joint may be cleansed and loosely closed under local anesthesia with fine synthetic sutures. Absorbable sutures may be convenient to use in anxious young patients, but they are somewhat more reactive than monofilament nylon and may leave a more prominent scar. Deeper lacerations with apparent muscle or tendon involvement should be referred for surgical evaluation. Surgical consultation should be promptly obtained whenever joint contamination is suspected. Arthrotomy and debridement are necessary to prevent subsequent infection.

Puncture wounds of the knee often pose treatment dilemmas. Retained intra-articular foreign material may initiate a bacterial or chemical synovitis that persists until surgical debridement is performed. Unfortunately, many objects such as thorns, wood splinters, and fine pieces of pencil lead or glass may not be evident on clinical or x-ray examination. Surgical consultation should be obtained whenever the presence of a retained foreign object is suspected.

Superficial contusions about the knee are generally best treated with rest, ice, mild compression, and elevation. When contusions are associated with joint effusion, more serious intra-articular injury may be present. A severe contusion of the peripatellar region may indicate a chondral or osteochondral fracture of the patella. The presence of an effusion after acute injury is reason for orthopedic consultation.

Ligament Injuries

Treatment of acute knee injuries varies with severity. Patients with a full range of motion, little or no effusion, minimal tenderness, and no instability require only symptomatic care. Acute injuries may be treated by application of ice packs, elevation, and rest. The patients may be permitted to return to full activity when comfortable, provided they have a full range of motion and normal strength. Patients with acute instability, limitation of motion, deformity, or severe effusion should be promptly referred for orthopedic treatment. Ligament tears, intra-articular derangements and periarticular fractures are best treated immediately, before edema and muscle spasm obscure clinical findings.

Treatment of a ligament injury depends on the other associated injuries. An isolated medial collateral ligament sprain is usually treated with a hinged brace, allowing protected motion for 4 to 6 weeks while the ligament heals. Isolated lateral collateral injuries are much less common but may usually be treated similarly. Severe collateral ligament injuries combined with cruciate or capsular injury may require surgery.

Arthroscopic evaluation of acute injuries in children has led to an increased understanding of anterior cruciate ligament injuries in the immature knee. Isolated partial or complete anterior cruciate ligament injuries do occur but must be differentiated from avulsion fractures of the cruciate insertions. Anterior cruciate ligament tears are frequently associated with meniscal injury in children, so arthroscopic examination or possibly magnetic resonance imaging is indicated.

Partial tears of the anterior cruciate ligament may have some healing potential in a child, but many progress to complete rupture with a subsequent minor injury. The decision of whether to repair and/or reconstruct the anterior cruciate in a child or adolescent is difficult. To gain a stable knee with the best chance of avoiding further meniscal or chondral injury in a very active young person, reconstruction of the torn anterior cruciate ligament is often appropriate. However, the most anatomical anterior cruciate ligament reconstructions require violation of the physis about the knee, possibly causing premature physeal closure. These methods are frequently used for the adolescent who is nearing skeletal maturity but are best avoided in the younger child. Other less anatomical reconstruction methods may be used, or the child may be advised to rehabilitate the knee vigorously and observed for evidence of instability that may require surgery when the child is more skeletally mature.

Unlike the anterior cruciate ligament, the partially torn posterior cruciate ligament seems to have reasonable healing potential. Currently, knees with an isolated partial acute posterior cruciate ligament sprain are immobilized in extension for approximately 6 weeks. Associated intra-articular injuries should be treated appropriately.

Meniscal Injuries

Although long-term data are not yet available on the advantages of retaining as much meniscus as possible, most orthopedists now perform partial rather than total meniscectomy when appropriate. Some types of meniscal tears may even be repaired. Both meniscectomy and meniscal repair can be done arthroscopically. Although the ability of magnetic resonance imaging to accurately diagnose meniscal injury is rapidly improving, arthroscopy is frequently indicated for the child or adolescent with suspected meniscal injury so the pathology can be both diagnosed and treated.

Discoid Lateral Meniscus

The normal meniscus is tapered at its central margin so that it is wedge-shaped in cross-section. The margin of the discoid meniscus is rounded and thickened, and the abnormal meniscal tissue may extend so far centrally that it prevents normal articulation between the femur and the tibia. Lateral menisci apparently develop the abnormal discoid shape due to hypermobility. The more firmly tethered medial menisci rarely are discoid. Discoid menisci usually become symptomatic between the ages of 4 and 12 years, causing locking, clicking, pain, or effusions. Symptomatic discoid menisci are treated by partial excision.

Extensor Mechanism Dysfunction

The extensor mechanism of the knee consists of the quadriceps muscle and its tendon, the patella and patellofemoral joint, the patellar ligament and the tibial tubercle. Most of the lower extremity overuse disorders seen in children and adolescents involve these structures, singly or in combination. As the knee becomes painful, quadriceps inhibition leads to muscle imbalance with resultant maltracking of the patella and subsequent patellofemoral joint pain. Therefore, the separate extensor mechanism dysfunction syndromes may exist singly or in combination.

Quadriceps

The quadriceps muscle is composed of four parts: the vastus lateralis, medialis, and intermedius, and the rectus femoris. They join in a common tendon to insert into the patella. With rapid growth, the muscle frequently becomes tight. When a child lies prone, the heel can normally be brought to the ipsilateral buttock with minimal pressure by the examiner. Limitation of excursion of the quadriceps is almost always found in younger patients who have painful extensor mechanism problems. In addition, the oblique portion of the vastus medialis (VMO) is frequently deficient so the patella tracks more laterally than normal as the knee is actively brought into full extension.

Quadriceps contusions are common among adolescents and are treated with some restrictions of activity, ice, compression, and elevation. Diagnostic ultrasound examination may be used to determine the presence of significant hematoma formation since the more serious injuries with larger hematomas require longer periods of rest and slower rehabilitation. Quadriceps strains near the knee are uncommon in this age group but are treated the same as deep contusions. Normal quadriceps strength must be regained before the patient is discharged from care. Particular attention is necessary to the vastus medialis obliquus, since the VMO strength usually returns last, and VMO deficiency frequently leads to maltracking syndromes.

Patellofemoral Joint

Diffuse aching retropatellar pain accentuated by stair climbing, bicycling, or prolonged sitting is a common adolescent complaint. Pain on patellar compression and tenderness along the medial border of the patella are often present. The clinical syndrome is known as *chondromalacia patellae*, but in reality the cartilage softening or fibrillation that is the hallmark of chondromalacia patellae is almost never present. In some cases the onset of pain is slow and insidious; in others, it follows direct trauma or acute lateral dislocation. Retropatellar tenderness elicited by compression of the patella with the knee slightly flexed is pathognomonic. The painful syndromes of the patellofemoral joint form a spectrum from minimally painful maltracking through recurrent subluxation to frank dislocation. Maltracking and minor subluxation disorders usually resolve spontaneously by adulthood and do not appear to be associated with premature development of degenerative arthritis. More severe subluxation and true dislocation are more serious conditions that may cause significant limitations in adolescence and possibly early degenerative joint disease.

Traumatic patellofemoral dislocation may be associated with osteochondral injury and may require surgical debridement and medial capsular repair. The initial dislocation is usually treated by reduction and immobilization with the knee extended for 4 to 6 weeks. However, a few patients have such shallow sulci on the anterior femur that the patella redislocates unless the knee is flexed enough to hold the patella firmly in the sulcus. Recurrent dislocation is much more common in this group than in patients who sustained traumatic dislocations but have normal patellofemoral joint contours.

Dislocation often results from a laterally directed force applied to the medial border of the patella while the knee is partially flexed. Acute pain and muscle spasm are intense. If the patient is seen prior to reduction, the patella is obvious on the lateral aspect of the knee. Spontaneous reduction often occurs if the knee is extended for splintage prior to transport to the hospital.

Radiologic evaluation should be done, if possible, before manipulative reduction is attempted, to exclude the possibility of other osseous damage. Parenteral sedation is often helpful in reducing spasm and pain prior to manipulation. Reduction can usually be achieved by extension of the knee combined with gentle pressure over the lateral border of the patella. Postreduction films are essential.

Traumatic effusion following dislocation may be quite severe and painful. Careful aspiration under local anesthesia using sterile technique may be performed to relieve pain if the knee is extremely tense. Often 100 to 200 ml of bloody fluid is obtained.

Significant damage to the medial retinacular ligaments of the patella and the cartilage surfaces of the patella and femoral condyles may occur in acute traumatic dislocation. Unless the knee is protected for a sufficient time to permit healing to occur, recurrent dislocation may develop. During the first few days after injury, the knee may be held in extension with a bulky soft dressing reinforced with plaster splints. After the initial swelling subsides, a cylinder cast is employed for 4 to 6 weeks. During the period of immobilization, isometric quadriceps exercises are essential to minimize muscle atrophy. Gentle, active range of motion exercises after cast removal ordinarily restore function in 3 to 4 weeks.

Patellofemoral joint subluxation occurs most often in adolescent females, presumably because the wider female pelvis causes the line of pull of the quadriceps muscle to lie lateral to the normal position of the patella. Often these patients have rotatory malalignment of the lower extremities as well as VMO deficiency. The usual direction of subluxation is lateral, but patients who have undergone surgical release of the lateral retinaculum of the knee joint may begin to subluxate medially, particularly if the femoral sulcus is shallow.

Less severe maltracking of the patella may also cause patellofemoral pain syndrome. The diagnosis of patellofemoral pain syndrome is made primarily from the patient's history. Most often it starts after a growth spurt, a minor injury, or a change in activity level. Pain is felt around the kneecap or in the popliteal region. Pain when ascending or descending stairs is common, as is pain after sitting with the knee flexed for a prolonged period. Pseudolocking (stiffness that causes the knee to feel locked) may occur, but the patient can actively extend the knee without performing any of the rotational movements at the tibiofemoral joint that are usually required to unlock a torn meniscus. Some patients complain of occasional buckling of the knee. The pain is frequently bilateral. Physical examination findings include tenderness in the peripatellar region and tenderness to gentle patellofemoral compression. If attempted medial or lateral displacement of the patella causes marked pain or guarding (positive apprehension test), the patient may have recurrent subluxation or recurrent dislocation rather than mild maltracking.

Initial treatment for mild patellofemoral maltracking, more severe recurrent subluxation, and recurrent dislocation is similar. Tight quadriceps and hamstring muscles must be stretched to normal flexibility while they are also being strengthened with an exercise program utilizing progressively increasing resistance. Active quadriceps extension exercises are best performed only over the last 30 degrees of extension since resisted extension in more than 30 degrees of flexion places large compressive forces across the patellofemoral joint and further irritates the knee. For the few patients whose femoral sulci are so shallow that the patella subluxates or dislocates when the knee is fully extended, the exercises are done with the knee flexed 20 to 30 degrees. Oral nonsteroidal anti-inflammatory medications and local application of ice are often helpful. A soft elastic brace with a laterally placed felt horseshoe that abuts the patella may provide extra support during the exercises and during other activity. The exercise program solves the patellofemoral pain problem in several months in 85% to 95% of complaint patients. Some patients who do not respond may be helped by subcutaneous lateral retinacular release, followed by continuation of the exercise program. However, the release may not change the natural history of the disorder and may even lead to recurrent medial patellar subluxation or dislocation. The efficacy of open patellar realignment procedures is also being questioned.

Patellar Tendinitis

Inflammation of the patellar tendon commonly occurs in young active individuals engaged in running and jumping sports. Adolescents with tight quadricep muscles are predisposed to this problem and may develop not only inflammation of the tendon but also irritation of its bony insertions. Tenderness at the inferior pole of the patella may be accompanied by development of a small ossicle and is known as jumper's knee or Sinding-Larsen-Johansson disease. Irritation at the tibial tubercle insertion is called Osgood-Schlatter disease, to be discussed below. The inflamed tendon is tender and may feel boggy to palpation, with loss of the usually firm borders of the tendon in severe cases. In some patients the peritendinous fat pad may also be quite inflamed, and these patients are much slower to rehabilitate. Treatment consists of strengthening and stretching the quadriceps and hamstring muscles utilizing the same program described above for patellofemoral pain syndrome.

OSGOOD-SCHLATTER DISEASE

Painful prominence of the tibial tubercle in adolescence is called Osgood-Schlatter disease after the investigators who independently described the lesion in 1903. Osgood-Schlatter disease is a common problem in active teenagers. Pain below the kneecap is the most frequent complaint. Symptoms usually are made worse by activity or kneeling and are relieved somewhat by rest. Tenderness on palpation over the tibial tubercle at the insertion of the patellar tendon is a consistent finding. The tubercle may be quite prominent.

When characteristic symptoms and clinical findings are present, roentgenograms should be obtained if symptoms or signs are atypical. Irregularity and prominence of the tibial tubercle are the usual radiologic findings; occasionally irregular ossicles within the substance of the tendon are present (Fig 4–12). Follow-up films during the course of the disease are not necessary.

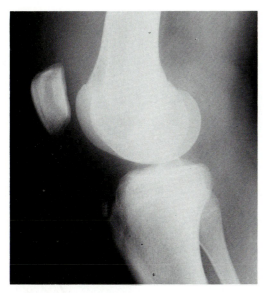

FIG 4–12.
Osgood-Schlatter disease. Note ossicle that persists
in patellar tendon after closure of the tibial tubercle
apophysis.

Trauma probably plays a role in the
etiology of Osgood-Schlatter disease. The
process was initially thought to result
from partial avulsion of the tubercle following violent quadriceps contracture.
More recently, periosteal inflammation at
the insertion of the patellar tendon secondary to repeated minor trauma has
been implicated. There is little evidence
that Osgood-Schlatter disease is a form of
avascular necrosis.

Osgood-Schlatter disease is self-limited. Symptoms can be expected to cease
when the proximal tibial epiphysis closes
between ages 14 and 16 years. Nonoperative, symptomatic care until that time is
almost always successful. Mild cases can
be treated by temporary restriction of activity, stretching exercises, and aspirin.
Ice packs may be helpful in controlling
acute symptoms. Immobilization of the
knee is rarely required, and even patients
with marked pain should be immobilized
only for short periods while allowing
some daily motion out of the immobilizer.

On occasion, bone fragments persist in
the patellar tendon after closure of the
proximal tibial growth plate. If these ossicles are symptomatic, surgical excision
may be necessary.

OSTEOCHONDRITIS DISSECANS

Roentgenograms of the knee in older
children and adolescents occasionally
show areas of rarefaction on the articular
surface of the femoral condyles (Fig 4–13).
Osteochondritis dissecans is the term generally applied to these lesions. The lateral
surface of the medial femoral condyle is
the most common location.

The etiology of osteochondritis dissecans is unclear. Traumatic subchondral
fracture and local ischemic necrosis of
bone have both been implicated. Histologic examination of available specimens
has shown that the lesion is composed of
a fragment of articular cartilage and subchondral bone separated from the underlying bone by a bed of fibrous tissue. In
those cases in which surgical exploration
has been performed, gross findings have
been variable. In some instances the articular surface is smooth, and the defect is
identified only by an area of softening
corresponding to the location of the lesion
on x-ray films. In other cases, the fragment is separate but lies firmly fixed in its
bed. Occasionally the fragment is displaced and lies within the joint, leaving a
shallow crater on the articular surface.

Many children with osteochondritis
dissecans are asymptomatic; the lesion is
an incidental radiographic finding in
these cases. In other instances, mild effusion and vague aching knee pain may be
present. If the lesion is small and symptoms are mild, restriction of activity may
be sufficient treatment. Most such cases
heal spontaneously. If the lesion is large
or symptoms more severe, immobilization
in a plaster cylinder for 1 or 2 months

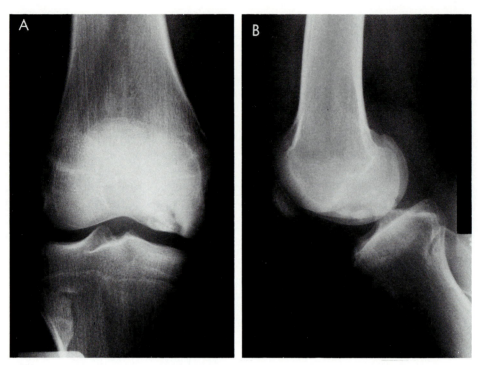

FIG 4–13.
Osteochondritis dissecans. **A,** note radiodense ossicles below articular surface of medial femoral condyle. **B,** several separate bone fragments are apparent on lateral view.

may be required. Joint locking may indicate an intra-articular loose fragment. Surgical exploration may be required in these instances. In some cases, the fragment may be replaced and fixed in position with thin wires or bone pegs; in others it must be removed. In most cases, however, osteochondritis dissecans of the knee in children is self-limited and heals without surgical treatment.

POPLITEAL CYSTS

Popliteal cysts, or Baker's cysts, are fluid-filled expansions of synovial tissue that arise between the semimembranous tendon and the medial head of the gastrocnemius muscle in the popliteal fossa. The cysts may arise from the semimembranosus bursa or from the synovial lining of the knee joint and are filled with clear gelatinous material.

Baker's cysts occur throughout childhood and adolescence. Boys are affected somewhat more often than girls. Large cysts may cause annoying pressure, but most patients are asymptomatic. The cysts are usually nontender and soft; transillumination is characteristic. Lesions that arise in other areas of the popliteal fossa or that are firm, tender, or pulsatile should be suspected.

Spontaneous resolution can be expected to occur in most patients within 2 years. Surgical excision is rarely required and is often followed by recurrence.

SUGGESTED READINGS
Structure and Function
Hsieh HH, Walker PS: Stabilizing mechanisms of the loaded and unloaded knee joint. *J Bone Joint Surg Am* 1976; 58:87.

Ozonoff MB: The lower extremity, in Ozonoff MB, *Pediatric Orthopedic Radiology*. Philadelphia, WB Saunders Co, 1979, chapter 4.

Teitz C, et al: Evaluation of the use of braces to prevent injury to the knee in collegiate football players. *J Bone Joint Surg Am* 1987; 69:2.

Chondromalacia Patellae

Goodfellow J, Hungerford DS, Woods C: Patellofemoral joint mechanics and pathology. *J Bone Joint Surg Br* 1976; 58:291.

Gruber MA: The conservative treatment of chondromalacia patella. *Orthop Clin North Am* 1979; 10:105.

Insall J, Falbo KA, Wise DW: Chondromalacia patellae: A prospective study. *J Bone Joint Surg Am* 1976; 58:1.

Recurrent Subluxation and Dislocation

Crosby EB, Insall J: Recurrent dislocation of the patella. *J Bone Joint Surg Am* 1976; 58:9.

Hughston JC: Subluxation of the patella. *J Bone Joint Surg Am* 1968; 50:1003.

Osgood-Schlatter Disease

Mital MA, Matza RA, Cohen J: The so-called unresolved Osgood-Schlatter lesion. *J Bone Joint Surg Am* 1980; 62:732.

Ogden JA, Tross RB, Murphy MJ: Fractures of the tibial tuberosity in adolescents. *J Bone Joint Surg Am* 1980; 62:205.

Osteochondritis Dissecans

Chiroff RT, Cooke CP: Osteochondritis dissecans: A histologic and microradiographic analysis of surgically excised lesions. *J Trauma* 1975; 15:689.

Green WT, Banks HH: Osteochondritis dissecans in children. *J Bone Joint Surg Am* 1953; 35:26.

Hughston J, Hergenroeder P, Courtenay B: Osteochondritis dissecans of the femoral condyles. *J Bone Joint Surg Am* 1984; 66:1340.

Zeman SC, Nelson MW: Osteochondritis dissecans of the knee. *Orthrop Rev* 1978; 7–9:101.

Popliteal Cysts

Dinham JM: Popliteal cysts in children: The case against surgery. *J Bone Joint Surg Br* 1975; 57:69.

MacMahon EB: Baker's cysts in children: Is surgery necessary? *J Bone Joint Surg Am* 1973; 55A:1311.

5

The Hip

Victoria M. Dvonch, M.D.
Wilton H. Bunch, M.D., Ph. D.
Peter V. Scoles, M.D.

The hip is one of the major weight-bearing joints of the body. Mechanical analysis of the hip joint indicates that forces greatly exceeding body weight are generated by the muscles that cross the joint during routine walking, sitting, and stair climbing. The articular surfaces of the proximal femur and acetabulum must fit concentrically and glide smoothly if the hip is to function normally throughout a lifetime. A number of conditions that occur during the neonatal period or that may arise during childhood can alter the shape of the femoral head or affect its position with respect to the acetabulum. Permanent malformation may follow. Even minor irregularities in joint configuration that develop during childhood predictably result in premature and disabling degenerative arthritis. In many instances, if the normal relationship of the femoral head to the acetabulum can be restored before the growth plates of the hip close, remodeling will occur. Early recognition and prompt treatment of childhood hip disease may forestall or prevent disabling arthritis.

EMBRYOLOGY

The hip joint differentiates during the first 3 months of gestation. During the sixth embryonic week, condensations of primitive chondrocytes form a block of cartilage that will later differentiate into the acetabulum and the proximal femur. By 8 weeks, the general shape of the future joint is identifiable, and cartilaginous anlagen of the femoral head and greater trochanter have developed. The joint cavity does not appear until the 11th week when a cleft develops in the primitive model and the true hip joint is formed. Articular cartilage lines both sides of the joint, and the passive restraints of the capsule and ligaments are present by the end of the first trimester (Fig 5–1).

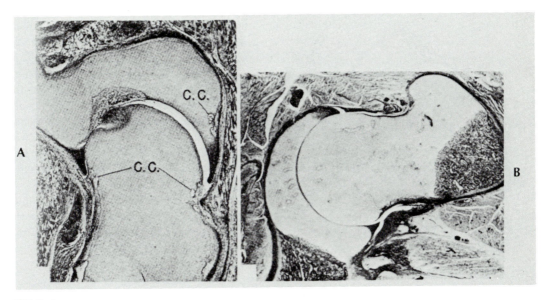

FIG 5–1.
The components of the fetal hip joint at 13 weeks' gestational age (length, 70 mm). **A,** the capsular structures became better defined, and the acetabular roof more completely covers the femoral head. Vascular channels *(C.C.)* are evident at the junction of the femoral head and femoral neck, and at the junction of the acetabulum with the acetabular labrum. **B,** the zona orbicularis is also evident, and the cartilage of the head and neck and trochanters, along with the acetabulum, are well vascularized. (From Gardner E, Gray DJ: Prenatal development of the human hip joint. *Am J Anat* 1950; 87:163. Reproduced by permission.)

During the second and third trimesters, the acetabulum increases in height and width. Concentric enlargement of the proximal femoral epiphysis occurs, and the acetabulum increases in depth in response to the presence of the femoral head. Ossification centers appear in the femoral shaft, ilium, ischium, and the pubis during the first trimester. The secondary ossification center of the proximal femoral epiphysis does not develop until the fifth to seventh month after birth. Asymmetric appearance of the secondary ossification centers of the proximal femur is common and does not imply underlying abnormality of the hip in the absence of other clinical or radiographic signs of dysplasia.

VASCULAR SUPPLY

The vascular pattern of the proximal femur is established by the end of the first trimester. An anastomotic ring derived from the medial and lateral femoral circumflex vessels surrounds the capsule of the hip joint at the base of the femoral neck (Fig 5–2). Branches of this ring penetrate the capsule and ascend along the femoral neck to form a second intracapsular ring at the base of the articular surface of the proximal femur. Penetrating branches supply the metaphysis of the femoral neck and the epiphysis of the proximal femur. The medial femoral circumflex artery is the principal component of the vascular network. Most of the posterior, lateral, and superior portions of the head and neck appear to depend on flow from this vessel. The lateral femoral cir-

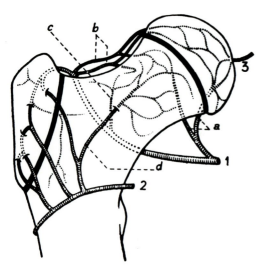

FIG 5–2.
The vascular supply of the proximal femur. *1*, medial femoral circumflex artery: *a*, posteroinferior arteries to the femoral head; *b*, posterosuperior ones; and *c*, a posterior one to the neck. *2*, lateral femoral circumflex artery: *d*, anterior branch to the neck. *3*, artery of the ligament of the head. (After Nussbaum and Funck-Brentano, from Mathieu P: Lesions traumatiques du hanche: Fractures du col du femur, in Ombredanne L, Mathieu P (eds): *Traité de Chirurgie Orthopédique.* Paris, Masson et Cie, 1937, vol 4. Reprinted in Hollinshead WH: *Anatomy for Surgeons,* ed 2. New York, Harper & Row, 1969, vol 3, p 654. Reproduced by permission.)

cumflex artery provides blood flow to the anterior medial aspects of the proximal femur.

The growth plate is a barrier to intraosseous flow between the femoral neck and femoral head until closure occurs late in adolescence. The lower parts of the physis, including the zone of cell proliferation, are supplied by the vessels of the epiphysis. Occlusion of these vessels may therefore result in necrosis of the secondary ossification center of the femoral head and the germinal layers of the proximal femoral physis, and irreversible damage to the growth plate may occur.

The bones of the hip joint grow and remodel throughout childhood and adolescence. The acetabulum increases in diameter by epiphyseal growth at the junction of the iliac, ischial, and pubic bones and in depth by periosteal bone formation around its rim (Fig 5–3). Epiphyseal growth also enlarges the femoral head and neck. Initially, the head and neck form a single epiphyseal region. With increasing age, this separates into two zones, with separate growth centers for the femoral head and the greater trochanter.

Normal muscle balance and a stable femoral head—concentrically, congruently, and completely seated in the acetabulum—set the stage for normal hip development during the growing years. If any component is missing, normal development will not occur. If the hip is well seated but the muscles are unbalanced, as in myelomeningocele or cerebral palsy, late subluxation or dislocation may occur. If the muscle forces are normal but the hip is not well seated, subluxation is present, and deformity will result. Untreated dislocations, while often functional for many years, eventually lead to late degenerative joint disease.

CONGENITAL HIP DISEASE

Complete, concentric, and congruent fit of the femoral head in the acetabulum is essential for continued normal growth and development of the hip joint after birth. Hip dislocation and subluxation alter this relationship and result in abnormal forces acting on the growing skeleton. These forces can change the shape of the growing bones around the hip and cause permanent joint deformity. Initially, this deformity may not interfere significantly with function, but with time, the abnormal wear will result in joint degeneration and pain.

The extent of deformity and corre-

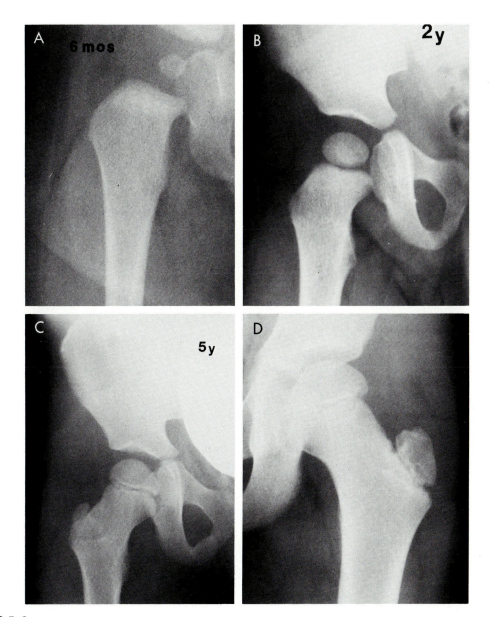

FIG 5–3.
Secondary ossification centers of the proximal femur. **A,** age 6 months. **B,** age 2 years. **C,** age 5 years. **D,** age 10 years.

spondingly the ease and success of treatment of congenital hip disease is directly related to the age at which the diagnosis of dislocation is made. If the diagnosis is made early and the degree of deformity is mild, with proper positioning, growth alone can remodel the hip joint. In the older child, when the deformity is greater, the potential for remodeling during growth is less, and surgery is often necessary to re-establish the joint relationship.

Terminology

In theory, terminology should be standard and should help to clarify issues. In practice, however, terms used in congenital hip disease can have varied meanings and frequently confuse physician and family alike. In conversations with a colleague (be it a radiologist, orthopedist, or pediatrician), agreement on the definition of terms increases the likelihood of a meaningful discussion. In this section, the following conventions are used:

Dysplasia is the most commonly used (and abused) term describing neonatal hip disease. It is sometimes used to refer to the predisposing factors such as ligamentous laxity and acetabular shallowness found in a significant percentage of infants with hip disease. Preferably, the term is used to describe the sequelae of the abnormal relationship of the proximal femur with the acetabulum. Abnormal bony modeling resulting in a steep acetabular roof (acetabular dysplasia) and a small femoral head (femoral dysplasia) are signs of dysplasia. Dysplasia is the result of congenital hip disease and results in later degenerative disease.

Dislocation of the hip exists when the femoral head lies outside the acetabulum with no contact between articular surfaces. The most common or *typical dislocations* occur at or around the time of birth in otherwise normal children. There is no obvious underlying pathology present to explain the dislocation. Radiographs of the hips reveal no abnormal bony development. In contrast are children whose hips dislocate early in intrauterine life. These dislocations, called *teratologic dislocations*, result in severe joint deformity and are frequently associated with a genetic or congenital neuromuscular disorder such as arthrogryposis. Radiographs taken at birth reveal the distorted anatomy of the hip. The distinction between typical and teratologic dislocation is significant; in most instances, patients with typical dislocation are easier to treat and have a far better prognosis than those with teratologic dislocation.

Subluxation of the hip exists when there is partial contact between the two articular surfaces but the femoral head is not completely, concentrically, or congruently reduced. In this sense, subluxation is essentially a radiographic diagnosis and implies a pathologic relationship between the acetabulum and femoral head of long enough duration to produce bony abnormality. Subluxation is sometimes seen in infants carried in abnormal intrauterine positions. At birth, asymmetric soft tissue contractures may be present around the hip. Even though these resolve spontaneously, the bony relationship can remain abnormal. This partial displacement or subluxation of the femoral head results in an alteration in joint mechanics leading to abnormal joint development. Subluxation can also occur as a sequel to treatment for dislocation of the hip.

Subluxation is also used at times to describe the clinical finding of hip joint instability, and its use in this sense implies that the femoral head can be partially displaced on examination. Such instability is not normal, and some children with instability on neonatal examination will later show clinical and radiographic signs of hip dislocation.

Incidence

The reported incidence of congenital hip dysplasia varies. Differences in screening techniques and diagnostic criteria account for some of the variation; genetic characteristics and cultural habits of each population may account for the rest of the difference. In western Europe and white North American populations, the incidence of frank dislocation of the hip in the newborn is about 0.1%. Instability on neonatal examination is much more common and has been reported to range from approximately 0.2% to 2.0%. Congenital hip dislocation appears to occur less frequently in Chinese, Korean, and black populations and is more common in North American Indian, Lapp, Japanese, and central and southern European groups. Traditional child care techniques may account for much of this discrepancy. A position of flexion and abduction encourages stability. In many of the populations with a high incidence of congenital hip disease, however, infants are swaddled with their hips and knees in extension. Infants with unstable hips nursed in this manner may subsequently develop frank dislocation.

Dislocation occurs 4 to 6 times more often in female infants than in male infants. Girls may be more susceptible to the effects of the maternal estrogen hormones that cause pelvic relaxation at the time of delivery. Some investigators have found increased estrogen levels in infants with congenital hip dysplasia. Since excessive ligamentous laxity is often the only abnormal finding in infants with congenital hip dysplasia, any genetic factor that increases susceptibility to hormones causing ligamentous laxity might be associated with an increased incidence of hip dislocation.

Most studies have shown a high familial incidence of congenital hip dysplasia. The incidence of dysplasia in first-degree relatives of affected children is ten or more times higher than that in the population in general. Sibs and siblings of affected males appear to be especially at risk. Nonidentical twins do not appear to have a higher rate of dislocation than nontwin siblings. Identical twins are both affected in nearly half the cases in some studies.

Mechanical factors play a significant role in the development of congenital hip dysplasia. Wrapping a susceptible infant's hips in extension probably results in frank dislocation. There is a high incidence of dislocation in infants who are the products of breech delivery. In these infants, the hips have been acutely flexed and the knees extended during development. Since both iliopsoas and rectus femoris are shortened, hip extension at delivery may predispose to dislocation. Congenital hip dislocation has been noted in association with other congenital deformities such as torticollis, clubfoot, and metatarsus adductus. Infants with congenital hyperextension deformities of the knees are especially at risk. In these conditions, increased intrauterine pressure may restrict fetal movement or impose an abnormal position that leads to subsequent hip dysplasia, as well as other deformities in which fetal position plays a role.

In summary, it appears that congenital hip disease is a multifactorial problem, partly genetic and partly mechanical. Instability occurs much more frequently than dislocation and often spontaneously subsides. In a genetically susceptible infant, abnormal posturing or restriction of motion in utero or immediately after delivery may result in frank dislocation.

Diagnosis

Identification of the child with hip dislocation requires an understanding of the changing nature of the signs of congenital hip disease. Physical examination findings and radiographic abnormalities vary with age in patients with congenital hip disease. Tests designed to elicit instability in the neonatal period are of little value later in infancy and childhood when soft tissue contractures hold the hip in an abnormal position. Roentgenographic abnormalities are usually not present in the neonatal period in infants with typical dislocation but are characteristic in older infants. Clinical signs and roentgenographic findings in the neonatal period and in later infancy are considered below.

Dislocation in the Neonatal Period

A high index of suspicion is the first requirement for early diagnosis of congenital hip disease. As previously noted, there are two major categories of congenital hip disease: typical and teratologic dislocations. Neonates with marked asymmetry or limitation of hip abduction or pronounced shortening of one lower limb may well have congenital hip dislocation, but this is more likely teratologic than typical dislocation. Although such findings will develop in time in the untreated infant with typical dislocation, they are rarely present at birth. A careful search for other abnormalities should be made in infants with teratologic dislocation.

Diagnosis of typical congenital hip disease in the neonatal period requires identification of the subset of infants with hip instability (approximately ⅟₆₀) and gleaning from that group the neonate with hip dislocation (approximately ⅟₁,₀₀₀). A high index of suspicion should be present for any neonate who is at risk for dislocation. Infants who present in breech position, especially female infants, infants with excessive ligamentous laxity, and infants who have a family history of dislocation have a higher than average incidence of dislocation. As noted above, infants with torticollis, knee hyperextension, and possibly congenital foot anomalies have a predisposition for hip disease.

The diagnosis of hip instability in the neonatal period is made by physical examination. The predominant physical finding is that of instability. In 1937, Ortolani, an Italian pediatrician, described a clinical test that, when carefully performed on the newborn, identified a high percentage of infants with congenital hip dislocation (Fig 5–4). Ortolani noted that

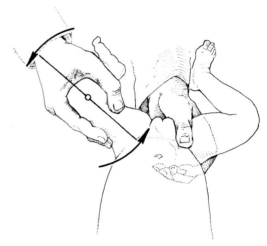

FIG 5–4.
Ortolani test. The pelvis is held steady with one hand while the limb to be examined is grasped with the other. The hip and knee are flexed. While gently pulling the femur forward, the examiner abducts limb under examination, using the greater trochanter as a fulcrum. Reduction of dislocation is manifested by a sudden shift in position of the proximal femur, often accompanied by a palpable or audible click. Sufficient ligamentous laxity must be present to permit relocation of the proximal femur into the acetabulum; the test is therefore principally useful in the neonatal period.

as the flexed hip was slowly and gently abducted in an infant with congenital hip dislocation, a sudden shifting sensation, often accompanied by an audible click, could be felt in the hip joint. The *segno dello saccato*, as Ortolani called the phenomenon, has been translated into English as a "click," "clunk," and "shift." Ortolani presumed that the sensation was produced as the dislocated hip passed over the rim of the acetabulum and sank into a reduced position in the hip socket. Subsequent anatomical studies have indicated that occasionally the acetabulum may be biconcave, like a tea saucer, and that in some instances, the Ortolani sign may be produced as the femoral head glides over the ridge between the concavities in neonates who have unstable rather than frankly dislocated hips.

Subsequent investigators have noted that the Ortolani test, although a valuable diagnostic tool, does not identify all neonates with hip instability. Some neonates with ligamentous laxity and reduced but unstable hips have normal Ortolani test results but subsequently develop hip subluxation or dislocation. In 1962, to improve the reliability of neonatal screening, Barlow described a provocation test for neonates with unstable hips (Fig 5–5). By exerting gentle downward pressure over the lesser trochanter with the hip in flexion and adduction, a sensation similar to the Ortolani sign was produced. Abduction shifted the unstable hip back into position. Barlow noted instability in almost 2% of infants examined within the first week of life. Although instability spontaneously resolved in most instances, a small percentage progressed to true dislocation.

The contributions of Ortolani and Barlow are significant, but it must be emphasized that tests are not perfect. Even in the most comprehensive screening programs, with early examination by experienced pediatricians and pediatric orthopedists, there is a definite limit to the accuracy of physical examination. In 1981, Mackenzie and Wilson reported the results of a 10-year screening program involving more than 50,000 infants in Aberdeen, Scotland. The overall incidence of instability at birth was approximately 5%; at 1 month, approximately 3% were considered abnormal. Dislocation was subsequently noted in 59 patients who were considered normal at initial screening examination. Similar findings have been noted by others. There appears to be an irreducible minimum level of accuracy of neonatal screening. This has led some to conclude that dislocation may develop later in infancy in infants whose hips were stable at birth and in whom acetabular dysplasia rather than ligamentous laxity is responsible for dislocation.

Although it is possible that some infants may develop late dislocation, in most instances, the diagnosis of dislocation can be made early in infancy. Careful and repeated evaluation is necessary; these clinical evaluations are not easy to do correctly, and many factors can produce false negatives. Even conscientious examiners can miss dislocated hips in the neonatal period. For greatest accuracy, the baby must be warm, quiet, and relaxed (not a common state for some newborns). If the baby is cold, hungry, or just plain ornery, tightening of the muscles around the hip can result in a false negative examination. Because the examination of the infant is not foolproof, it is important that a hip examination be done on *all* well-baby visits, not just for those infants at risk.

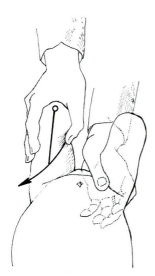

FIG 5–5.
The Barlow test permits the early diagnosis of hip instability. It is a provocation test for dislocatability. The pelvis is steadied with one hand while the leg to be tested is grasped with the other. The thumb of the examiner's hand should lie over the lesser trochanter and the tip of the middle finger over the greater trochanter. With the hip and knee in flexion, gentle pressure is exerted with the thumb over the lesser trochanter. Dislocatability is manifested by a sudden shift of the proximal femur. Dislocation may be reversed with the Ortolani test.

Diagnosis of Hip Disease After the Neonatal Period

By 6 weeks of age, the Ortolani and Barlow signs are present in fewer than 30% of infants with hip dislocation. Physiologic tightening of the soft tissue around the hip replaces the ligamentous laxity of the neonate, and the movement necessary for these tests is lost. The abnormal relationship between the femoral head and the acetabulum, however, results in other signs that allow a diagnosis to be made (Fig 5–6).

Incomplete or asymmetric abduction of the hips resulting from a contracture of the adductor group replaces instability as the cardinal sign of hip dislocation in the older infant. It is normally possible to abduct both hips to 90 degrees in a position of 90-degree hip flexion. One of the difficulties in diagnosing bilateral hip disease is that the examination relies on a comparison of one side of the body with the other—a presumed normal with an abnormal. The asymmetry allows a diagnosis. In the case of bilateral dislocations, however, the child's body may be essentially symmetrical and still not be normal. Any child who has symmetrical but limited abduction undergoes radiologic evaluation. As the child approaches 3 months, the hip examination should be performed in hip extension as well as in hip flexion as a further evaluation of abduction.

When dislocation persists, contracture of the primary hip flexor, the iliopsoas, results in superior migration of the dislocated proximal femur, producing apparent shortening of the limb. Initially, the shortening can be misdiagnosed as a leg-length inequality rather than a sign of hip disease. Parents are frequently quick to pick up on an apparent length discrepancy. When apparent leg-length inequality is noted in infancy, thorough evaluation of the hip motion is indicated. If asymmetric abduction is found in association with leg-length inequality, hip roentgenograms should be ordered.

When a child with hip dislocation begins to walk, other signs of hip disease become apparent. The proximal migration of the femur shortens the abductors of the hip, the gluteus medius and minimus. This weakens these muscles, producing the waddling or Trendelenburg's gait associated with hip dislocation. In the stance portion of this gait, the child leans over the side of abductor weakness to keep the pelvis level.

Congenital hip dislocation, although clinically quite striking, produces few symptoms in early childhood. Despite appearance, pain is uncommon in childhood, and functional limitations are slight. Later in adolescence, fatigue and pain on exercise may develop, and by early to midadult life, most patients with untreated congenital hip dislocation experience significant pain and disability.

Radiologic Findings

The radiologic findings of congenital hip disease vary with the age of the patient and the effects of treatment. In infants with teratologic dislocations associated with conditions such as arthrogryposis multiplex congenita, roentgenograms made at birth may be abnormal, reflecting abnormal intrauterine development of the hip. In typical dislocations, however, early roentgenograms may be normal or may show only subtle changes. When dislocation persists, abnormal development soon becomes manifest, so that after 3 months of age, roentgenograms are valuable diagnostic aids.

A number of roentgenographic criteria have been devised to identify hip dysplasia and to estimate the severity of secondary changes around the hip. An anteroposterior view of the pelvis with both legs extended and in neutral abduc-

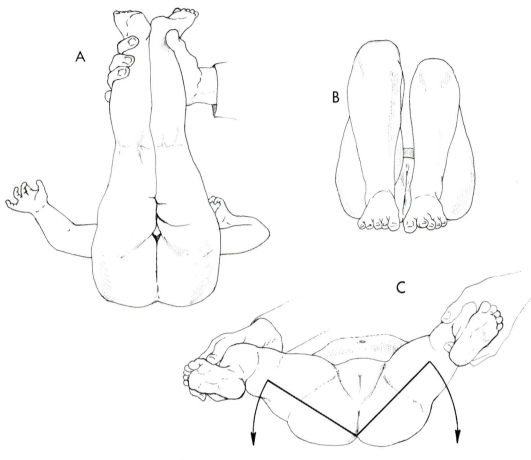
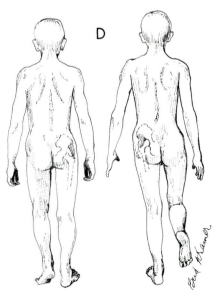

FIG 5–6.
Physical findings in congenital hip dislocation. **A,** thigh fold asymmetry is often present in infants with unilateral hip dislocation. An extra fold can be seen on the abnormal side. The finding is not diagnostic, however. It may be found in normal infants and may be absent in children with hip dislocation or dislocatability. **B,** leg length inequality is a sign of unilateral hip dislocation. It is not reliable in children with dislocatable but not dislocated hips or in children with bilateral dislocation. **C,** limitation of hip abduction is often present in older infants with hip dislocation. Abduction of greater than 60 degrees is usually possible in infants. Restriction or asymmetry indicates the need for careful radiologic examination. **D,** Trendelenburg's sign. In single-leg stance, the abductor muscles of the normal hip support the pelvis. Dislocation of the hip functionally shortens and weakens these muscles. When the child attempts to stand on the dislocated hip, the opposite side of the pelvis drops. When bilateral dislocation is present, a wide-based Trendelenburg limp will result.

tion-adduction position is adequate; lateral views are not necessary. Gonadal shields should be used on boys and, if possible, on girls. Care must be taken not to obscure the hips with the shields.

The landmarks used for reference include the center of the triradiate cartilages, the outer edge of the acetabulum, and the medial metaphyseal beak of the proximal femur. In older infants, the secondary ossification center of the proximal femoral epiphysis is also a valuable reference point. A reference grid is constructed on the pelvis by drawing a horizontal line through the centers of both triradiate cartilages; this is known as Hilgenreiner's line (Fig 5–7). Next, perpendiculars, called Perkins' lines, are

dropped from the outer edges of the acetabulum. Four quadrants are thus marked on each hip. The medial metaphyseal beak of the proximal femur and the secondary ossification center of the femoral head, if present, should lie within the inner lower quadrant on each side.

Another measurement used to evaluate the hip is a line traced along the curved inferior aspect of the proximal femoral metaphysis, continuing along the inferior surface of the superior pubic ramus. A break in Shenton's line, as this line is called, indicates superior displacement of the proximal femur (Fig 5–8).

If there is a high index of suspicion that the hip is truly dislocated (Ortolani positive) and not just unstable (Barlow

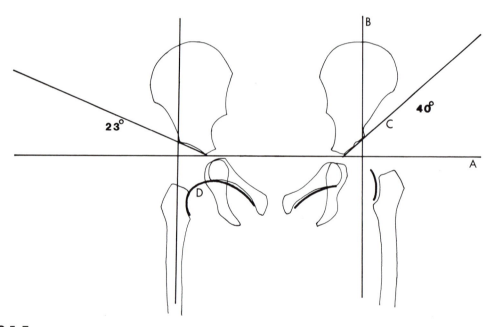

FIG 5–7.
Radiologic signs of congenital hip dislocation. A horizontal line *(A)* is drawn through the junctions of of the iliac, ischial, and pubic bones at the center of the acetabulum (Hilgenreiner's line). A perpendicular line *(B)* is next drawn through the outer border of the acetabulum (Perkins' line). The secondary ossification center of the femoral head, or, in its absence, the medial metaphyseal beak of the proximal femur should lie within the inner lower quadrant formed by the intersection of these lines. The acetabular index, a measure of acetabular depth, can be estimated by inscribing a line *(C)* joining the inner and outer edges of the acetabulum. The angle formed by this line and Hilgenreiner's line is normally less than 30 degrees. Increased angles indicate acetabular hypoplasia. Shenton's line *(D)* is inscribed along the inferior border of the femoral neck and inferior border of the superior pubic ramus. It is ordinarily smooth and unbroken. Proximal displacement of the femoral head in congenital hip dislocation result in interruption of Shenton's line.

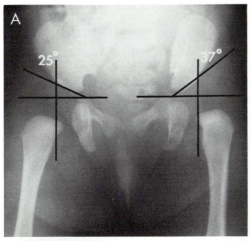

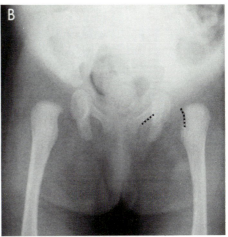

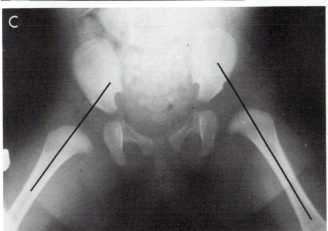

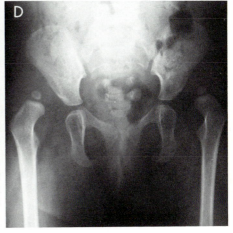

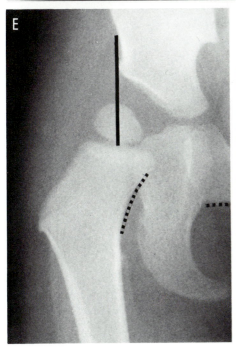

FIG 5–8.
Radiologic appearance of congenital hip disease in various age groups. **A,** 1-week-old child with bilateral positive Ortolani tests. Both hips were judged clinically to be dislocated. Hilgenreiner's and Perkins' lines have been drawn in on the right, and the right acetabular index has been measured. **B,** 1-week-old child with bilateral positive Barlow tests. Lateral displacement of the proximal femur is more subtle. This roentgenogram was interpreted as normal, even though Shenton's line was broken. **C,** Von Rosen's view of the hips demonstrates left dislocation. A line drawn along the femoral shaft falls outside the confines of the acetabulum. **D,** bilateral hip dislocation in an 18-month-old child. **E,** subluxation of the hip as a result of incompletely treated dislocation is manifested by lateral displacement of the femoral head. The angle inscribed between the center of the femoral head and acetabulum edge may be 5 degrees or less.

151

positive), Von Rosen's lateral views of the hips are sometimes useful. They are only valuable, however, when obtained properly. This requires a well-trained assistant who can position the patient correctly. An anteroposterior view of the pelvis is obtained with each hip extended, internally rotated, and abducted 45 degrees. In this position, a line drawn along the femoral shaft normally passes through the acetabulum below its outer edge. In hip dislocation, the line lies above the acetabulum. Full internal rotation and 45 degrees of abduction are essential; a false appearance of dislocation may be present if the hip is not fully abducted. A hip that dislocated with a Barlow maneuver may appear normal when a Von Rosen's view is taken.

An index of acetabular depth can be obtained by inscribing a line through the outer edge of the acetabulum and the center of the triradiate cartilage on each side. The angle formed by the intersection of this line and Hilgenreiner's horizontal line is commonly used to estimate the adequacy of the acetabulum in hip dysplasia and to follow the acetabulum's response to treatment. Normally, the acetabular index is less than 30 degrees; an increased index implies a shallow socket. There are limits to the accuracy of this measurement, however. Roentgenograms are two-dimensional representations of three-dimensional phenomena. Pelvic tilt and pelvic rotation at the time of the study will alter acetabular angles and may mask or exaggerate dysplasia.

When the dislocation persists past infancy, more evidence of the abnormal relationship is visible on the radiograph. The ossification of the femoral head, which normally appears on the x-ray between 5 and 7 months of age, is delayed. This delay in appearance reflects the abnormal growth that is occurring throughout the hip as a result of the altered joint mechanism. Acetabular development is affected by this alteration as well. With time, the true acetabulum becomes progressively more shallow, and its roof becomes more steep. A false acetabulum develops in the ilium in response to the pressure of the dislocated femoral head. Successful treatment of the underlying dislocation gradually corrects this altered relationship. The extent of correction possible depends on the degree of distortion and the growth potential of the child at the time of treatment.

Treatment

The goals of childhood treatment of congenital hip dislocation are to restore as closely as possible the anatomical alignment of the hip while maintaining pain-free function. Objectives, methods, and results vary with the age of the child at the time of diagnosis. In general, the younger the patient at the time of diagnosis, the greater the chance of obtaining a good clinical and radiologic result with minimum risk. The complexity of treatment and the risk of complications increase with age.

Prompt recognition is the key to successful treatment of congenital hip disease. The hip examination should be a routine part of the neonatal examination and the results recorded in the hospital chart for later reference. Infants with a positive Ortolani test result should be referred promptly for treatment. In theory, treatment could be postponed in infants who have hips that are dislocatable on a Barlow provocation test since many children with unstable hips spontaneously become normal. In practice, however, some of these infants may not return for repeat examination at age 1 month, and the golden opportunity may be lost. It is probably prudent to initiate treatment in all neonates with positive Barlow and Ortolani tests.

Neonatal Period

Treatment of typical hip dysplasia in the neonate usually consists of splintage in flexion and abduction. A variety of braces and splints are currently in use, including plastic-covered metal splints, abduction pillows, and cloth harnesses (Fig 5–9). Spica casts are occasionally employed. For treatment to be successful, an appliance must fit comfortably, hold the hips reduced, and not interfere with diapering or sponge bathing. Triple diapers are not a reliable form of treatment. The amount of flexion and abduction achieved is inconsistent; and often only the uninvolved hip is held in the correct position. Reduction, if obtained, may be lost at the time of diaper changes. In addition, the cost of the required course of treatment with triple diapers often equals or exceeds the cost of brace treatment.

Patients with easily reduced congenital dislocation or hip instability are usually treated with continuous wear of abduction-flexion braces for 2 to 4 months. A night splint is sometimes prescribed for an additional 2 to 6 months after continuous bracing is complete to insure proper

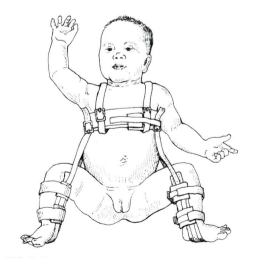

FIG 5–9.
The Pavlik harness is a safe, reliable means of treatment of hip instability and dislocation in the neonate.

remodeling. Mothers are not usually permitted to remove the braces during the first weeks of treatment of frank dislocation. They are sometimes allowed to remove the appliance briefly for bathing in later phases of treatment for dislocation and in infants with dislocatability.

The primary physician can greatly facilitate treatment by being aware of the orthopedist's instructions and by reinforcing them on routine well-baby visits. He can also alert the family that frequent visits to the orthopedist will be necessary because careful supervision is required to insure that the hips are reduced throughout the treatment period.

Treatment complications are rare in neonates with typical dislocation. On occasion an infant may develop avascular necrosis of part or all of the capital femoral epiphysis. When this happens, roentgenograms may show delayed appearance, fragmentation, or arrested growth of the secondary ossification center, or irregularity of the proximal femoral metaphysis (Fig 5-10). Avascular necrosis in the infant can lead to severe hip joint deformity. Gentle reduction and splintage in the "human" position of 90-degree to l00-degree flexion and 50-degree abduction usually prevent this iatrogenic complication.

Teratologic dislocation in the neonate is more difficult to treat and is associated with a much higher complication rate. Closed reduction may be difficult to obtain and maintain because of soft tissue contractures and hypoplasia of bony elements. Preliminary muscle release and traction are usually necessary, and open reduction is often necessary. Although careful preoperative and operative techniques lower the high incidence of avascular necrosis following treatment of teratologic dislocation, results are too often disappointing. The prognosis for normal joint development in teratologic dislocation is poor.

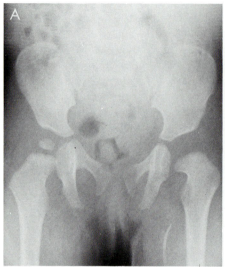

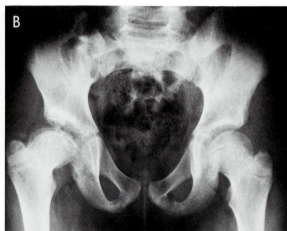

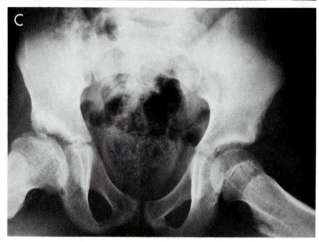

FIG 5–10.
Avascular necrosis of the femoral head. **A,** delayed appearance of the secondary ossification center of the femoral metaphysis, as well as widening of the proximal femoral metaphysis, are early manifestations of avascular necrosis of the left femoral head in this 13-month-old child. **B** and **C,** avascular necrosis in this 8-year-old patient is manifested by lateral displacement and right femoral head deformity.

Ages 3 to 18 Months

Treatment of the older infant with undetected congenital hip dislocation is much more difficult. By age 2 to 3 months, the period of ligamentous laxity in the neonate has passed, and contractures of soft tissues around the dislocated hip are usually present. Fibrous and fatty tissue may fill the acetabulum, and the capsule of the hip joint may be interposed between the femoral head and the hip socket (Fig 5–11). Acetabular dysplasia is usually present in older children in this age group, and the femoral head may be dysplastic as well. In most instances, a false acetabulum develops in the ilium above the true acetabulum in response to pressure from the femoral head.

Concentric reduction of the femoral head in the true acetabulum ordinarily reverses the dysplastic process. Considerable remodeling of the bony elements of the hip can be expected if reduction is carefully achieved and held for a sufficient period. Closed reduction can be safely attempted in most of these infants after a preliminary period of traction to gently stretch the tissues around the hip.

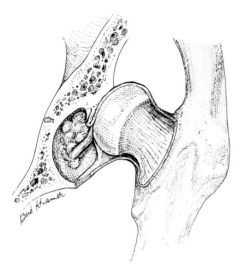

FIG 5–11.
Interposition of soft tissues between the femoral head and acetabulum may block reduction of hip dislocation. Fatty and fibrous tissue often fills the acetabulum. The ligamentum teres is often hypertrophic. The capsule of the hip may fold against the labrum and obstruct reduction, and the tendon of the iliopsoas muscle may form an hourglass constriction of the capsule.

A Pavlik harness provides this for children under 6 months of age. Skin traction is usually used for infants between ages 6 months and 1 year. Skeletal traction may be necessary in older or larger patients. Traction is continued until the femoral head is at or below the level of the acetabulum. This may require 10 days to 3 weeks. Preliminary release of tight adductor muscles may be necessary. Little or no force should be required to place the femoral head in the acetabulum, and the hip should be stable in flexion and mild abduction. An arthrogram may be required to check the adequacy of reduction.

Open reduction of the hip is usually performed if closed reduction cannot be obtained gently or if there is radiologic evidence of soft tissue interposition blocking stable reduction. Following reduction, immobilization in a series of spica casts is necessary to permit remodeling. Four to 8

months of cast treatment may be required, and a night splint may be necessary for an additional 4 to 6 months.

A high percentage of children in whom concentric closed reduction is achieved by preliminary traction and gentle manipulation develop clinically and radiologically normal hips. Even after careful treatment, however, 10% to 20% of these infants develop avascular necrosis in part or all of the femoral head. Many more develop avascular necrosis if adequate prereduction traction is not employed. Primary open reduction has been advocated by some authorities in an attempt to decrease the rate of avascular necrosis, but most authors believe that a trial of closed reduction after preliminary traction is still the most acceptable method of treatment.

Ages 18 Months to 4 Years

Surgical treatment is almost always required for children over 18 months old at the time of diagnosis. Soft tissue contractures are usually severe, and capsular and ligamentous obstructions block reduction. Significant acetabular and femoral deformities are usually present, and remodeling cannot be reliably expected to occur even with prolonged immobilization. A combination of muscle release, skeletal traction, open reduction, and pelvic or femoral osteotomy may be required to obtain a stable hip. Treatment is technically demanding, and the complication rates are high (Fig 5–12).

When a stable, well-contained hip can be achieved without secondary avascular necrosis, the prognosis for acceptable long-term function is good. Although the affected hip may always show radiologic evidence of surgical treatment for dislocation, clinical results are often excellent. Many children successfully treated at this age can expect a lifetime of normal function, although some children with early

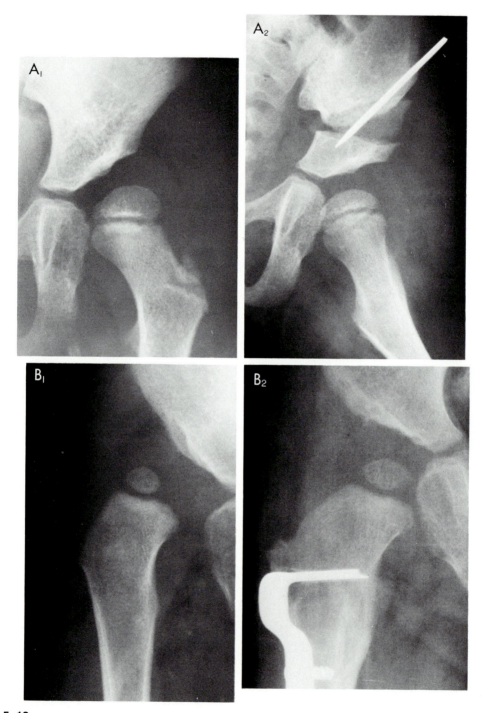

FIG 5–12.
A₁, A₂, open reduction and femoral osteotomy for treatment of congenital hip dislocation in a 15-month-old patient. **B₁, B₂,** pelvic osteotomy for treatment of persistent lateral displacement of the femoral head following nonoperative treatment of congenital hip dislocation.

good results may later develop degenerative joint disease and require reconstructive hip arthroplasty.

As in children treated in infancy, avascular necrosis and residual subluxation are the principal complications of treatment of children aged 2 to 4 years. Partial necrosis of the lateral portion of the epiphysis usually leads to valgus deformity of the femoral neck; necrosis of the medial portion predisposes to varus deformity of the femoral neck. Complete necrosis usually results in a short, broad femoral neck and a mushroom-shaped, large femoral head. Continued growth at the greater trochanteric epiphysis accentuates the deformity. Children with complete avascular necrosis usually develop leg-length inequality with continued growth; a difference of 2 cm or more may be present by age 10 years. Trochanteric overgrowth functionally shortens the abductor muscles of the affected side, producing a Trendelenburg limp. Passive and active abduction may be restricted because of femoral head deformity, and a mild flexion contracture is often present. Radiologic evidence of degenerative joint disease may develop during the second decade; hip pain and progressive disability often occur earlier in these patients than in those with untreated dislocation.

Persistent lateral displacement of the femoral head shown on a roentgenogram obtained after treatment is a sign of incomplete reduction or failure of the hip to remodel. A subluxed hip is not mechanically sound; altered force transmission across the joint accelerates premature wear. Degenerative arthritis is a frequent sequela. Surgical attempts to center the head in the acetabulum or provide additional acetabular coverage for the child with residual subluxation are often justified. A number of operative procedures are available, depending on the severity of dysplasia, the age of the child, and the preference of the surgeon. Although a satisfactory radiologic and early clinical result can often be achieved, hip stiffness and functional limitation are more frequent with each operative procedure a patient undergoes.

Ages 4 to 5 Years and Older

Occasionally a child with congenital hip dislocation will escape diagnosis until his fourth or fifth year. Fortunately, this is now a rare occurrence. Leg-length inequality and Trendelenburg limp are usually present with unilateral dislocation; a broad pelvis and wide-based waddling gait are signs of bilateral dislocation. Pain is usually not present, and function is ordinarily good. Benefits and risks must be carefully considered before beginning treatment in these cases. Extensive surgical reconstruction is necessary to obtain a stable hip. Preliminary muscle releases, prolonged skeletal traction, and pelvic and femoral osteotomies are often required. The risks of avascular necrosis, residual subluxation, and hip stiffness are high. Unless a near-perfect surgical result is obtained, the patient may have significantly more disability than he did preoperatively. Nevertheless, in skilled hands a satisfactory result can be obtained in many of these children. Even when it is not possible to provide a lifetime of normal function, operative treatment in childhood can set the stage for later replacement arthroplasty.

SUGGESTED READINGS

Development of the Hip Joint
Chung SMK: The arterial supply of the developing proximal end of the human femur. *J Bone Joint Surg Am* 1976; 58:961.

Ponseti I: Growth and development of the acetabulum in the normal child. *J Bone Joint Surg Am* 1978; 60:575.

Trueta J: The normal vascular anatomy of the human femoral head during growth. *J Bone Joint Surg Br* 1957; 39:358.

Watanabe RS: Embryology of the human hip. *Clin Orthop* 1974; 98:8.

Congenital Hip Dysplasia: Terminology, Etiology, and Incidence

Carter CO, Wilkinson JA: Genetic and environmental factors in the etiology of congenital dislocation of the hip. *Clin Orthop* 1964; 33:119.

Coleman SS: *Congenital Dysplasia and Dislocation of the Hip*. St Louis, CV Mosby Co, 1978.

Ponseti I: Morphology of the acetabulum in congenital dislocation of the hip. *J Bone Joint Surg Am* 1978; 60:586.

Stanislavjevic S, Mitchell CL: Congenital dysplasia, subluxation, and dislocation of the hip in stillborn and newborn infants. *J Bone Joint Surg Am* 1963; 45:1147.

Diagnosis

Barlow TG: Early diagnosis and treatment of congenital dislocation of the hip. *J Bone Joint Surg Br* 1962; 44:292.

Bialik V, et al: Clinical assessment of hip instability in the newborn by an orthopedic surgeon and a pediatrician. *J Pediatr Orthop* 1986; 6:703.

Davies SJM: Problems in the early recognition of hip dysplasia. *J Bone Joint Surg Br* 1984; 66:479.

Mackenzie IG, Wilson JG: Problems encountered in the early diagnosis and management of congenital dislocation of the hip. *J Bone Joint Surg Br* 1983; 63:38.

Von Rosen S: Diagnosis and treatment of congenital dislocation of the hip joint in the newborn. *J Bone Joint Surg Br* 1962; 44:284.

Treatment

Ishii Y, Ponseti I: Long-term results of closed reduction of complete congenital dislocation of the hip in children under one year of age. *Clin Orthop* 1978; 137:167.

Ponseti I: Non-surgical treatment of congenital dislocation of the hip. *J Bone Joint Surg Am* 1966; 48:1392.

Salter RB: Role of innominate osteotomy in the treatment of congenital dislocation and subluxation of the hip in the older child. *J Bone Joint Surg Am* 1966; 48:1413.

Complications

Cooperman DR, Wallenstein R, Stulberg DS: Postreduction avascular necrosis in congenital dislocation of the hip. *J Bone Joint Surg Am* 1980; 62:247.

Gage JR, Winter RB: Avascular necrosis of the capital femoral epiphysis as a complication of closed reduction of congenital dislocation of the hip. *J Bone Joint Surg Am* 1972; 54:373.

Weiner DS, Hoyt WA, O'Dell HW: Congenital dislocation of the hip: The relationship of pre-manipulation traction and age to avascular necrosis of the femoral head. *J Bone Joint Surg Am* 1978; 59:306.

6

Developmental Disorders of the Hip

The hip joint is susceptible to a number of disease processes during childhood and adolescence. Conditions that result in incongruity of the femoral head and acetabulum at the end of growth subject the individual to premature degenerative joint disease and adult disability. In most instances, prompt diagnosis and early treatment minimize the late sequelae of childhood hip disease. Because early symptoms of hip disorders in children are often vague and nonspecific, a high index of suspicion is necessary to ensure recognition. Infections and trauma around the pelvis are covered in other chapters; in this chapter, transient synovitis of the hip, Legg-Calvé-Perthes disease, slipped capital femoral epiphysis, and chondrolysis will be discussed.

TRANSIENT SYNOVITIS OF THE HIP

In growing children, the most common cause of hip pain not directly related to injury is transient synovitis of the hip, also known as toxic synovitis, transient arthritis, irritable hip syndrome, viral synovitis, phantom hip, and observation hip. The syndrome is characterized by arthritis of brief duration that almost always resolves without long-term sequelae.

The etiology of transient synovitis is unclear. Transient synovitis has long been recognized as an entity distinct from tuberculous and bacterial septic arthritis. Prodromal tonsillar and upper respiratory infections have been implicated by those who thought that septic embolization to the synovium of the hip was responsible for the inflammation, but the absence of systemic signs of sepsis and the results of joint fluid analysis in patients who have undergone aspiration of the hip do not support this contention. Inflammation of viral or allergic origin has been cited as a possible cause, but again there is little supporting evidence for these theories. Trauma has been implicated in some studies, but minor trauma is so common in the age group involved that it is difficult to causally relate transient synovitis to injury. Synovial biopsy, when performed, has shown nonspecific synovitis. It is likely that the clinical syndrome of transient synovitis is the common end result of a number of benign disease processes.

Transient synovitis occurs most often in children between ages 2 and 12 years; the peak incidence is between 6 and 7 years. In most studies, boys have been affected more often than girls. Most patients have symptoms less than 1 week in duration, although occasionally chronic or recurrent hip pain is the presenting complaint. Severely affected children present with hip pain of acute onset, refuse to walk, and have markedly restricted active and passive hip motion. Less severely involved children may complain of thigh or knee pain as well as hip pain, limp while walking, and have restricted hip extension and internal rotation on examination. Low-grade fever may be present, and a history of prodromal upper respiratory tract infection or otitis media may be noted. A history of mild trauma may be present.

Laboratory and roentgenographic findings are nonspecific. Mild leukocytosis and elevated erythrocyte sedimentation rates have been reported in some series but are not consistent findings. Immunologic studies when performed are most often normal. Aspiration of the hip joint may produce clear or blood-tinged fluid that is always sterile. Intracapsular pressure is variable; some investigators have reported elevations of pressure within the hip joint in affected patients, but others have failed to confirm this finding.

Hip roentgenograms are usually normal. Distortion of the soft tissue planes around the hip and capsular distension have been reported in some studies, but these findings may be artifacts of positioning. Slight widening of the joint space has been reported in some patients who have undergone arthrography. This may represent proliferation of chondrocytes at the surface of the joint in response to synovitis. Radioisotope bone scans usually show diffuse mild increase in uptake in the affected hip consistent with joint inflammation. Magnetic resonance imaging to date has not shown abnormalities of subchondral bone or surrounding soft tissues, but experience with this technique is limited.

The relationship of transient synovitis to Legg-Calvé-Perthes disease is unclear. Both conditions may produce similar acute clinical syndromes, but few patients with transient synovitis subsequently develop radiologic evidence of Legg-Calvé-Perthes disease. The incidence of Perthes disease following transient synovitis is reported as between 2% and 6%; children with recurrent synovitis appear more at risk for the development of avascular necrosis.

Accurate diagnosis is the most important step in the treatment of transient synovitis. Hospitalization is justified if symptoms are acute and if fever is present. Blood counts, sedimentation rates, and hip roentgenograms should be obtained. Infection is unlikely in the absence of fever and leukocytes, but aspiration of the hip joint should be performed if there is any suggestion of septic arthritis. If cloudy joint fluid with a white blood cell count greater than 100,000 cells/cu mm is obtained or if bacteria are present on Gram stain, infectious arthritis must be assumed to be present, and surgical drainage is mandatory.

In the absence of sepsis, patients with presumed transient synovitis should be placed on bed rest. Most patients can be managed at home, but if pain and muscle spasm are severe, hospitalization may be necessary. In such cases, light skin traction in hip flexion relieves pain and muscle spasm. Most children with synovitis recover within 3 to 5 days. After symptoms have subsided, a child may be permitted to resume full activity gradually. Most patients are back at school within 2 weeks. There is little evidence that transient synovitis is related to subsequent femoral head deformity or late degenerative joint disease.

Prolonged pain or muscle spasm makes a diagnosis of transient synovitis less likely. Early Legg-Calvé-Perthes disease or acute monarthric rheumatoid arthritis must be considered if synovitis persists. Follow-up roentgenograms obtained 6 to 8 weeks after the episode may be indicated in children with severe or prolonged symptoms to exclude subsequent avascular necrosis.

LEGG-CALVÉ-PERTHES DISEASE

In the early part of this century, Arthur T. Legg in the United States, Georg Perthes in Germany, and Jacques Calvé in France separately described a form of arthritis of the hip in children that was clinically and radiologically distinct from juvenile tuberculous arthritis. According to Calvé, affected patients presented with transitory arthritis and radiologic signs of fragmentation of the secondary ossification center of the femoral head. In contrast to tuberculous arthritis, suppuration and abscess formation around the hip joint were not present, and systemic signs of tuberculosis were absent. The duration of symptoms was short, although severe, permanent alterations in the femoral head often developed.

Legg-Calvé-Perthes disease has been extensively studied since its original description, and although many of the changes seen are better understood now, there remains a great deal of controversy regarding etiology, natural history, and treatment. The radiologic findings reflect a temporary interruption of blood flow to the proximal femoral epiphyseal region, with resultant necrosis, collapse, and regeneration of bone in the secondary ossification center. The extent of involvement of the epiphysis varies widely, as does the severity of both acute and chronic symptoms. The precise etiology of the disease was unclear to Calvé in 1910 and remains uncertain today. The clinical symptoms and signs and roentgenographic findings associated with Legg-Calvé-Perthes disease may well be the result of a number of pathologic processes that cause interruption of blood supply to the femoral head in the growing child.

Pathophysiology

Normal development of the proximal femur is the result of coordinated growth and remodeling at several sites. The femoral neck elongates by endochondral growth at the proximal physis. Appositional bone growth around the neck increases its diameter. Enlargement of the femoral head occurs by endochondral bone formation around the periphery of the femoral head. Greater trochanteric enlargement occurs by both endochondral ossification at the base of the trochanter and by appositional growth at its surface.

The medial femoral circumflex artery is the principal vessel of the anastomotic network that supplies the femoral head and neck; lesser contributions come from the lateral femoral circumflex artery and, at times, from the artery of the ligamentum teres femoris. Most of the blood supply of the active regions of the proximal femoral growth plate and the secondary ossification center of the proximal epiphysis is derived from branches of the medial and lateral femoral circumflex arteries, which penetrate the capsule of the hip at the base of the femoral neck and ascend along the surface of the femoral neck to form a second ring at the base of the articular surface of the femoral head.

The articular and growth cartilage of the femoral head receives nourishment by diffusion from both the synovial fluid of the hip joint and the underlying endochondral bone of the secondary ossification center of the epiphysis. The superficial layers of cartilage cells, including the zone of cell proliferation, are principally dependent on joint fluid. Deeper within the growth plate of the epiphysis, in the zones of cell hypertrophy and provisional calcification of the chondroid matrix, diffusion from the vessels that supply the secondary ossification center becomes more important.

The zone of provisional calcification of the proximal femoral growth plate is a dividing line between blood flow in the femoral head and neck. Distal to this zone, blood supply is provided by metaphyseal vessels of the femoral neck. Proximal to it, blood flow depends on the ring of vessels at the base of the femoral head. Prior to skeletal maturity, there is little vascular communication across the physis between the proximal femoral metaphysis and the secondary ossification center of the femoral head. The germinal layer of the proximal femoral physis receives its blood supply from the same anastomotic network that supplies the proximal femoral secondary ossification center. Occlusion of major portions of this network may result in necrosis of portions of both the secondary ossification center and the proximal femoral physis.

There are few gross specimens available for study of the sequence of events in Legg-Calvé-Perthes disease, and much of the available information is based on experimental animal models or biopsy specimens obtained at surgery. These studies indicate that if a section of the femoral head is deprived of blood flow for a sufficient period of time, the cells within it die. When circulation is reestablished, healing occurs through a gradual process of substitution of new bone for old bone. Immediately after infarct, the osteocytes within the lacunae of trabecular bone in the affected region undergo necrosis.

When circulation is reestablished, vascular ingrowth occurs and primitive granulation tissue lines the dead trabecular bone. Osteoblastic cells differentiate from this tissue, and osteoid is laid down on top of dead trabeculae. Osteoclastic resorption of necrotic bone occurs, and at the termination of the healing process, the bony architecture of the secondary ossification center is restored.

Experimental studies by Salter and others suggest that in patients with infarction of significant portions of the femoral epiphysis, subchondral fracture within the epiphysis may occur during the process of revascularization of the femoral head. When subchondral fracture complicates avascular necrosis, the architecture of the secondary ossification center is altered, and a second infarct may occur as the microfracture lines pass through provisional vessels. The area beneath the subchondral fracture is weakened and subject to deformation as healing occurs.

Etiology and Incidence

The precise etiology of Legg-Calvé-Perthes disease is unknown. Metabolic bone diseases, thrombotic vascular insults, trauma, infection, and transient synovitis have all been implicated. Any one of these causes may be responsible for avascular necrosis in a particular patient, but in most instances no underlying abnormality can be identified. Experimental animal studies have suggested that increases in intracapsular pressure may result in tamponade of vessels that supply the proximal femoral epiphysis, but the results have not been consistently reproducible. Recent studies suggest that in most patients with Legg-Calvé-Perthes disease, it is doubtful that intracapsular pressures are high enough for a long enough period to produce avascular necrosis. Although the incidence of avascular necrosis in patients with transient synovitis is low, it rises in patients with recurrent synovitis, and it may well be that recurrent elevations of intracapsular pressure are a factor in some patients with Legg-Calvé-Perthes disease.

Trauma has been implicated in some patients with Legg-Calvé-Perthes disease. Avascular necrosis could theoretically be produced by direct damage to femoral vessels or by synovitis secondary to damage to the hip capsule. In epidemiologic studies from Great Britain and New England, less than 20% of affected patients reported a clear episode of antecedent trauma, suggesting that in most patients trauma plays a minor role in the production of avascular necrosis.

There is no clear genetic pattern in Legg-Calvé-Perthes disease, although retarded growth and delayed skeletal maturation have been statistically significant findings in some epidemiologic studies. Boys are affected four to five times as often as girls. Children between ages 2 and 13 years are at risk, with the risk peaking at age 6 to 7 years. The proportion of affected children with bilateral disease is estimated at 12% to 20%. An increased familial incidence has been reported by some investigators, but this has not been confirmed in larger incidence surveys. There is little evidence at present to suggest a multifactorial pattern of inheritance in Legg-Calvé-Perthes disease.

Symptoms and Signs

Clinical findings in Legg-Calvé-Perthes disease are quite variable. Clinical findings and radiographic changes often correlate poorly. Some children with roentgenographic signs of significant head involvement of long duration have few symptoms at initial evaluation, while others have symptoms and signs of acute inflammation of the hip joint with little roentgenographic evidence of change within the femoral head. Salter and Thompson have postulated that the initial episode of infarction of the femoral head is asymptomatic. In their opinion, it is the subchondral fracture and resulting synovitis that initiate symptoms.

In the early stages of the disease, children may complain of hip pain and refuse to walk. A limp and restriction of voluntary motion are often present. Adductor and iliopsoas spasm are frequently present, and passive motion may be painful and limited. Tenderness may be present over the anterior groin and adductor muscles. These findings are identical to those seen in children with transient synovitis. Later in the disease process, after the acute synovitis has subsided, vague thigh and knee pain may be present. Medial rotation and abduction of the affected hip are often restricted, and hip flexion contracture may be present. A positive Trendelenburg sign, reflecting weakness of the hip abductor muscles on the affected side, is common.

In patients with long-standing disease and significant damage to the femoral head, passive abduction and rotation may be markedly restricted. Leg-length inequality secondary to damage to the proximal femoral growth plate may be present. Relative overgrowth of the greater trochanter is common in patients with physeal damage, and the trochanter may be quite prominent. A positive Trendelenburg sign and limp reflecting abductor weakness are common findings in such cases. Often, however, clinical symptoms are much less severe than hip roentgenograms might suggest. Patients with Legg-Calvé-Perthes disease often have few complaints in adolescence and early adult life regardless of the radiographic appearance of their hips. Some patients may complain of hip pain or fatigue after exercise, but most function well despite severe residual deformity.

Radiologic Findings

The changes on the hip roentgenogram in Legg-Calvé-Perthes disease reflect the histologic events that occur after infarction (Fig 6–1). The disease process has been divided into stages on the basis of radiologic findings, and attempts have been made to correlate the degree of involvement and stage of healing with the ultimate radiologic outcome. Such characterization is difficult, and variability between observers is high. Arthrography, radioisotope bone scanning, and more recently magnetic resonace imaging have improved imaging reliability and permitted more careful selection of patients for treatment.

Few changes are apparent on roentgenograms obtained in the first few weeks after the onset of Legg-Calvé-Perthes disease. The zone of cartilage cell proliferation that lies below the articular surface of the proximal femoral epiphysis is not seriously affected by underlying infarction since most of its nutrient supply is derived from synovial fluid. The preliminary phases of endochondral growth continue in the femoral head even though provisional calcification does not occur. For this reason, the secondary ossification center of the infarcted femoral head may appear smaller than on the contralateral normal side. This relative difference in size may be one of the earliest radiologic changes of Legg-Calvé-Perthes disease. Arthrographic studies have suggested that joint-space thickening may occur as superficial chondrocytes proliferate in response to chronic synovitis.

Later in the disease process, the affected secondary ossification center may appear more radiodense than the normal side. Mild disuse osteopenia may develop in the surrounding pelvic bones as a re-

sult of restriction of activity. No bone resorption occurs in the avascular secondary ossification center, and the area may be relatively radiodense. Precipitation of calcium salts in the dead marrow spaces between trabeculae, subchondral fracture, and impaction of bone within the secondary ossification center of the femoral head further increase the density of the epiphysis.

When new vessels invade the secondary ossification center from the periphery of the head, healing begins. With the simultaneous resorption of old bone and deposition of new bone, the secondary ossification center may take on a fragmented appearance. Healing occurs over many months; on standard anteroposterior and lateral x-ray films, healing zones may be superimposed on vascular necrotic areas. This accounts for much of the variation seen in the healing phases of Legg-Calvé-Perthes disease.

Irregularity in the growth plate below the secondary ossification center may become evident in the early healing phases. This is a reflection of damage to the germinal layers of the physis, which depend on diffusion from the proximal epiphysis for nutrition. At times, this irregularity is focal and of little significance; at other times, large portions of the growth plate may be irreversibly damaged. The radiolucent metaphyseal "cyst" occasionally seen in Legg-Calvé-Perthes disease is a manifestation of such physeal damage.

The final radiologic picture in Legg-Calvé-Perthes disease depends on the degree of initial infarction, the extent of subchondral fracture, and the effects of treatment. Patients with initial infarction of only a small portion of the epiphysis, or in whom secondary subchondral fracture involves less than half of the epiphysis, may show significant healing with little or no residual deformity within 12 to 18 months of infarction.

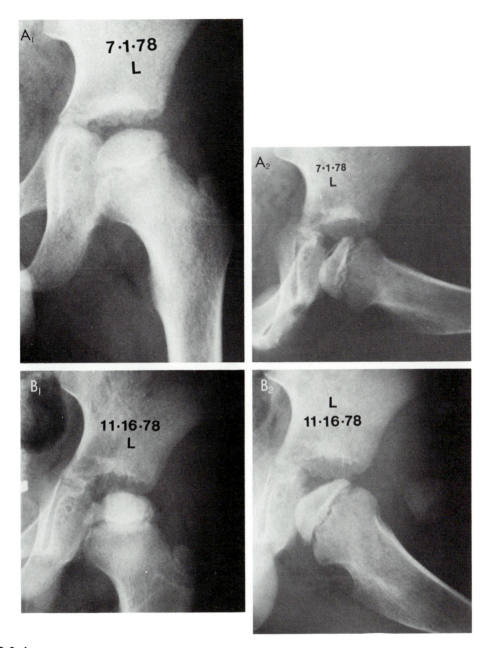

FIG 6–1.
Radiologic evolution of Legg-Calvé-Perthes disease. **A₁,** anteroposterior view of left hip in a 7-year-old boy with hip pain of 4 weeks' duration. No abnormality is obvious. **A₂,** frog-leg lateral view demonstrates area of microfracture and compaction of the anterolateral portion of the secondary ossification center of the proximal femur. Treatment with an abduction brace was started. **B₁,** 4 months later, increased radiodensity is noted in the infarcted segment. **B₂,** slight collapse of the infarcted area has occurred, but no further extension into the remainder of the epiphysis has taken place. *(Continued.)*

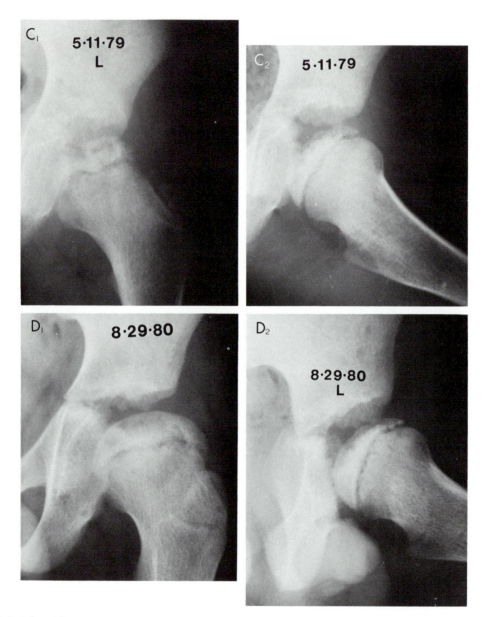

FIG 6–1 (cont.).

C₁, healing is progressing by resorption of dead bone and replacement with new osteoid through a process called "creeping substitution." Mild involvement of the lateral portions of the growth plate may be present. **C₂,** although the femoral neck is widened, the spherical contour of the femoral head has been preserved. Treatment was discontinued 4 months later. **D₁,** healing is nearly complete 2 years after infarction. **D₂,** contour of the femoral head is preserved, and the hip joint is congruent. The long-term prognosis for this hip is excellent.

In patients with more extensive infarction and in whom secondary fracture involves more than half of the secondary ossification center, healing is much less predictable. The necrotic epiphysis is vulnerable to deformation from forces across the hip joint, and persistent spasm of hip musculature may result in extrusion of portions of the head beyond the confines of the acetabulum. As healing progresses, the femoral head may become irregular and mushroom-shaped, with large extra-articular prominences that restrict motion. Spherical enlargement of the femoral head, termed *coxa magna*, develops presumably from stimulation of the germinal layers of the epiphysis by increased vascularity in the synovial tissue lining the joint capsule. If large areas of the growth plate in the femoral neck have been damaged, growth of the proximal femur may be seriously affected, with consequent shortening and varus deformity of the femoral neck (Fig 6–2). As previously mentioned, greater trochanteric overgrowth may be pronounced.

Radioisotope imaging techniques are useful in identifying infarction early in the course of the disease process, before secondary radiographic changes have developed. In addition, scans are sometimes helpful in determining the extent of epiphyseal infarction. Decreased uptake within a suspect epiphysis indicates avascularity; isotope uptake increases during healing phases. The resolution of the bone scan is limited to about 0.5 cm, and it suffers from the same two-dimensional handicap as the standard roentgenogram. The development of coincident scanning techniques using specific radiopharmaceutical agents to trace revascularization and ossification within the epiphysis may be useful in the near future, but at present radioisotope scanning is most helpful in the early diagnosis of infarction in chil-

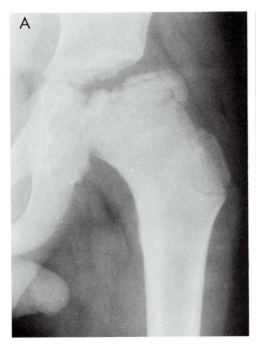

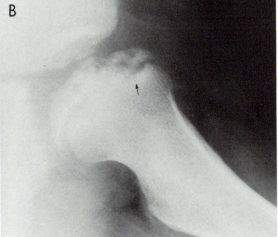

FIG 6–2.
A, Legg-Calvé-Perthes disease with poor prognosis. The entire epiphysis is involved, and the femoral head appears extruded laterally on the anteroposterior roentgenograms. **B,** involvement of the anterolateral corner of the growth plate *(arrow)* is obvious. The femoral head is flattened, and the hip joint is not congruent. Treatment is likely to fail, and premature arthritis is likely.

dren with symptoms suggestive of Legg-Calvé-Perthes disease.

Magnetic resonance scanning has recently been demonstrated to be of significant value in early diagnosis and treatment planning in avascular necrosis. Although the cortical bone of the femur and acetabulum produce very weak signals in magnetic resonance scanning, strongly positive images are generated by the cancellous bone of the normal proximal femoral metaphysis, the acetabulum, and the secondary ossification center of the proximal femoral epiphysis. This strong signal is lost at the time of infarction and permits early identification of the area of infarction of the proximal femur. Because image reconstruction is possible in transverse, frontal, and sagittal planes, a more clear picture of the extent of infarction can be obtained than possible with conventional radiography or with isotope scanning techniques. In addition, the cartilage surfaces of the hip are well imaged, permitting estimation of congruency and coverage previously possible only through invasive techniques such as hip arthrography (Fig 6–3). No ionizing radiation exposure is involved, and image quality is improving dramatically as experience with the technique grows.

Diagnosis and Treatment

A number of disease processes produce symptoms, signs, and laboratory findings similar to those of acute Legg-Calvé-Perthes disease. If the characteristic radiologic signs of epiphyseal collapse and fragmentation are present, a diagnosis can be easily established. Most often, however, initial roentgenograms are not diagnostic, and it may be difficult to separate children who will eventually develop Legg-Calvé-Perthes disease from children with other causes of hip pain.

Septic arthritis and proximal femoral osteomyelitis must be considered in the differential diagnosis when fever, leukocytosis, and increased erythrocyte sedimentation rates are present. Roentgenograms may be normal, and bone scanning may not show focal changes in uptake necessary for diagnosis. Aspiration of the hip joint is essential if infection is suspected.

Proximal femoral fracture and acute or chronic slippage of the proximal femoral epiphysis may produce signs and symptoms that mimic avascular necrosis. Roentgenograms usually can be used to separate these diseases from Legg-Calvé-Perthes disease.

Signs and symptoms in acute Legg-

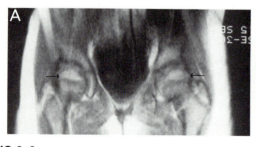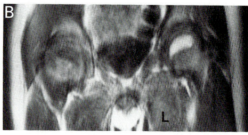

FIG 6–3.
Magnetic resonance scans of the pelvis and hip joints. **A,** normal hips in a 7-year-old girl. Note the strong signal from the secondary ossification centers of the proximal femurs *(arrows).* The articular surfaces of the hip joints are clearly visible. **B,** Legg-Calvé-Perthe's disease of the right hip. Normal signal intensity is present on the left side, but there is little or no signal from the right proximal femur.

Calvé-Perthes disease and transient synovitis are identical. Hip and groin pain, adductor muscle spasm, tenderness around the hip joint, and restriction of motion are present in both conditions. Mild leukocytosis and increased sedimentation rates are common. Roentgenograms in both instances may be normal. Bone scanning and magnetic resonance imaging are helpful in establishing a diagnosis in such cases. If focal decrease in radioisotope uptake is found within the epiphysis, or if the normally strong magnetic resonance signal generated by the secondary ossification center of the proximal femur is absent, a tentative diagnosis of avascular necrosis is warranted. If the bone scan or magnetic resonance scan is normal, circulation to the head was intact at least at the time of scanning, and a diagnosis of transient synovitis is more likely. Presently available evidence is not sufficient to permit the assumption that a child with synovitis and a normal radioisotope or magnetic resonance scan will not subsequently develop infarction, however. Although the incidence of avascular necrosis following one episode of transient synovitis is low, radiologic follow-up is advisable 6 to 8 weeks after the acute episode subsides.

Initial treatment of a patient with suspected acute Legg-Calvé-Perthes disease entails hospitalization for evaluation and planning. Bed rest and skin traction in balanced suspension usually relieve spasm and tenderness around the hip joint while diagnostic studies are under way. Traction with the hip in extension increases pressure on the capsular vessel and should be avoided; mild hip flexion is a more comfortable and safer position. When acute symptoms have subsided, good quality anteroposterior, lateral, and abduction views of the affected hip should be made. If these are normal and bone scanning or magnetic resonance im-

aging shows no abnormalities, a diagnosis of transient synovitis is more likely than Legg-Calvé-Perthes disease, and the child may be discharged.

If a diagnosis of Legg-Calvé-Perthes disease is established, consideration must be given to long-term treatment after the initial synovitis has subsided. Selection of patients for treatment is complicated by evidence that not all patients with Legg-Calvé-Perthes disease do poorly without treatment and that treatment does not affect the outcome in other patients. As in congenital hip disease, patients with a poor radiologic result often function quite well for much of their young adult life. Most authorities agree, however, that patients with significant head deformity eventually will develop degenerative arthritis. Treatment of children with Legg-Calvé-Perthes disease is based on the following premises:

1. Some children with avascular necrosis will develop significant deformity of the femoral head.
2. Patients with femoral head deformity will develop premature degenerative arthritis.
3. Appropriate treatment can preserve the contour of the femoral head and delay or prevent degenerative arthritis.

There appears to be a relationship between the extent of head involvement on radiologic examination early in avascular necrosis and ultimate radiologic outcome. Catterall, Salter, Thompson, and others have divided patients into prognostic groups based on the extent of head involvement and the apparent phase of healing on roentgenograms. In general, patients with minimal head involvement do well without treatment, and patients with whole head involvement often develop significant deformity in spite of treatment. Patients with intermediate degrees of involvement in early phases of healing benefit most from treatment; permanent deformity is likely to develop in these children unless the femoral head is protected while reossification occurs.

Factors other than extent of involvement have been identified in the outcome of affected patients. Most investigators have concluded that patients under the age of 5 or 6 years at the time of disease onset generally, but not always, do well regardless of extent of involvement or nature of treatment. Patients older than 10 years at the time of infarction often do poorly in spite of treatment. Patients with loss of containment of the femoral head by the acetabulum are at higher risk for development of subsequent deformity than patients in whom the femoral head is well contained. Finally, Salter and Thompson have indicated that patients with persistent restriction of hip motion are at significant risk for hip subluxation and deformity.

Current treatment of Legg-Calvé-Perthes disease is based on relief of muscle spasm, restoration of motion around the hip, and containment of the femoral head within the acetabulum during the revascularization and reossification stages in patients with high risks for deformity. In these patients, spasm in the iliopsoas and adductor muscles tends to compress and displace the femoral head anteriorly and laterally, uncovering vulnerable areas of the proximal epiphysis. Unprotected weight bearing may deform the epiphysis and produce an irregular femoral head.

In the past, prolonged periods of bed rest or spica cast immobilization were used in the treatment of avascular necrosis. Many children were hospitalized for 1 to 3 years while healing occurred. This is no longer standard. Bed rest and traction for 1 to 4 weeks early in the course of the disease are appropriate to relieve spasm and permit accurate assessment, but after the acute phase, other methods of treatment are now usually employed.

Most authorities believe that if the femoral head can be well centered within the acetabulum, the danger of eventual deformity can be minimized. In effect, the acetabulum is used as a mold for the healing femoral head. Both operative and nonoperative techniques are employed; the choice of a particular method depends on the extent of femoral head involvement, the experience of the physician in charge, and the preferences of the patient and his or her parents. If abduction roentgenograms indicate that the femoral head can be centered in the acetabulum, abduction bracing may be employed. A variety of braces have been designed; all attempt to hold the hip in abduction during the weight-bearing phases of gait. In a cooperative patient, excellent results can be obtained with brace treatment. However, there are some disadvantages to bracing. Twelve to 18 months of brace use may be necessary. Although the patients are independent in most orthoses, the braces are awkward and inconvenient. Compliance is often difficult to monitor and enforce.

Operative management of Legg-Calvé-Perthes disease is indicated when brace treatment is not feasible or when coverage of the femoral head in abduction is not possible. Most investigators feel that a spherical femoral head is a prerequisite for surgical treatment; hip arthrography may be necessary to document this. If significant femoral head deformity exists, the results of surgical attempts at containment are mixed.

Both femoral and pelvic osteotomies are employed in the surgical treatment of Legg-Calvé-Perthes disease. At times, both procedures may be necessary to achieve satisfactory coverage of the hip. The choice of a particular technique depends on the characteristics of the particular patient and the experience of the surgeon. Surgical treatment has the advantages of directly covering the femoral head. Unprotected weight bearing may be permitted when the pelvic or femoral osteotomies have healed, usually within 12 weeks of surgery. The disadvantages of surgery include the magnitude of the procedure itself, the need for a second operative procedure to remove internal fixation devices, and the risks attendant on general anesthesia and possible blood transfusion.

SLIPPED CAPITAL FEMORAL EPIPHYSIS

Pathophysiology

The first description of the deformity produced by posterior displacement of the proximal femoral epiphysis on the femoral neck is credited to Ambroise Paré in 1572. The disorder, also called epiphysiolysis, has been extensively studied since that time. The incidence, natural history, effects of treatment, and complications have been carefully documented. To date, however, the etiology of the disease remains unclear.

In most patients with slipped capital femoral epiphysis, the femoral head displaces posteriorly and inferiorly with respect to the femoral head. Slip occurs through what would normally be the zones of cartilage cell hypertrophy and provisional calcification. Examination of core biopsy specimens obtained at the time of surgical treatment of patients with varying degrees of slip shows disorganization of the growth plate. The orderly sequence of cell columnation, matrix production, provisional calcification, and metaphyseal remodeling is disrupted. Cartilage columns in the growth plate are irregular, and islands of cartilage are pres-

ent within the metaphysis. The fibrous tissue content of the plate is increased, and endochondral ossification appears to occur in a random fashion.

From studies on patients with bilateral disease, growth plate abnormality apparently precedes slippage. Superimposition of acute trauma in some patients or the chronic stresses of weight bearing in others may initiate displacement. Once slippage has begun, it will continue until the growth plate is stabilized by either natural or surgical closure.

Deformity develops slowly in patients with chronic slip. As the slip progresses, bone resorption occurs at the anterosuperior border of the femoral neck, and bone deposition occurs in the posteroinferior corner. If growth ceases or the slip is stabilized before significant displacement occurs, minimal deformity and restriction of motion result. If slippage continues, however, grotesque proximal femoral deformity may develop. Limitation of motion and early degenerative arthritis follow.

Acute trauma may initiate displacement in some patients with a growth plate abnormality prior to the slip or may cause further sudden displacement in patients with a history of chronic slippage. Slipped capital femoral epiphysis is, however, clinically and pathologically distinct from type I physeal fracture of the proximal femoral growth plate. There are a number of significant differences between the two entities. In acute fracture, failure occurs through the hypertrophic zones of a normal growth plate; preexistent abnormalities of the growth plate occur in patients with slipped capital femoral epiphysis. Fracture of the proximal femoral physis is much less common than slipping of the epiphysis and is usually the result of violent trauma; the traumatic episode that precedes acute slippage is usually minimal. Although many patients with slipping of the capital femoral epiphysis report a recent history of injury, the injury is usually much less severe than that which causes physeal fracture. Finally, there is a high incidence of subsequent avascular necrosis of the secondary ossification center as a result of damage to the network of vessels that surround the femoral head in patients with type I femoral neck fractures. Avascular necrosis is uncommon even in severe slips unless secondary damage occurs during treatment.

Etiology

The etiology of slipped capital femoral epiphysis is unclear. Most investigators believe that although trauma plays a role in the progression of deformity, it is not solely responsible for the pathologic changes found in the growth plate. The disorder can be produced experimentally in laboratory animals by the administration of chemical compounds that interfere with collagen cross-linkage; other investigators have proposed that slipped capital femoral epiphysis is due in part to defective chondroid matrix production. In biopsy specimens obtained at the time of surgical fixation of the physis in a large number of patients with slipped capital femoral epiphysis, Agamanolis, Weiner, and Lloyd in 1985 reported gross distortion of the architecture, collagen deficiency, and chondrocyte degeneration and death in the proliferative and hypertrophic zones of the growth plate and suggested that abnormalities of chondrocyte metabolism, perhaps hormonally induced, might be responsible for alterations in the strength of the growth plate.

Endocrine abnormalities of several types have been implicated in the etiology of slipped capital femoral epiphysis. Many patients are obese and appear clinically to have delayed sexual maturation. Skeletal age is often below chronological age. No clear hormonal abnormalities have been identified, however.

Incidence

The precise incidence of slipped capital femoral epiphysis is not known. Epidemiologic studies by Kelsey and Southwick in Connecticut indicate that approximately 10 of 100,000 adolescents between ages 8 and 17 years are hospitalized yearly for treatment of slips. Most studies indicate that boys are affected two to three times as often as girls. An age range of 10 to 17 years with a peak incidence at age 13 to 14 years is commonly reported for boys. Girls are at risk between ages 8 and 15 years, with a peak incidence at about 11 years.

Many studies have reported a higher frequency of slipped capital femoral epiphysis in blacks. It is not clear whether this represents a true increase in risk or whether it is the result of sampling bias. Complications of slippage appear to be more common in blacks. Genetic factors may be involved in some patients. A 5% familial incidence has been found by some investigators, and there are several reports of slipped capital femoral epiphyses in identical twins. This has led to the hypothesis that the condition may be transmitted as an autosomal dominant trait with variable penetrance, but this has not been established to date.

Trauma appears to be a factor in the initiation or propagation of displacement in one fourth to one half of patients. Obesity is reported in as many as 75% of patients in some series. Once growth plate disorganization occurs, the chronic stresses imposed on the femoral neck by obesity may initiate and perpetuate displacement until the growth plate is stabilized by skeletal maturation or surgical intervention. Bilateral disease occurs in about 25% of cases. Often slip may begin and progress without symptoms in the second hip. Young patients, black patients, and obese patients are at special risk for development of bilateral disease.

Clinical Findings

Symptoms in patients with slipped capital femoral epiphysis are quite variable. Patients with slowly progressive chronic slip often, but not always, complain of leg pain; it may be vague and difficult to localize. Many have hip pain, but others experience aching thigh and knee pain. Hip pain is more common in patients with acute traumatic slip and in patients in whom acute slip is superimposed on chronic slip.

Slippage may also occur without hip or thigh pain. Some researchers estimate the incidence of silent slip to be as high as 20%. Asymptomatic slip is often seen in children with bilateral involvement; radiologic signs of displacement of the capital femoral epiphysis of the contralateral hip may develop without pain during or after treatment of the first hip.

The nonspecific nature of complaints in many patients with slipped capital femoral epiphysis often leads to prolonged delay in diagnosis. Too frequently patients with early slips are assumed to have muscle strains, ligament sprains, Osgood-Schlatter disease, or growing pains. The opportunity for early treatment before significant deformity occurs is often lost.

Limitation of active and passive motion is a constant finding in slipped capital femoral epiphysis. Medial rotation of the hip joint is restricted, and at rest the limb usually lies in a laterally rotated position. Flexion of the hip is accompanied by further lateral rotation of the limb. Full flexion and extension may be impossible in patients with more than minimal degrees of slip; abduction of the hip may be markedly restricted by impingement of the femoral neck upon the acetabulum.

Most patients have a limp, and the Trendelenburg test result is often positive. Leg-length inequality of 1 to 3 cm may be present.

Tenderness over the involved hip and in the groin on the involved side is present more often in patients with acute slips than chronic slips. Spasm of the adductor muscles of the involved leg is usually present in patients with acute slip. Patients with chronic slips may have no tenderness on palpation around the hip joint.

Radiologic Findings

The radiologic changes in patients with slipped capital femoral epiphysis reflect the extent of femoral head displacement, the duration of the disease, and the effects of remodeling on the contour of the femoral head and neck (Fig 6–4). Good quality anteroposterior and frog-leg lateral roentgenograms are essential for proper evaluation; obesity and restriction of motion may make them difficult to obtain. Inadequate roentgenograms should not be accepted, since early slips may be missed. Both hips should be studied since 20% to 25% of cases are bilateral.

Irregularity and widening of the growth plate of the proximal femur is the earliest radiologic change in epiphysiolysis. It is a subtle finding and is most often seen in children who develop contralateral disease while under treatment for unilateral slips. Usually displacement of the femoral head has already occurred at the time of diagnosis. In acute slips, the contours of the femoral neck and head are sharp and easily defined. In chronic slips, remodeling occurs simultaneously with displacement, and outlines may be blunted (Fig 6–5).

A number of methods have been devised to grade the degree of slip. For diagnostic purposes, an adequate assessment of displacement can be obtained

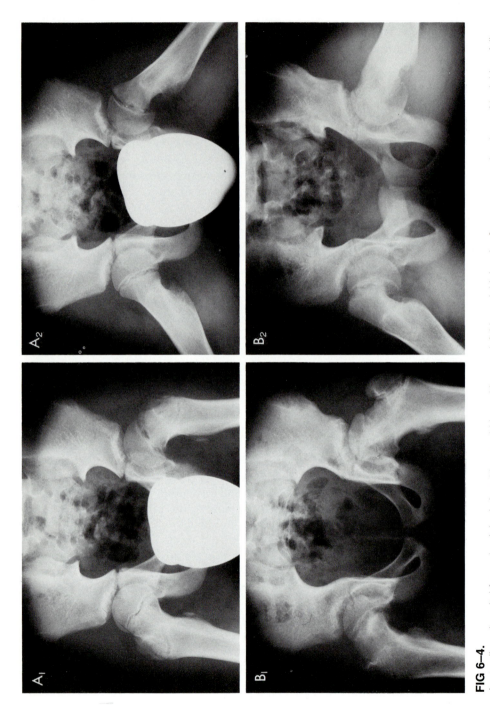

FIG 6–4.

Acute slipped capital femoral epiphysis in a 10-year-old boy with acute left hip and thigh pain. **A₁,** anteroposterior views of both hips. A line drawn along the superior surface of the femoral head, as seen on the right side, should intersect a corner of the femoral head. The left femoral head has slipped inferiorly. **A₂,** frog-leg lateral roentgenograms of both hips demonstrate the mild displacement of the left femoral head more clearly. There is no evidence of remodeling in this acute slip. **B₁,** the left hip was treated by open epiphysiodesis; the bone graft placed across the growth plate is evident and the left growth plate has closed. At this time, 2 years after the onset of left hip pain, the patient presented with slight right hip pain of 3 months' duration. **B₂,** lateral roentgenograms demonstrate moderate to severe slip of the right femoral head.

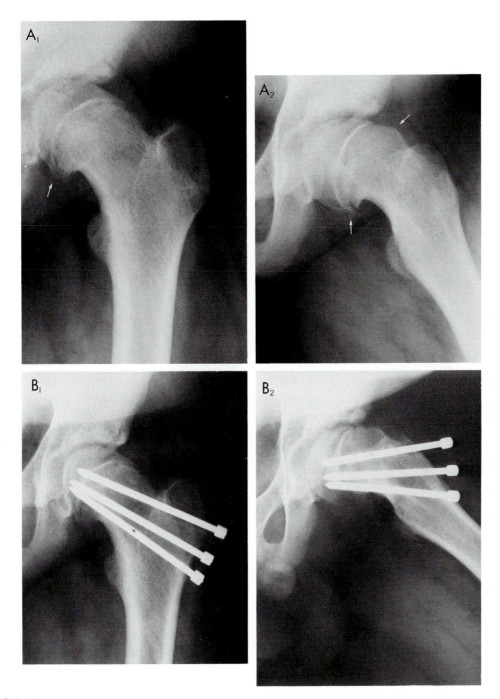

FIG 6–5.
Chronic slipped capital femoral epiphysis. **A₁, A₂,** anterior and lateral roentgenograms of the left hip in a 14-year-old boy with hip pain of 6 months' duration. Remodeling changes are present at the inferior and posterior portions of the growth plate, and resorption of the anterior superior corner of the proximal femoral metaphysis is occurring. **B₁, B₂,** patient was treated by in situ fixation with three pins, which will be removed after growth plate closure.

from the lateral roentgenogram. Displacement of less than one third the diameter of the femoral neck is termed "minimal slip"; displacement between one third and one half, "moderate slip"; and displacement greater than one half, "severe slip." The remodeling that occurs in chronic slips may make judgment of the degree of slip quite difficult. The angular relationship of the epiphysis to the femoral neck on the anteroposterior and lateral roentgenogram are more precise measurements of the degree of slip useful when surgical intervention is planned.

Treatment

Once slip of the femoral head on the femoral neck has begun, it will continue until the growth plate is stabilized either by skeletal maturation or by surgical intervention. Treatment should be started immediately after diagnosis to prevent further slip from occurring; patients with minimal slips have much better long-term results than patients with severe slips. Significant residual displacement at the termination of growth limits function and predisposes the patient to early degenerative arthritis.

Prevention of further slip is the basic goal of treatment; nonoperative methods such as bed rest or crutch walking do not reliably achieve this goal and are not recommended. Immobilization in a spica cast has been used in a few centers for treatment, but most investigators believe that the period required for plate closure in patients treated this way is excessive.

Surgical stabilization is the treatment of choice for patients with slipped capital femoral epiphysis. A variety of techniques are employed with the common goals of preventing further slip by closure of the growth plate. Patients with mild and moderate chronic slips do well with in situ stabilization, without efforts to realign the femoral head and neck. Plate

closure can be obtained most rapidly by open grafting of bone across the physis. Alternatively, stabilization may be accomplished by transfixing the plate with surgical pins. In either case, unprotected weight bearing must be delayed until radiologic evidence of physeal closure is present.

More severe slips limit function and predispose to early degenerative arthritis. Surgical attempts to realign the femoral head are justified. To achieve this, osteotomies performed at the level of the femoral neck or in the intertrochanteric and subtrochanteric regions have been developed. These are technically demanding procedures with complication rates higher than those experienced with stabilization in situ. Chondrolysis, an inflammatory disease of the hip joint characterized by pain, restriction of hip motion, and loss of joint space, and avascular necrosis of the femoral head may occur after any procedure in patients with slipped capital femoral epiphysis, but they are more common in patients who have undergone extensive realignment osteotomies or manipulative reductions for treatment of severe slips. In general, the results of realignment are never as good as those obtained with in situ fixation after early diagnosis of minimal slip.

Premature degenerative arthritis can be expected to occur in many patients with moderate to severe slips, even after successful surgical stabilization of the growth plate. Joint incongruity and alterations in force transmission across the hip predictably result in joint degeneration during adult life. Early diagnosis and treatment minimize but do not eliminate this complication.

Avascular necrosis of the femoral head may complicate slipped capital femoral epiphysis if the vessels that supply the secondary ossification center are damaged during treatment. Manipulative closed reduction, open reduction, and osteotomies performed through the femoral neck all carry the risk of producing avascular necrosis. The outcome is usually poor.

Limitation of motion sometimes follows in situ fixation of moderate to severe slips. Surgical realignment of the proximal femur is sometimes indicated if disability is severe.

CHONDROLYSIS

Chondrolysis, sometimes called acute cartilage necrosis, is a a poorly understood process characterized by progressive loss of articular cartilage on both sides of the hip joint. Most often chondrolysis occurs as a complication of slipped capital femoral epiphysis, but it may also develop in previously normal individuals with no clinical or radiographic signs of slip. In both instances, the condition is characterized by pain and limitation of motion, often terminating in fibrous ankylosis of the hip joint.

The reported incidence of chondrolysis in patients with slipped capital femoral epiphysis varies from 1% to almost 30% in follow-up studies of large series. Dark-skinned races appear to be at greater risk, although this has not been firmly established. Females may be at higher risk than males. No consistent immunologic abnormalities have been noted in affected patients. It appears that at least some cases of chondrolysis have a mechanical etiology; the condition occurs more frequently in those cases of slipped capital femoral epiphysis treated by pin fixation in which the pins protrude across the surface of the femoral head into the joint. Trauma probably plays a role in many cases; patients with severe slips have a higher incidence of acute cartilage necrosis than patients with mild slips, and the incidence of chondrolysis rises with the vigor of treatment attempts. Manipulative

reduction, open reduction, and prolonged immobilization are followed more often by chondrolysis than is in situ fixation.

The etiology of idiopathic acute cartilage necrosis is unknown. White cell counts, sedimentation rates, and rheumatoid studies are normal. Joint aspirations have most often produced little or no joint fluid. Cultures have been sterile in all cases, and immunologic studies when performed have been normal. The disorder has been reported in both males and females and in white and black races but appears to be most severe in black females, although the total number of reported cases is still relatively small.

Affected patients manifest insidious onset of hip and thigh pain and progressive loss of motion. Flexion and adduction contractures of the involved hip are common. No other systemic or musculoskeletal signs of inflammatory disease are present. Progressive joint-space narrowing on radiologic examination in the absence of signs of slipped capital femoral epiphysis is diagnostic. Narrowing of the articular cartilage space to less than 2 mm, compared to normal widths of 3 to 5 mm is common. When progression continues, the joint space may be completely obliterated, and changes resembling advanced degenerative joint disease may develop.

In patients with either idiopathic chondrolysis or chondrolysis following slipped capital femoral epiphysis, treatment is directed toward relief of pain during the acute phases. There is no known method of reversing the disease. Bed rest and anti-inflammatory agents are usually employed. In some cases, the clinical and radiographic signs may improve dramatically, with restoration of joint spaces and return to normal function. In other instances, progressive joint destruction occurs in spite of rest and anti-inflammatory agents. In these patients, painless ankylosis of the hip in good position is considered a fortunate outcome. Joint arthroplasty or arthrodesis may be necessary to improve function or position in some patients.

SUGGESTED READINGS

Transient Synovitis

Adams JA: Transient synovitis of the hip joint in children. *J Bone Joint Surg Br* 1963; 45:471.

Gershuni DH, Axer A, Hendel D: Arthrographic findings in Legg-Calvé-Perthes disease and transient synovitis of the hip. *J Bone Joint Surg Am* 1978; 60:457.

Haueisen DC, Weiner DS, Weiner SD: The characterization of "transient synovitis of the hip" in children. *J Pediatr Orthop* 1986; 6:11.

Nachemson A, Scheller S: A clinical and radiologic follow-up study of transient synovitis of the hip. *Acta Orthop Scand* 1969; 40:479.

Sharwood F: The irritable hip syndrome in children. *Acta Orthop Scand* 1981; 52:633.

Valderrama JAF: The observation hip syndrome and its late sequelae. *J Bone Joint Surg Br* 1963; 45:462.

Legg-Calvé-Perthes Disease

Catterall A: The natural history of Perthes disease. *J Bone Joint Surg Br* 1971; 53:37.

Clarke TE, et al: Legg-Perthes disease in children less than four years old. *J Bone Joint Surg Am* 1978; 60:166.

Gershuni DH: Preliminary evaluation and prognosis in Legg-Calvé-Perthes disease. *Clin Orthop* 1980; 150:16.

Salter RB: The present state of surgical treatment for Legg-Perthes disease. *J Bone Joint Surg Am* 1984; 66:961.

Salter RB, Bell M: The pathogenesis of deformity in Legg-Perthes disease: An experimental investigation. *J Bone Joint Surg Br* 1968; 50:436.

Salter RB, Thompson GH: Legg-Calvé-Perthes disease: The prognostic significance of the subchondral fracture. *J Bone Joint Surg Am* 1984; 66:479.

Scoles PV, et al: Nuclear magnetic resonance findings in Legg-Calvé-Perthes disease. *J Bone Joint Surg Am* 1984; 66:135–137.

Wynne-Davies R, Gormly L: The aetiology of Perthes disease. Genetic, epidemiological, and growth factors in 310 Glasgow and Edinburgh patients. *J Bone Joint Surg Br* 1978; 60:6.

Slipped Capital Femoral Epiphysis

Agamanolis DP, Weiner DS, Lloyd JK: Slipped capital femoral epiphysis: A pathological study. Parts I and II. *J Pediatr Orthop* 1985; 5:40, 47.

Bishop JO, et al: Slipped capital femoral epiphysis: A study of 50 cases in black children. *Clin Orthop* 1978; 135:93.

Boyer DW, Mickleson MR, Ponseti I: Slipped capital femoral epiphysis: Long-term follow-up study of one hundred and twenty-one patients. *J Bone Joint Surg Am* 1981; 63:85.

Jacobs B: Diagnosis and natural history of slipped capital femoral epiphysis, in American Academy of Orthopaedic Surgeons: *Instructional Course Lectures*. St Louis, CV Mosby Co, 1972, vol 221, p 167.

Kelsey J, Southwick WO: Etiology, mechanism, and incidence of slipped capital femoral epiphysis, in American Academy of Orthopaedic Surgeons: *Instructional Course Lectures*. St Louis, CV Mosby Co, 1972, vol 221, p 182.

Mauer RC, Larsen IJ: Acute necrosis of cartilage in slipped capital femoral epiphysis. *J Bone Joint Surg Am* 1970; 52:39.

Ponseti IV, McClintok R: Pathology of slipping of the upper femoral epiphysis. *J Bone Joint Surg Am* 1956; 38:71–83.

Wattleworth AS, et al: Pathology of slipped capital femoral epiphysis, in American Academy of Orthopaedic Surgeons: *Instructional Course Lectures*. St Louis, CV Mosby Co, 1972, vol 221, p 174.

Wilson PD, Jacobs B, Schecter L: Slipped capital femoral epiphysis: An end result study. *J Bone Joint Surg Am* 1965; 47:1128.

Chondrolysis

Bleck EE: Chondrolysis of the hip. *J Bone Joint Surg Am* 1985; 65:1266.

Duncan JW, Nasca R, Schrantz J: Idiopathic chondrolysis of the hip. *J Bone Joint Surg Am* 1979; 61:1024

Eisenstein A, Rothschild S: Biochemical abnormalities in patients with slipped capital femoral epiphysis and chondrolysis. *J Bone Joint Surg Am* 1976; 58:459.

7 _____

The Spine

The vertebral column provides a frame around and upon which the major organ systems of the body can be suspended and supported. Its stability permits heavy loads to be borne in the upright position; its flexibility permits balance to be maintained while the trunk and upper extremities are positioned for function. The vertebral arches protect the spinal cord and permit segmental exit of spinal nerves to the extremities and trunk.

Spine deformities have a profound effect on the entire body. Neuromuscular, cardiopulmonary, and psychological complications often accompany severe deformity. Some spinal disorders begin in the embryonic period as a result of malformations of vertebrae. In other instances, spine deformities result from muscle imbalance in paralytic disease. In most cases, however, spine deformities develop during late childhood or early adolescence in otherwise healthy children for reasons that are incompletely understood.

Progressive spine deformities lead to significant adult disability; in many cases, early diagnosis and prompt treatment can limit or prevent late disastrous complications.

THE NORMAL SPINE

Embryology

Development of the spinal cord and vertebral column begins during the third week of gestation. The neural components of the spine evolve from the ectodermal layer of the embryonic disk. The neuroectodermal cells that will form the cord thicken into a neural plate. This plate invaginates into the dorsal aspect of the embryo and curls to form the neural tube before the end of the third week. Incomplete closure of the neural tube is a serious defect that results in the spectrum of disorders grouped together as myelomeningocele.

The vertebral column, which surrounds and protects the developing cord, develops from primitive mesenchymal cells on either side of the neural plate. Formation of the spinal column begins a short distance below the cranial region of the embryo at the end of the third week of gestation and proceeds cranially and caudally. The first manifestation of vertebral column development is thickening of the mesenchyma on either side of the notochord. Segmentation of this paraxial mesoderm into discrete units called somites begins on the 20th day of gestation. At the end of the fifth embryonic week, 42 bead-like somites are visible on the dorsal aspect of the embryo. The limb buds and trunk musculature develop from the dorsal and lateral mesenchymal cells of each somite. The ventral and medial cells develop into the vertebral column.

Early in the fourth week of gestation, mesenchymal cells from the medial portion of each column of somites migrate medially and begin to surround the notochord (Fig 7–1). Additional mesenchymal cells migrate posteriorly to begin formation of neural arches around the develop-

ing neural tube. A third group of mesenchymal cells migrates laterally to form primitive ribs. The process begins in the cranial portion of the embryo even as further somites are differentiating below. The caudal portion of the column lags behind the cranial portion in development.

Resegmentation occurs shortly after the mesenchymal elements have surrounded the notochord (Fig 7–2). Fissures develop in each somite, separating them into cranial and caudal halves. Definitive vertebral bodies are formed by fusion of the caudal portion of one somite with the cranial portion of the somite below (Fig 7–3). The notochord within each vertebral segment atrophies; the notochord between segments gives rise to the nucleus pulposus of the intervertebral disk. Growth of the posterior neural arches continues until the tips of the neural elements from each side meet. Closure of the arches occurs during the third month of embryonic life.

The primitive mesenchymal spine is replaced first with chondroid and then with osteoid during early growth and development. Ossification centers are pres-

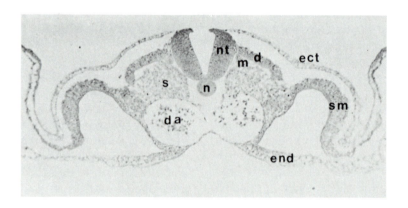

FIG 7–1.
Cross section of the thoracic somite of the chick embryo of the 20-somite stage. The notochord *(n)* underlies the neural tube *(nt)*. The somite is divided into dermatomal *(d)*, myotomal *(m)*, and sclerotomal portions *(s)*. The ectoderm *(ect)* lies posterior to the neural tube; the somatic mesoderm *(sm)* lies lateral to the somite. The dorsal aorta *(da)* lies anterior to the notochord. *end* indicates endoderm. (From Parke WW: Development of the spine, in Rothman RH, Simeone FA (eds): *The Spine*. Philadelphia, WB Saunders Co, 1975, p 3. Reproduced by permission.)

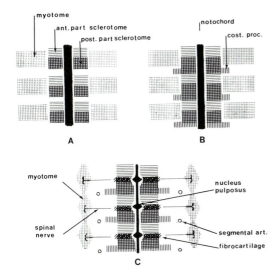

FIG 7–2.
Schematic representation of vertebral development. (From Parke WW: Development of the spine, in Rothman RH, Simeone FA (eds): *The Spine.* Philadelphia, WB Saunders Co, 1975, p 3. Reproduced by permission.)

ent at birth in each vertebral body and in each half of each neural arch. The ossification centers of the neural arches join posteriorly during the first year of life. Fusion of the arches with the vertebral bodies occurs between the second and sixth year of life. Fusion occurs first in the thoracic region of the spine and later in the cervical, lumbar, and sacral areas.

Anatomy

The spinal column normally consists of 24 distinct vertebrae—7 cervical vertebrae, 12 thoracic vertebrae, and 5 lumbar vertebrae—and 2 fused vertebral segments. The sacral and coccygeal segments are respectively composed of 5 and 4 fused segments.

At birth, each vertebra, with the exception of the first and second cervical vertebrae and the sacral and coccygeal vertebral segments, consists of an anterior body and a posterior vertebral arch (Fig 7–

4). Paired articular facets arise from the superior and inferior aspects of the vertebral arches; synovial joints link the superior articular facets of one vertebra with the inferior facets of the vertebra superior to it. Transverse processes extend laterally from the arches. In addition to providing sites of origin and insertion for paraspinal muscles, the transverse processes provide articulation sites for the ribs in the thoracic spine. The spinous processes extend posteriorly at the junction of each side of the neural arch and provide sites for ligament and muscle attachment.

Adjacent vertebral bodies are separated by intervertebral disks. Each disk consists of a gelatinous central portion, the *nucleus pulposus*, and a fibrous outer portion, the *annulus fibrosis*. The nucleus pulposus is a remnant of the primitive notochord and serves to distribute stress between vertebral segments evenly. The annulus fibrosis is composed of alternating oblique layers of dense fibrous connective tissue that contain the nucleus and permit intervertebral motion. The peripheral lay-

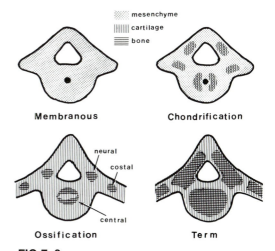

FIG 7–3.
Sequential development of chondrification and ossification centers in the fetal spine. (From Parke WW: Development of the spine, in Rothman RH, Simeone FA (eds): *The Spine.* Philadelphia, WB Saunders Co, 1975, p 4. Reproduced by permission.)

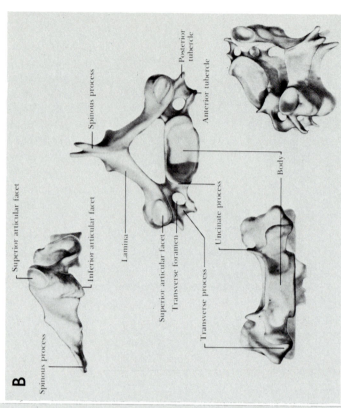

Atlas

Sup.

Anterior tubercle
Anterior arch

Axis

Ant.

Superior articular surface
Dens
Anterior articular surface
Body
Inferior articular process

Lateral mass
Posterior tubercle

Superior articular fovea

Inferior articular fovea

Transverse foramen

Transverse process

Dens
Posterior articular surface
Transverse process
Lamina
Spinous process

Post.

Inf.

The atlas and the axis.

A

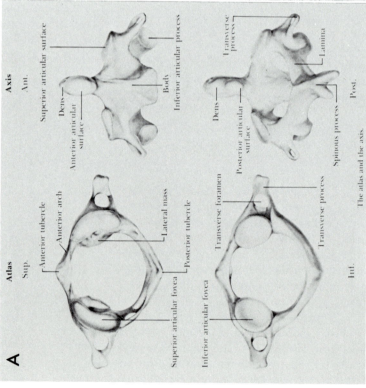

Spinous process
Superior articular facet
Inferior articular facet
Lamina
Superior articular facet
Transverse foramen
Transverse process

Spinous process
Posterior tubercle
Anterior tubercle
Uncinate process
Body

B

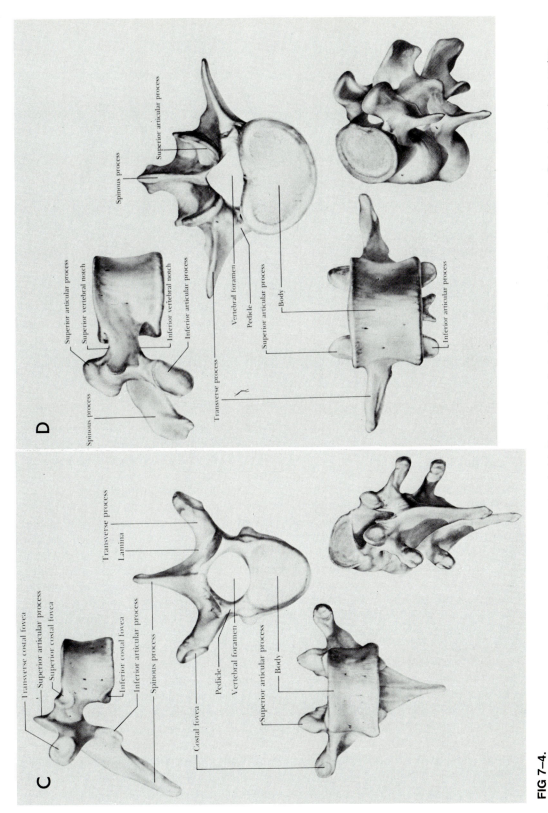

FIG 7-4.
A, the first cervical vertebra (atlas) and second cervical vertebra (axis). **B,** typical cervical vertebra. **C,** typical thoracic vertebra. **D,** typical lumbar vertebra. (From DePalma AF, Rothman RH: *The Intervertebral Disc.* Philadelphia, WB Saunders Co, 1970. Reproduced by permission.)

ers insert firmly into the periosteum of adjacent vertebral bodies. Dense longitudinal anterior and posterior spinal ligaments reinforce the insertion of annular fibers into the vertebral bodies.

The blood supply of the spinal column is derived from segmental vessels that lie along the midportion of each vertebral body. In the cervical region, the segmental arteries are branches of the vertebral artery; in the thoracic and lumbar regions, the segmental arteries are aortic branches. Branches of these vessels perforate the vertebral cortex to supply the underlying cancellous bone. It has been suggested that branches of the segmental vessels penetrate the vertebral endplates to supply the intervertebral disk in the neonate and infant. If present at all, these vessels atrophy by midchildhood. Throughout most of life, the intervertebral disk is nourished by diffusion across the vertebral end-plates from adjacent vertebral bodies.

Growth and Development

In early embryonic development, the vertebral column is curved in a concave anterior position (Fig 7–5). This is termed *kyphosis*. By the time of birth, posterior concavities have developed at the cervicothoracic and lumbosacral junctions. These are called *lordotic curves.* Accentuation of thoracic kyphosis and cervical and lumbar lordosis occurs with growth until adult spine configuration is achieved in the second decade.

In early childhood, the portion of total height attributable to the spinal column is greater than at skeletal maturity. At age 2 years, the vertebral column has reached approximately 50% of its ultimate length. The lower limbs at the same point have reached less than 40% of their ultimate length, and the young child appears top-heavy compared to the adult. Spinal growth occurs at a slower rate than

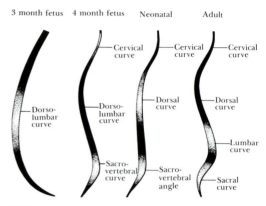

FIG 7–5.
Development of normal anterior and posterior curves in the spine. The early fetal spine is entirely kyphotic. By the time of birth, lordotic curves have developed at the cervicothoracic and lumbosacral areas. The normal adult spine is kyphotic in the thoracic and sacral regions and lordotic in the cervical and lumbar regions. (From DePalma AF, Rothman RH: *The Intervertebral Disc.* Philadelphia, WB Saunders Co, 1970, p 6. Reproduced by permission.)

lower limb growth, and with continued normal development, adult proportions are reached by the end of the adolescent growth spurt.

Overall increase in height occurs at a rate of 4 to 6 cm/year in both boys and girls from approximately age 2 years until the onset of the adolescent growth spurt. This occurs between the 11th and 12th years in girls and between the 13th and 14th years in boys. The velocity of growth may double at that time, and during the period of adolescent growth, height may increase by 6 to 12 cm. Growth ordinarily slows 1½ to 2 years after the onset of the adolescent growth spurt and is usually completed 2 years later. The onset of adolescent growth is said by Tanner to roughly correspond to the onset of testicular and penile enlargement in boys. In girls the adolescent spurt precedes the development of secondary signs of sexual maturation and is nearly complete by menarche. This is of great significance in predicting the natural history of spinal deformity since the greatest risks of progression occur during the adolescent period.

The vertebral column increases in height by endochondral growth at the cartilage end-plates of vertebral bodies. Secondary ossification rings appear around the periphery of the vertebral end-plates early in the second decade and unite with the underlying vertebral bodies by the end of the second decade. It has been estimated that each vertebral segment will add 0.07 cm/year to total height from age 2 years until skeletal maturity. This is of great significance in the treatment of spinal deformities by surgical fusion since successful fusion stops growth across the involved segment of the spine. Although growth rates vary in different individuals and in different portions of the spine, it is possible to calculate roughly the loss in height that will occur after fusion by multiplying the estimated number of years remaining until skeletal maturity times the number of segments involved times 0.07 cm/year. Thus, a six-segment fusion in a child with 10 years' growth remaining would result in a loss in height of only 4.2 cm. This is far less than the loss in height that would occur with progressive spine curvature. In older children, the increase in height gained by correction and stabilization of spine curvature often is greater than the predicted loss from growth arrest across the fusion.

There are numerous radiologic signs of skeletal maturation. The radiologic appearance of the growth plates of the hand, wrist, and knee is commonly used to determine skeletal age. The Greulich and Pyle atlases of normal skeletal development can be used to estimate the relative skeletal age of a given individual; this is more accurate than chronological age in determining skeletal maturity. The appearance of the iliac crest apophysis, Risser's sign (Fig 7–6), is also valuable. A secondary ossification center develops in the anterior section of the apophysis 2 to 3 years before the cessation of growth; it extends along the apophysis and fuses with the iliac crest with increasing maturation. The iliac crest apophysis first appears in girls between ages 13 and 14 years, around the time of the onset of menses. In boys it appears approximately 2 years later. Most of the adolescent growth spurt has passed by the time of appearance of the iliac crest apophysis; overall increase in height after its appearance is approximately 4 cm in girls and 5 cm in boys.

Closure of the vertebral end-plate epiphyseal centers is the most reliable indication of spinal maturation. Closure occurs first in the lumbar spine and progresses cranially. By age 17 to 18 years in girls and 18 to 19 years in boys, the vertebral epiphyses have closed.

SPINE DEFORMITY

Spine deformity may occur in either the anteroposterior or the lateral direction. Mild kyphosis is normal in the thoracic spine; lordosis is normal in the cervical and lumbar regions. The limits of normal are hard to define precisely, but excessive lordosis and kyphosis in adolescence may cause significant adult disability. Lateral deviation of the spine, or *scoliosis*, is always abnormal.

There are many causes of spine deformity in children and adolescents. Some curves are potentially far more disabling than others. Progressive scoliosis is predictably associated with severe cardiopulmonary compromise. Progressive kyphosis may cause spinal cord compression and paralysis. Excessive lumbar lordosis, especially if associated with abnormalities of the lower lumbar vertebrae, may lead to nerve root compression and premature degenerative disk disease. Grotesque deformity, psychological complications, early fatigability, and back pain are common

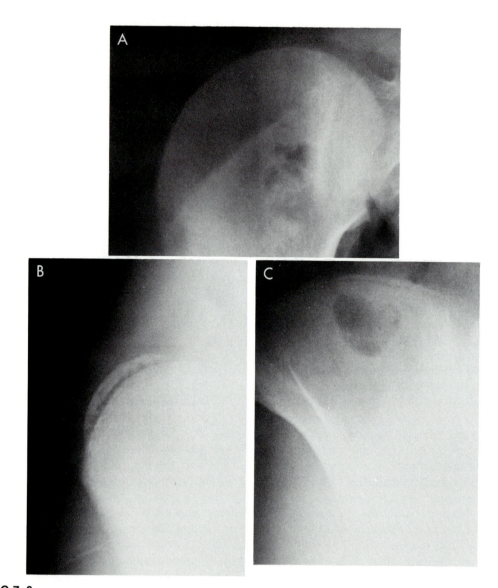

FIG 7–6.
Risser's sign: The iliac crest apophysis. **A,** absence of the secondary ossification center of the iliac crest apophysis indicates that skeletal maturity is not yet near. **B,** the iliac crest apophyseal center appears first over the anterior portion of the iliac crest and advances posteriorly during adolescence. **C,** closure of the apophysis occurs about 2 years after its appearance. Skeletal maturation is near.

with severe kyphotic, lordotic, and scoliotic curves.

Precise definitions permit the complex subject of spine deformity to be broken down into more easily considered divi-

sions. A comprehensive system of terminology has been developed by the Scoliosis Research Society to permit classification, measurement, and study of the many types and causes of spinal curvature. A glossary of selected terms is included at the end of this chapter (see Table 7–3).

Radiographic Evaluation

High-quality roentgenograms are essential in the evaluation and treatment of spine deformity. In most instances, initial radiologic evaluation of suspected spinal curvature should consist of standing posteroanterior and lateral views. Special views to determine flexibility and bone age should be made only if screening films are abnormal.

Routine school screening examination has increased the number of children referred for roentgenographic evaluation and has resulted in longer follow-up for those patients with potentially progressive curves. Nash et al. in 1979 estimated that the average total radiation dose absorbed by breast tissue over a 3-year observation period during which 22 exposures were made was approximately 14 rads. Other workers have estimated that the incidence of breast cancer in women irradiated between ages 13 and 20 years rises by a factor of 162 cases per million women exposed to one rad of radiation. The risk drops with increasing age; for women more than 20 years old, the risk falls to 78 cases per million exposed cases per rad. Unfortunately, the incidence of scoliosis is highest in the immature female. The risks of radiation to other tissues must be considered as well; thyroid and bone marrow tissues appear to be especially vulnerable. Gonadal tissue as well is exposed during spine radiography and can only be partially shielded.

A number of techniques have been suggested to reduce the radiation exposure of children with suspected scoliosis. First, careful selection of individuals referred for radiographic evaluation is necessary. Secondary physician screening of patients identified by primary screening is recommended. Second, appropriate selection of radiographic views is necessary. For individuals suspected of having scoliosis, a single coronal plane view will suffice. For individuals with suspected excessive kyphosis or lordosis, a sagittal plane view alone is sufficient. Several technical modifications in radiographic technique have been developed to reduce exposure of vulnerable tissues. These suggestions, outlined by Gray et al. in 1983, include:

1. The use of the posteroanterior (PA) projection instead of the anteroposterior projection for coronal views.
2. The use of specially designed lead-loaded acrylic filters and nongradient intensifying screens.
3. Specially designed cassette holders that eliminate grid cassettes and ensure better alignment.
4. Breast shields.
5. Additional filtration in the x-ray tube collimator.

Such modifications can result in 50- to 70-fold reductions in exposure of sensitive tissues without adversely affecting film quality. The routine use of PA films, breast shields, and avoidance of multiple unnecessary views are perhaps the simplest and most readily applicable modifications for scoliosis evaluation. Finally, competent radiography technicians are essential. Multiple exposures to obtain a properly penetrated film are unwarranted.

In the normal spine, vertebral bodies appear squarely stacked one upon another in anteroposterior or posteroanterior roentgenograms. Vertebral end-plates are parallel, and intervertebral disks are symmetric. When scoliosis develops, vertebral bodies tilt, and end-plates are no longer horizontal. The intervertebral disks appear narrower on the concave side of the curve than on the convex side. Vertebral bodies also rotate along the long axis of the spinal column toward the convexity of the curve; posterior elements appear rotated into the concavity.

The degree of lateral curvature present is determined by measuring the angular difference between vertebral end-plates at each end of the curvature. The Cobb-Lippman technique is usually employed (Fig 7–7). Although originally described for scoliosis, it can be used for kyphosis and lordosis as well. In this technique, the vertebrae at each end of a curve are defined as those whose end-plates deviate most from horizontal. This can be simply determined by drawing light pencil lines along the superior end-plates of two or three bodies at the apparent upper limit of a curve and along the inferior end-plates of several bodies at the lower limit of the curve. The superior and inferior vertebrae whose end-plates are most tilted are the end points of curvature. Next, perpendiculars are drawn from the end-plates of the most tilted bodies. The angle formed by the intersection of the perpendicular lines is the degree of curvature. Kyphosis and lordosis can be measured in the same manner.

The *location* of a curvature is defined by the location of the *apex* or *center vertebra*. The apical vertebra is usually the least tilted and most rotated vertebra in the curve. If the apex lies in the thoracic spine, the curve is said to be thoracic; if the apex lies in the lumbar spine, a lumbar curve is present. When apical vertebrae lie at the junction of two major segments of the spine, the curves are termed cervicothoracic, thoracolumbar, or lumbosacral, according to the location of the apex.

By convention, the *direction* of lateral curvature is indicated by the side of convexity. Curves convex to the right are right curves; curves convex to the left are left curves. Curves convex posteriorly are kyphotic; curves convex anteriorly are lordotic.

Lateral spine curvature can be divided into two major groups based on flexibility (Fig 7–8). *Flexible* or *nonstructural* curves straighten or overcorrect as the patient bends toward the convexity of the curve. *Nonflexible* or *structural* curves persist during bending, although some correction occurs in all but the most rigid deformities.

Single lateral curves are uncommon. In most instances, the curve of greatest magnitude is surrounded superiorly and

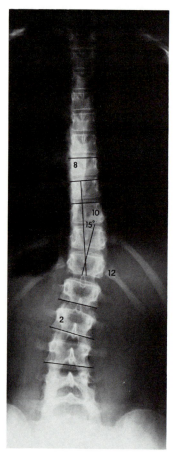

FIG 7–7.
The Cobb-Lippman method of curve measurement in scoliosis. Perpendicular lines are constructed from the end vertebral bodies of each curve (in this illustration, T-9 and L-2). The angle of intersection is the degree of curvature present.

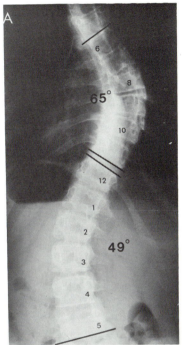

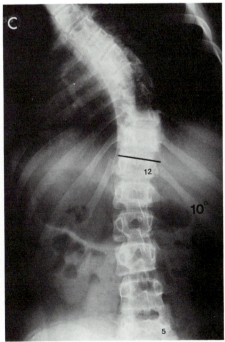

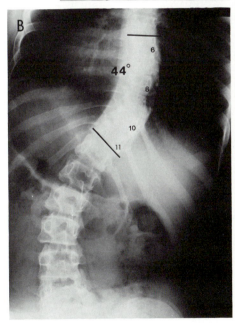

FIG 7–8.
Structural thoracic and lumbar idiopathic curves. **A,** the thoracic curve measures 65 degrees from T-6 to T-11 by the Cobb-Lippman method. The apex vertebra is T9; it is the least tilted vertebra in the curve, but it is the most rotated body. Note the asymmetry of the outlines of its pedicles. The lumbar curve extends from T-12 to L-5 and measures 49 degrees. The apex is L-3. Rotation is present, but not as pronounced. **B,** on supine bending toward the right, the thoracic curve corrects to 44 degrees. Rotation is still pronounced. Note the appearance of the iliac crest apophysis—Risser's sign. The patient is still skeletally immature, and curve progression is likely. **C,** the lumbar curve corrects to 10 degrees on supine left bending. Both curves are structural by definition since neither completely corrects.

inferiorly by curves of lesser magnitude in the opposite direction. Such curves are called *compensatory* curves and serve to maintain overall alignment of the spine. The curve of greatest magnitude is called the *major curve;* lesser curves are called *minor* curves. In most instances, the major curve develops structural changes first and is termed the *primary* curve. Compensatory curves are then known as *sec-*

ondary curves. Often, however, structural changes are present in both the major and minor curves, and it is impossible to determine accurately which curve developed structural changes first. For that reason, the terms "primary" and "secondary" curve are rarely used.

The terms *fractional curve, half curve,* and *hemicurve* are sometimes used to designate incomplete compensatory curves that occur in the upper thoracic or lumbosacral region. The end vertebral bodies of these curves are horizontal rather than tilted; they may be structural or nonstructural and must be considered in treatment planning.

Vertebral rotation is an important component of structural scoliosis and is responsible for the prominence of the rib hump on the convex side of a thoracic curve. Shift in position of vertebral pedicles is sometimes used to estimate the amount of rotation present in a curve. On anteroposterior roentgenograms of the normal spine, the vertebral pedicles appear as symmetric oval outlines on each side of the vertebral bodies. With vertebral rotation, the pedicles appear asymmetric. The pedicles on the convex side of the curve shift toward the midportion of the vertebral body. Pedicles on the concave side appear to move off the edge of the corresponding body.

Scoliosis

There are many causes of lateral spine curvature. At times scoliosis may be the result of poor posture, leg-length inequality, or hip or knee flexion contractures. Such curves are almost always nonstructural; often they disappear when the patient is seated or supine. Structural changes rarely develop, and late complications are uncommon.

Flexible scoliosis also may accompany the acute phases of back injury. Muscle spasm results in imbalance, and spine curvature results. Intervertebral disk her-

niations in older patients may cause nerve root compression and back pain, with listing of the spine to the side. Such curves resolve with healing of the underlying disorder.

Structural scoliosis can be grouped into three broad etiologic categories: (1) congenital, (2) neuromuscular or paralytic, and (3) idiopathic. Congenital malformations of the spine such as hemivertebrae and unsegmented vertebral bars often produce structural curves that are present at birth. Curve progression may occur very early in congenital curves, and extraordinarily severe deformities may develop. Paralytic diseases, whether the result of primary muscle or primary nerve pathology, often cause scoliosis. Neuromuscular curves usually begin as flexible deformities, but progression commonly occurs with growth, and structural changes develop rapidly. Severe cardiopulmonary compromise is common in untreated cases. Children with myelomeningocele may develop spinal curvature from either vertebral abnormalities or from associated paralysis. Progressive spine deformity is one of the most difficult management problems in myelodysplasia.

Most patients with scoliosis have no obvious cause for deformity. These patients are said to have *idiopathic scoliosis.* The curves of idiopathic scoliosis usually begin as nonstructural deformities and develop into structural deformities with further growth.

Idiopathic Scoliosis

Idiopathic scoliosis is the most common type of lateral spine curvature. Although it differs in origin from congenital and paralytic scoliosis, it shares many clinical and radiologic features. It is the model upon which most of the principles of diagnosis and treatment of spine curvature have been developed.

Idiopathic scoliosis begins in the growing spine. It can be subdivided into three groups according to age at onset of curvature. *Infantile idiopathic scoliosis* is present at birth or develops during the first 3 years of life. *Juvenile idiopathic scoliosis* develops after age 3 years but before puberty. *Adolescent idiopathic scoliosis* has its onset at or about the onset of puberty, but before maturity. The principles of diagnosis and the complications of progression are similar in each group, but the natural history of disease and prognosis vary.

Presentation.—The early manifestations of idiopathic scoliosis are subtle. Patients have no symptoms, and deformity is often not obvious. Many patients with slight curves are unaware of the presence of spine deformity. Shoulder height may be unequal, and leg-length inequality may seem to be present (Fig 7–9). Shirts and blouses fit poorly, and hemlines may be difficult to adjust. When progression occurs, more severe deformity develops. The trunk is proportionately short, and a prominent rib hump develops. The head and shoulders usually appear to be shifted to one side, and the distance between the elbows and flanks is asymmetric. If a curve extends into the upper thoracic or cervical regions, severely disfiguring alterations in the neckline or shoulder levels may be present. Pelvic obliquity and apparent leg-length inequality may complicate uncompensated lumbar or lumbosacral curves.

The most consistent finding in patients with idiopathic scoliosis is caused by vertebral rotation that accompanies lateral deviation of the spine. As progression occurs, vertebral bodies within a curve rotate into the convexity of the curvature. This is most pronounced at the apex of a curve and least prominent at its end points. The vertebral transverse processes, ribs, and paraspinal muscles on the convex side of the curve are drawn posteriorly; the ribs on the concave side of the curve are thrust anteriorly. This rotation is most obvious when a patient with scoliosis bends forward; a rib hump appears on the convex side of thoracic curves, and a hump caused by displacement of transverse processes and paraspinal muscles appears on the convex side of the lumbar curves. The forward-bending test used in screening examinations for scoliosis is based on the vertebral rotation that accompanies lateral deviation; it will detect flexible and small structural curves of 5 degrees or less.

Apparent breast asymmetry is common in adolescent girls with scoliosis. This, too, is a consequence of vertebral rotation. The anterior chest wall on the convex side of a curve is recessed because of posterior rib displacement. The breast on the convex side of the curve often appears smaller than that on the concave side, which is displaced anteriorly along with its underlying ribs.

Idiopathic scoliosis causes few symptoms in childhood and adolescence; idiopathic adolescent structural curves are not painful. Pain does not occur even in patients with severe idiopathic curvature until secondary degenerative arthritis develops in later adult life. Nerve root compromise and spinal cord compression are uncommon even in patients with very severe idiopathic curves. Alterations in sensation, muscle weakness, reflex changes, and asymmetry of foot size in patients with apparent idiopathic spine curvature suggest other pathologic processes. Cutaneous lesions such as hairy patches, café au lait spots, and sacral dimpling may be signs of underlying neurologic disorders. Other warning signs in patients with apparent idiopathic scoliosis include thoracic curves that are convex toward the left instead of toward the right, short sharp angular deformities in the midthoracic region, long, sweeping, poorly compensated curves, and rapid progression of deformity in spite of treatment. Careful evaluation is essential before treatment of the scoliosis is started. Bone scans, computed tomography, laminography, and myelog-

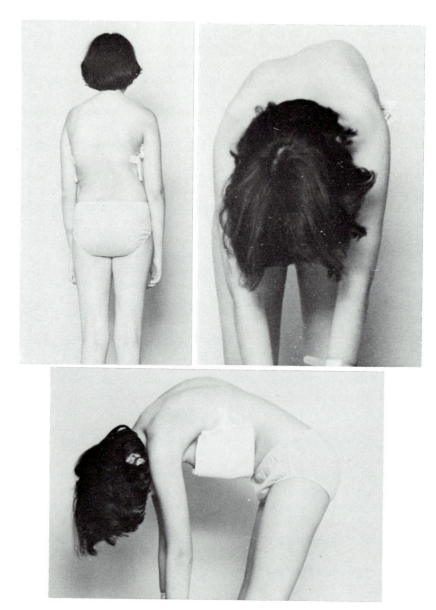

FIG 7–9.
Adolescent idiopathic scoliosis. Mild shoulder asymmetry is present on the posterior view in the upright position. A significant rib hump is present on forward bending.

raphy may be necessary to establish the cause of symptoms and exclude neural malformation or tumor.

Etiology.—The cause of idiopathic scoliosis is unknown. No consistent bio-chemical, neurologic, muscular, or trau-matic abnormalities have been found in extensive studies of idiopathic scoliosis. There is no analogous animal model of spontaneous idiopathic scoliosis, although spine deformity can be produced experimentally in animals by a number of techniques. Hormonal factors have been implicated because of the increased incidence of severe curves in girls, but no definite relationship has been established. Recent studies have demonstrated abnormalities of proprioception and vibratory sense in patients with even small degrees of idiopathic scoliosis and may implicate abnormalities of posterior column function as a cause of idiopathic scoliosis.

Genetic influences appear to be important in the etiology of idiopathic scoliosis. Curves occur more frequently in individuals with affected parents or siblings than in the population at large, but the relationship is not mendelian. Like other musculoskeletal diseases such as clubfoot and congenital hip dysplasia, idiopathic scoliosis appears to be inherited in a multifactorial manner. It is likely that a combination of genetic predisposition and other influences produce spine deformity in affected individuals.

Incidence.—The precise incidence of idiopathic scoliosis is difficult to determine. Many patients with slight curves are unaware of the presence of spine deformity. Since small curves cause no symptoms, scoliosis may be detected only as an incidental finding on chest roentgenograms made for other reasons. School screening studies based on the forward-bending test indicate that slightly more than 5% of older juveniles and adolescents have spine asymmetry. Follow-up radiologic studies indicate that some, but not all, of these children have small flexible or structural curves. Approximately 1% to 2% will have curves of 15 to 20 degrees, and 0.1% to 0.2% will have curves greater than 20 degrees. Retrospective reviews of several large series of tuberculosis screening examinations in the United States indicate that about 2% of adults have spinal curves of 10 degrees or more; 0.5% have curves of greater than 20

degrees. The majority appear to be idiopathic in origin. A smaller percentage are congenital or neuromuscular. The majority of idiopathic curves appear to have begun during adolescence.

Infantile Idiopathic Scoliosis.—Idiopathic curves that begin before puberty are uncommon in the United States and probably account for less than 10% of idiopathic curves. Idiopathic curves that begin during the first 3 years of life have been a much more common problem in Europe. Studies conducted in Edinburgh in 1968 indicated that approximately 50% of new cases of idiopathic scoliosis seen were infantile in origin. In contrast, however, infantile idiopathic scoliosis is rare in North America, even in populations of recent European descent. Incidence studies conducted in Boston in 1972 indicated that less than 1% of new cases of idiopathic scoliosis were infantile in origin.

Many of the clinical and genetic aspects of infantile idiopathic scoliosis differ significantly from those of juvenile and adolescent-onset spine deformity, and it may represent a different disease process. The majority of patients are male, in contrast to adolescent-onset curvature. Most curves occur in the thoracic region and are convex toward the left. The incidence of associated anomalies such as congenital hip dysplasia, congenital heart disease, and inguinal hernia is higher than in the normal population, and mental retardation has been reported in about 10% of infants with progressive infantile curvature. Most significantly, spontaneous resolution occurs in a high percentage of children with idiopathic scoliosis. The majority of curves that develop within the first 6 months of life resolve without treatment. Curves that begin later in infancy are less likely to resolve and almost always require treatment to prevent the complications common to other forms of progressive spine deformity.

Head molding or plagiocephaly is a peculiar but common finding in infantile scoliosis. It is usually not present at birth but develops within the first 6 months of life. The skull of affected infants appears asymmetric when viewed from above. The head seems flattened on the concave side of the curve and prominent on the convex side. The cause of the deformity is unclear; it has been suggested that the forces of gravity acting on the plastic skull of the supine infant positioned slightly toward the right tend to cause flowing of the bones of the cranium, flattening the anterior aspect of the left side of the skull and the posterior aspect of the right side of the skull. The same forces may flatten the posterior aspects of the ribs on the right side of the thorax and cause vertebral rotation toward the left. British investigators have reported that in past years, it has been common practice to nurse infants in the supine position, facing right, with the left side of the body propped higher than the right. In this position, gravitational forces might mold both the skull and the thorax. In contrast, infants in the United states are almost always nursed supine, and it has been proposed that this accounts for the difference in incidence of infantile scoliosis in the two otherwise similar populations. In most cases, plagiocephaly, like the accompanying scoliosis, resolves spontaneously once the infant becomes mobile, usually correcting by age 6 years. Recent British studies have indicated a marked fall in the number of infants presenting with idiopathic scoliosis to levels that now approach the incidence of infantile idiopathic scoliosis in the United States. This has coincided with a effort to encourage mothers to nurse infants in the prone position, lending support to postural theories of etiology.

Juvenile Idiopathic Scoliosis.—Scoliosis that is discovered after age 3 years but before puberty is termed juvenile idiopathic scoliosis. Some juvenile curves are probably in reality previously undetected infantile idiopathic curves. Other juvenile curves, particularly those that occur later in childhood, may be early manifestations of adolescent idiopathic scoliosis. Early in childhood the number of boys presenting with juvenile-onset curves exceeds the number of girls, but by late childhood, girls outnumber boys. Some juvenile curves remain small and may resolve spontaneously. Others progress either during childhood or at the onset of the adolescent growth spurt (Fig 7–10). There is no reliable method to predict either radiologically or clinically what the behavior of an individual juvenile curve will be; careful follow-up is essential, and treatment must be started if progression occurs.

Adolescent Idiopathic Scoliosis.—Approximately 85% to 90% of cases of idiopathic spine deformity in North America occur in adolescents. Most begin around the time of the adolescent growth spurt in previously normal children. Minor degrees of curvature occur with nearly equal frequency in boys and girls, but curves in girls progress five to six times more often. Most curves begin in the thoracic or thoracolumbar region and are convex toward the right. Compensatory left lumbar and upper thoracic curves develop to maintain trunk balance. Primary left thoracic curves are quite rare and should raise suspicions of underlying neurologic disorders or neoplastic disease. As noted above, early signs of adolescent idiopathic scoliosis are subtle, and symptoms are rare. Once again, back pain, reflex changes, sensory disturbances, lower extremity weakness, or alterations in bowel or bladder function are strong indications that spine deformity is not idiopathic in origin.

School screening surveys for spine deformity are now common in North Amer-

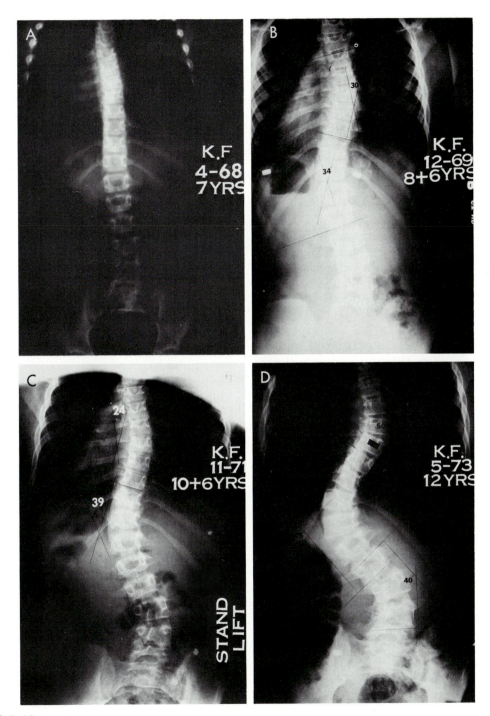

FIG 7–10.
Progression of curvature in juvenile idiopathic scoliosis. **A,** spine asymmetry was first noted at age 7 years. **B,** a right thoracic–left thoracolumbar curve pattern developed by age 8½ years. Treatment was refused. **C,** little progression occurred over the next 2 years. **D,** rapid progression occurred during the adolescent growth spurt. (Courtesy of C.L. Nash, M.D.)

ica. Most programs concentrate on children in the late juvenile and early adolescent years. Girls in the sixth, seventh, and eighth grades and boys in the seventh, eighth, and ninth grades benefit most from screening examination.

Follow-up radiologic evaluations indicate that most children and adolescents with clinical spine asymmetry have curves of at least 5 degrees. Most such curves are of little significance, require no treatment, and may in fact resolve spontaneously. Others, however, progressively worsen and may lead to serious adult complications. At present there is no way to predict at the time of discovery which idiopathic adolescent curves will worsen. The magnitude of the rib or paraspinal hump does not correlate well with the degree of underlying scoliosis. Although patients with large humps often have severe curves, the relationship is not absolute.

There is probably no single "natural history" for the adolescent with idiopathic scoliosis. Some patients with curves of 20 to 25 degrees at the time of initial screening evaluation never experience progression. Other patients gradually worsen throughout adolescence but end growth with acceptable amounts of spine deformity. In other individuals, progression of curvature after discovery is more rapid, and nonoperative treatment may be indicated. Other patients show rapid progression of curvature despite nonoperative care and require surgical intervention. At this time, factors that appear to be associated with an increased risk for progression are age at onset less than 12 years, absence of signs of secondary sexual maturation, absence of the secondary ossification center of the iliac crest apophysis (Risser's sign 0), and initial curve magnitude greater than 30 degrees. Factors that do not appear to be associated with an increased risk for progression include a positive family history of scoliosis, degree of accompanying kyphosis or lordosis, and

trunk balance. Although the magnitude of the rib hump present on examination does not correlate well with the magnitude of underlying curvature, it has been reported that patients whose angle of rib inclination is greater than 5 degrees show progression more frequently than patients with lesser degrees of inclination.

The behavior of curves after skeletal maturity is variable as well. Patients who reach skeletal maturity with thoracic curves of less than 40 degrees usually have little or no difficulty throughout life. Although cosmetic deformity persists, it is usually not severe. Back pain is no more likely to occur than in unaffected individuals. Significant progression of curvature is uncommon in these patients. The behavior of lumbar curves is less predictable, but patients who reach maturity with curves less than 30 degrees are probably not at serious risk. Pregnancy does not appear to cause progression of minimal curves but may adversely affect marginal curves.

The behavior of larger curves after skeletal maturity depends on the location and magnitude of curvature at the end of growth. Thoracic curves of less than 40 degrees rarely progress after adolescence; thoracic curves greater than 60 degrees at the end of growth most often continue to worsen throughout adult life at the rate of at least 1 degree per year (Fig 7–11). Thoracic curves between 40 and 60 degrees are unpredictable; although some show little progression, others may significantly increase. Curves of greater than 40 degrees in the thoracolumbar region and the lumbar spine commonly worsen with age.

Complications of Progression.—Uncontrolled progression causes serious problems in patients of all ages. Decreased vital capacity is a consistent finding in patients with thoracic curvatures greater than 60 degrees, although significant decreases in vital capacity do not oc-

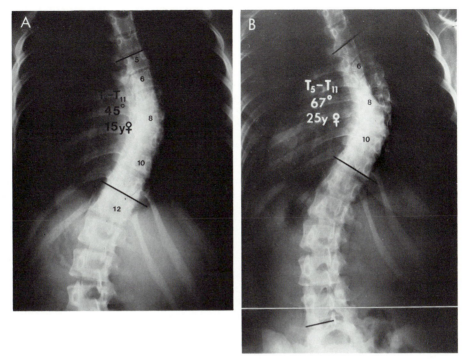

FIG 7–11.
Progression of curvature in adolescent idiopathic scoliosis. **A,** age 15 years. A 45-degree right thoracic curve is present. Surgical treatment was recommended but refused. **B,** age 25 years. Progression to 67 degrees has occurred. Easy fatigability and aching back pain were present.

cur in most cases until curves exceed 80 degrees. Pulmonary hypertension is common in patients with thoracic curves greater than 80 degrees; patients with the combination of thoracic scoliosis and decreased thoracic kyphosis are especially affected. Vital capacity and maximal breathing capacity continue to decrease with curve progression. Atelectasis, altered regional lung perfusion, and arteriovenous shunting have been demonstrated in patients with curves greater than 60 degrees, and arterial hypoxemia is almost always present in patients with curves greater than 100 degrees. In some studies, the mortality of patients with progressive untreated scoliosis after age 40 years has been twice that expected. Most deaths occur from cardiopulmonary failure.

There are other serious complications of progressive spine deformity. Back pain, chronic fatigue, and decreased work tolerance are common complaints in adults with severe untreated spine deformity. Premature degenerative arthritis is common. Spinal cord compression is rare in pure scoliotic curves, but nerve root impingement caused by deformity and secondary arthritic degeneration may occur. Scandinavian studies indicate that a high proportion of adult scoliosis patients are unemployed, unmarried, and psychologically disturbed by their deformities. Careful analysis of studies from North American centers suggests slightly lower morbidity and mortality for adults with untreated spine deformity but confirms suggestions that spine deformity is an unnecessary cause of premature death and disability.

Treatment.—Effective treatment of spine deformity depends on early detection and prompt referral. Evaluation of spine and head asymmetry should be part of neonatal physical examinations, and forward-bending tests should be included in routine examinations during childhood and adolescence. Brothers, sisters, and children of scoliosis patients should be especially carefully examined. School screening programs should be actively encouraged.

When spine asymmetry is identified on physical examination, radiologic evaluation is necessary. Initial reontgenographic examination of children and adolescents with clinical signs of scoliosis should consist of a single standing posteroanterior roentgenogram from the first thoracic level to the first sacral level. Those with excessive kyphosis or lordosis should have lateral films made as well. Infants should have supine anteroposterior roentgenograms. Special views to determine curve flexibility and bone age should be obtained after clinical suspicions of curvature are confirmed radiologically and when treatment appears necessary. Measurement of curvature is critical and should be performed by a specialist in spinal disorders. Most children's hospitals and crippled children's centers have scoliosis clinics where patients with scoliosis can be referred for evaluation and treatment if no local facilities are available.

When spine asymmetry is identified clinically and confirmed radiologically, a search for its cause is necessary. Although idiopathic scoliosis is the most common variety of spine deformity, it is not the only cause of spine asymmetry. Structural abnormalities of other parts of the musculoskeletal system, neurologic diseases, neoplasms of the spinal column, back trauma, and inflammatory disorders must be excluded before treatment of apparent idiopathic scoliosis is started.

Physical examination should include measurement of lower extremity lengths from anterosuperior iliac spines to corresponding medial malleoli. Contractures of the hip, knee, and ankle should be noted if present. Signs of neurologic impairment, such as asymmetric lower extremity muscle strength, thigh or calf asymmetry, unequal reflexes, or sensory deficits should be carefully assessed. Café au lait spots, cutaneous neurofibromas, hairy patches over the spine, and sacral dimples may indicate underlying abnormalities of the spinal cord. Back pain is uncommon in idiopathic scoliosis, but when it is present, a careful search for neoplasms or infections of the spine is necessary. Roentgenograms should be carefully examined for evidence of congenital, neoplastic, and infectious spinal abnormalities. A diagnosis of idiopathic scoliosis is indicated only when there is no other obvious cause of spine deformity.

The goals of treatment of scoliosis are to enable a patient to enter adult life with a balanced and stable spine with maximum flexibility, and acceptable residual deformity with the lowest possible morbidity. Progression and its attendant complications must be prevented during the years of active growth, and the risks of progression in adult life should be held as low as possible. It is not necessary to reduce all curves to less than 10 degrees.

The options for the child or adolescent with scoliosis include the following:

1. No treatment
2. Observation
3. Orthotic treatment
4. Electrical stimulation
5. Surgical intervention

Each has a role in management of spine deformity in the growing patient.

The adolescent with minimal rib asymmetry, cosmetically acceptable kyphosis and lordosis, and no symptoms or signs of underlying neurologic or musculoskeletal disease, and who is in the late phases of growth needs no treatment beyond initial radiographic evaluation. Girls in this category are 1½ to 2 years past the onset of menses and have changed little in height over the preceding 6 months. Boys in this group have completed voice change, have axillary, facial, and pubic hair, full genital development, and are no longer growing taller. Radiographically, curves in this group measure less than 30 degrees, and the iliac crest apophysis has completed its excursion.

Less fully mature individuals must be followed clinically and radiographically throughout remaining growth. Juvenile and adolescent patients with curves that measure less than 10 or 15 degrees radiographically most often can be followed at intervals of 6 to 12 months. Patients with curves in the range of 15 to 25 degrees usually must be followed at minimum intervals of 6 months, and patients with curves greater than 25 degrees usually must be seen at 4-month intervals.

Active treatment is usually started when idiopathic curves reach 30 degrees. Curves of lesser magnitude that have shown rapid progression on serial roentgenograms obtained after initial diagnosis are often treated as well, especially in younger patients with a long period of risk. Curves greater than 30 degrees can sometimes be followed closely without treatment in patients who are approaching skeletal maturity. In most cases, however, the risk of further progression is high enough to warrant treatment in immature patients with curves of more than 30 degrees.

At present, there are two principal nonoperative methods of treatment of idiopathic scoliosis: (1) orthotic or brace management and (2) electrical stimulation. Brace management has long been held to be effective for many idiopathic curves of moderate degree. Because of the impossibility of predicting the natural history of a given curve regardless of treatment at the time bracing is begun, it is difficult to definitively attribute the apparent success of bracing in a individual patient to a brace, but large series of reports have indicated that when carefully supervised and faithfully followed, spinal bracing throughout adolescence prevents progression in 75% to 85% of appropriate cases.

Many attempts to control spine deformity orthotically have been made throughout history. Most have failed, largely because they relied too heavily on intermittent passive distraction of the spine. It is impossible to exert enough pressure on the ribs and overlying skin or to pull long enough and hard enough on the head and pelvis to permanently correct spinal deformity. Modern spine braces combine passive control of the pelvis and trunk balance with active distraction of the spine. To achieve maximal benefit, brace patients are trained to actively twist away from lateral pressure pads and, when necessary, from throat molds. Bracing does not work in uncooperative patients or in patients with paralytic diseases.

The Milwaukee brace, introduced in 1946 by Blount and Schmidt, was the first spine orthosis demonstrated to be effective in idiopathic scoliosis, and it remains the standard against which other braces are evaluated (Fig 7–12). The Milwaukee brace, sometimes known generically as a cervico-thoracic-lumbo-sacral orthosis, or CTLSO, is now usually employed for midthoracic and upper thoracic curves whose apices lie between the ninth or tenth and fourth or fifth thoracic vertebrae.

A variety of underarm braces have been developed during the past decade. These braces, known as thoraco-lumbo-sacral orthoses, or TLSOs, are most often used for nonoperative treatment of curves

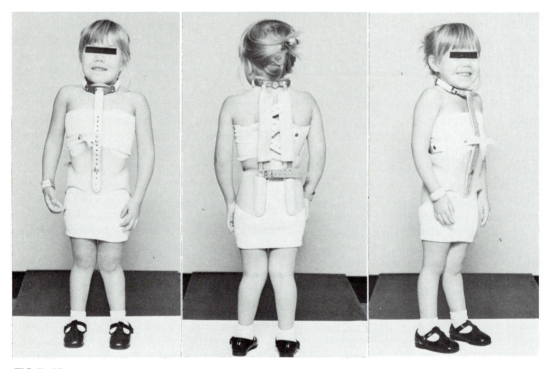

FIG 7–12.
The Milwaukee brace. The custom-molded pelvic girdle controls the pelvis and provides a base of support for the upright positions. The throat mold should not touch the mandible when the patient stands erect. The Milwaukee brace can be used for most idiopathic curves and is necessary for thoracic curves whose apex is above T-8.

whose apices lie below the ninth thoracic level (Fig 7–13). Patient acceptance of orthoses of this type is often much easier than with the CTLSO since it is easily covered by ordinary clothing. Anterior, posterior, and side-opening TLSOs have been designed, and each variety has its own applications.

The period of brace use can be as long as 3 to 4 years, and ordinarily braces are used 22 or 23 hours daily for most of this period. Part-time brace use, usually 12 to 16 hours/day, is under current study at a number of centers, and early results are encouraging, but more information is needed before conclusions can be drawn. Weaning from a brace usually is started after a curve has been stable for at least a year and skeletal maturation is evident radiologically. The weaning process usually

takes 2 to 3 years to complete. Many patients wear their braces to sleep until age 17 or 18 years. If signs of progression develop during the weaning process, full-time brace use is usually resumed.

In carefully selected patients, spinal bracing prevents progression of curvature in a high percentage of cases. Transient correction is often seen during the period of brace use, but relapse to within 5 degrees of initial curvature is common several years after bracing has been stopped. For maximum benefit, therefore, brace treatment must be started before significant deformity has developed. Not all curves can be controlled by bracing. Thoracic, thoracolumbar, and lumbar curves of 30 or 40 degrees that are moderately flexible and not associated with extreme rotational deformity respond best to brace

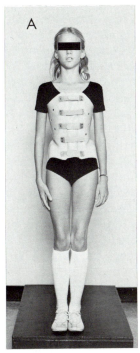
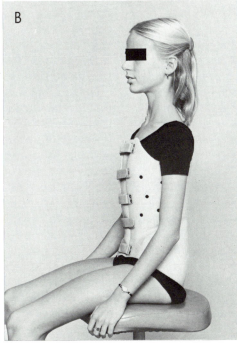
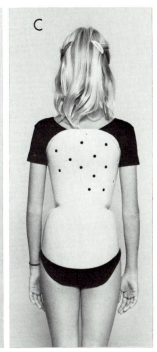

FIG 7–13.
The total contact orthosis is most appropriate for thoracolumbar and lumbar curves. When carefully fabricated and fitted, it is both comfortable and cosmetically acceptable. **A,** a properly fitting brace is cut high enough over the thighs to permit full hip flexion. **B,** the lower posterior margin of the brace should just clear a firm chair when seated. **C,** perforated holes are sometimes added to permit ventilation.

treatment. High thoracic and cervicothoracic curves respond poorly. Curves associated with loss of thoracic kyphosis or lumbar lordosis are difficult to treat with braces; bracing may increase pulmonary compromise and rib deformity in these patients.

Patients undergoing brace treatment should be encouraged to be as active as possible. Almost all routine school and athletic activities can be continued, with the exceptions of contact sports and trampoline exercises. Swimming is permitted if the patient wears the brace to the locker room and reapplies the brace promptly when finished. Cheerleading, band, and tennis can be encouraged. There are usually no restrictions on lifting, and track and field sports are permissible. Although

exercise programs designed to increase flexibility and strengthen abdominal and paraspinal muscles are important adjuncts to brace treatment of spine disorders, exercise alone has not been demonstrated to prevent progression of scoliosis.

The decision to undertake brace treatment involves significant emotional and financial investment. Excellent physician-patient rapport, a strong parent-patient relationship, and peer support are necessary. Emotionally disturbed or mentally retarded children and children from broken homes, ghettos, and Indian reservations rarely successfully complete brace treatment programs. A number of patient-parent organizations such as the National Scoliosis Association and its regional chapters actively provide guidance and support for scoliosis patients and their families, and participation should be strongly encouraged.

During the last decade, intermittent surface electrical stimulation of spinal musculature on the convex side of an idiopathic scoliotic curve has been extensively studied as an alternative to brace treatment of progressive curves. Two programs are currently under study. In the first, surface electrodes are positioned above and below the apex of a curve at the posterior axillary line on the convex side of a curve. In the second, surface electrodes are placed over the paraspinal musculature on the convex side of the curve. In both programs, intermittent bursts of low-voltage electrical current are used to stimulate contraction of muscles on the convex side of the curve, causing the spine to temporarily at least partially correct. Investigators hoped to strengthen muscles opposite the concavity of a curve and prevent further progression. The stimulation units are generally used part-time, in most cases 8 hours/night. Patients treated by electrical stimulation are permitted full activity without bracing during waking hours.

Electrical stimulation is most appropriate for idiopathic curves whose apices lie between the midthoracic and midlumbar regions and that are not associated with extreme sagittal-plane deformities. Nonstructural curves and structural curves that show some flexibility on side bending, and that are between 25 and 35 degrees at the time treatment is started, seem to respond best. Curves of greater magnitude and upper thoracic and low lumbar curves do poorly with intermittent electrical stimulation. The treatment program is continued throughout the growth period and is terminated when height is stable and there is radiographic evidence of skeletal maturation.

The program requires a great deal of medical and parental supervision, and there is a high rate of minor complications. Skin irritation from electrode paste and adhesive tape is common, and blistering beneath the electrodes is sometimes severe enough to force discontinuation of treatment. Electrode and battery failure occur on occasion and must be monitored. The position of the surface electrodes must be carefully followed between visits to prevent gradual migration and loss of correction force. Finally, patients and parents must be aware that when unacceptable progression occurs in spite of electrical stimulation, alternative methods of treatment such as bracing or surgery will be required.

The results to date of multicenter investigations of intermittent electrical stimulation are mixed. In carefully selected and compliant patients with mild to moderate curves, electrical stimulation appeared to be as successful or slightly less successful than bracing in preventing unacceptable progression. A few degrees increase in magnitude throughout treatment was common in most studies. As experience increases with electrical stimulation, results are less encouraging. Some recent studies fail to demonstrate any effect of electrical stimulation on curve progression in carefully controlled study groups. At this time, electrical stimulation must be considered experimental.

Surgical stabilization is necessary for patients who are not appropriate candidates for bracing (Fig 7–14). Idiopathic curves that exceed acceptable limits for adults at the time of initial evaluation in childhood are usually best treated operatively. Lesser curves associated with thoracic lordosis or extreme deformity are also most appropriately treated surgically. Documented progression in spite of nonoperative treatment is another indication for surgery, as is progression in children who cannot reliably participate in a brace program.

Techniques for the surgical treatment

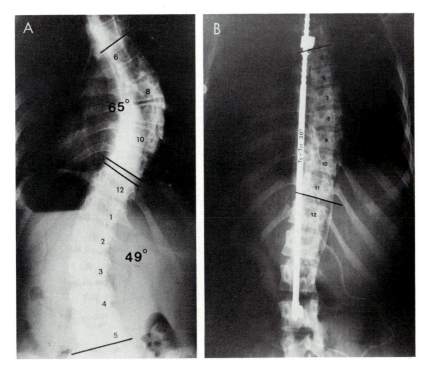

FIG 7–14.
A, preoperative roentgenogram of a curve too great to manage with bracing. **B,** postoperative roentgenogram demonstrates correction that can be obtained with Harrington instrumentation.

of spine deformities have evolved rapidly in the past two decades. Improved spinal instrumentation devices, intraoperative spinal cord monitoring, and advances in postoperative immobilization have made scoliosis surgery a safe and effective means of management of severe or progressive curvature and have dramatically changed the period of preoperative and postoperative disability. In the past, a period of preoperative casting or traction was sometimes employed to increase curve flexibility prior to surgery; this is no longer common. Advances in spinal instrumentation techniques have also changed the nature and duration of postoperative immobilization required. In most cases, patients can be placed in an ambulatory cast or postoperative orthosis 1 to 3 weeks after surgery and can begin to return to routine activities. Patients

usually return to school within 1 month of surgery and can begin to participate in noncontact sports within 2 months of surgery. Full resumption of activity can usually be permitted within 6 months.

Surgical treatment of spine deformity ordinarily consists of correction of the deformity and spine fusion (arthrodesis). Unless correction of the deformity is accompanied by meticulous fusion of the involved portion of the spine, eventual failure of instrumentation and loss of correction can be expected to occur. To obtain fusion, the posterior articulations of the involved vertebral bodies must be exposed, denuded of articular cartilage, and carefully grafted with autogenous or allograft bone. The posterior portion of the iliac crest is an excellent site from which to obtain autogenous bone and is the most common donor site. Sometimes a combination of autogenous and allograft bone is employed if insufficient autogenous graft can be obtained.

A variety of instrumentation systems are currently employed to achieve correction of spine deformity. Harrington distraction instrumentation was the first of the modern implants to become widely used and is currently probably the most frequently employed technique for correction of scoliosis, either alone or in combination with other implants. Harrington instrumentation has the advantages of simplicity, safety, and reliability but requires more restrictive postoperative immobilization than other techniques and provides poor correction of sagittal-plane deformity. The combination of distraction instrumentation on the side of curve concavity with compression instrumentation on the convex side of the curve is sometimes employed to increase the rigidity of fixation.

Attempts to improve the correction that can be obtained at the time of scoliosis surgery and to lessen the requirements for postoperative immobilization have led to a number of modifications in scoliosis surgery. Two mechanical principles are common to the wide variety of instrumentation systems currently employed in addition to Harrington distraction rods:

1. Transverse traction loads applied to vertebral segments involved in a curve greatly increase corrective forces.
2. The rigidity of fixation increases as the number of vertebral segments instrumented increases.

The first modern system to effectively employ transverse traction and segmental instrumentation for the treatment of paralytic scoliosis was developed in Mexico during the last decade by Eduardo Luque. In the Luque technique, stainless steel wires are passed beneath the lamina of in-volved vertebrae and then tightened and twisted around previously contoured stainless steel rods. Correction of both coronal and sagittal-plane deformities is excellent, and the strength of fixation is such that patients can be mobilized immediately postoperatively with little or no external support. As with other instrumentation techniques, meticulous arthrodesis must accompany the procedure. The potential for neurologic injury is much higher with the Luque technique than with Harrington instrumentation since segmental wires must be passed beneath the lamina and into the spinal canal. Furthermore, removal of the implants when necessary is both difficult and dangerous. Nevertheless, in experienced hands the technique is extremely useful, especially in treatment of neuromuscular scoliosis.

Combinations of Harrington distraction instrumentation with transverse wiring are often employed to improve correction and increase rigidity of fixation. Sublaminar segmental wiring, as in the Luque method described above, can be used, although it carries the risks of neurologic injury common to procedures that involve placement of implants within the spinal canal. A modification of segmental wiring developed by Drummond in which wires are passed through the base of the spinous process of involved vertebrae rather than through the sublaminar space is employed by some scoliosis surgeons to lower the risk of neurologic injury yet achieve secure segmental fixation.

Efforts to improve correction, lessen the need for postoperative immobilization, and lower risks in scoliosis surgery continue to lead to new surgical techniques. Yves Cotrel in France has developed a system that combines multiple points of laminar and pedicular fixation with transverse traction between rods implanted on both the convex and concave sides of a curve. The Cotrel method of spinal instrumentation is currently being used at a number of centers in the United States and is a valuable addition to the surgical armamentarium.

Regardless of the surgical technique employed, the segments of the spine spanned by successful fusion are rigid; further growth does not occur across a solid fusion mass. Although patients who have undergone spine fusion have less back motion than normal patients, they usually have little functional handicap. In all cases, decreased motion is a small price to pay to avoid the complications of progressive curvature.

It is a grave mistake to postpone surgical treatment of a patient with severe idiopathic scoliosis until skeletal maturity. In many cases, the increased height that results from surgical correction exceeds that which would be gained by spinal growth. It is usually impossible to regain ground lost while awaiting full growth, and respiratory compromise associated with increasing curvature increases the risks of surgery.

Although surgical treatment of scoliosis has become routine, it is not without risks. The magnitude of the operative procedures is large, and the surgery is technically demanding. Blood loss during surgery can be extensive. The possibility of neurologic damage at the time of surgery must be considered carefully when surgical treatment is recommended. Spinal cord or nerve root injury may result from traction applied to the spinal cord, nerve roots, or blood vessels supplying the cord at the time of curve correction or from impingement by sublaminar instrumentation. The incidence of paralysis is quite low, probably less than one case per thousand, but patients must be aware of the possibility of potentially irreversible neurologic damage. Transient weakness or temporary paresthesias in the legs has been reported much more commonly, especially when sublaminar

wiring is employed. Intraoperative monitoring of spinal cord function is presently in use in some scoliosis centers and promises to significantly decrease the risks of unrecognized spinal cord damage.

Pseudarthrosis, or local failure of complete fusion, is a recognized problem in scoliosis surgery. At times, pseudarthrosis is the result of displacement of internal fixation devices and subsequent loss of stability. At other times, failure of fusion at one or more segments of a curve places abnormal stresses on implants and causes secondary instrument failure. Pseudarthrosis is usually manifested by pain and loss of correction. When documented, pseudarthrosis must be surgically repaired to prevent further loss of correction.

Congenital Scoliosis

Defective vertebral formation during embryonic development often produces severe spine deformity. At times the anomalies are severe enough to produce a spine asymmetry that is obvious at birth. At other times, the outward manifestations of underlying spine deformity develop during childhood. Such curves are termed *congenital*; they are always structural, and they differ significantly from idiopathic curves in behavior, prognosis, and treatment.

Congenital vertebral anomalies can be grouped into three broad categories: (1) failure of vertebral formation, (2) segmentation errors, and (3) mixed abnormalities. Hemivertebrae and trapezoidal vertebrae are common examples of formation abnormalities. The hypoplastic segment may be located laterally—producing a scoliotic deformity, anteriorly—producing a kyphotic deformity, or anterolaterally—producing a combination deformity (Fig 7–15). At times a series of hemivertebrae or trapezoidal vertebrae may be present at various locations and on alternate sides of the vertebral column, producing compen-

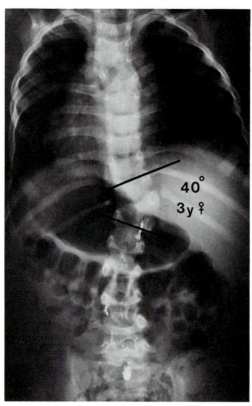

FIG 7–15.
Congenital scoliosis. A hemivertebra is present at T-12, producing a 40-degree curve over a short segment of the spine. Mixed formation and segmentation defects are present in the upper thoracic spine; they are balanced and so far have not produced a significant upper thoracic curve.

sating deformities. The fate of patients with formation defects depends on the nature of the vertebral deformity and its location in the spine. Some patients show little deformity and have nonprogressive curves; in others, the curves progress relentlessly unless treated early. All such patients must be carefully followed.

Segmentation defects are characterized by incomplete separation of vertebral bodies, posterior elements, or attached ribs into individual units. Affected vertebrae appear tethered together on radiologic examination. Unsegmented areas may lie in any location in the vertebral

column and produce corresponding spine deformities. Curves caused by segmentation errors are among the most malignant spine deformities and must be treated very aggressively.

Some patients with congenital scoliosis have mixed anomalies (Fig 7–16). Formation and segmentation defects may coexist in different areas of the spine. Hemivertebrae and unilateral unsegmented bars located close together on the same side of the spine may produce off-setting radiologic deformities with little clinical asymmetry. More often, however, segmentation and formation errors combine to produce spine deformities that are evident early in infancy and that rapidly worsen with growth. Such combination errors may be extremely difficult to treat, but unless controlled, they produce severe cardiopulmonary compromise and grotesque deformity.

Congenital abnormalities of the spine, like other congenital abnormalities, may result from a variety of embryonic mishaps. In some instances, exposure to x-irradiation or toxic drugs during the first trimester is responsible for defective vertebral formation. Congenital scoliosis may also occur as part of clinical syndromes associated with recognizable chromosomal aberrations. In most cases, however, the causes of congenital spine deformity are not apparent. Genetic influences appear to be significant in patients with myelomeningocele and in patients with multiple spine anomalies, but a family history is uncommon in patients with isolated vertebral anomalies.

Teratogenic influences that affect the developing spine may damage other organ systems as well. Congenital genitourinary tract anomalies are especially common in patients with congenital scoliosis. An overall incidence of 20% has been reported; patients with congenital abnormalities of the cervical spine have an even greater risk of associated renal

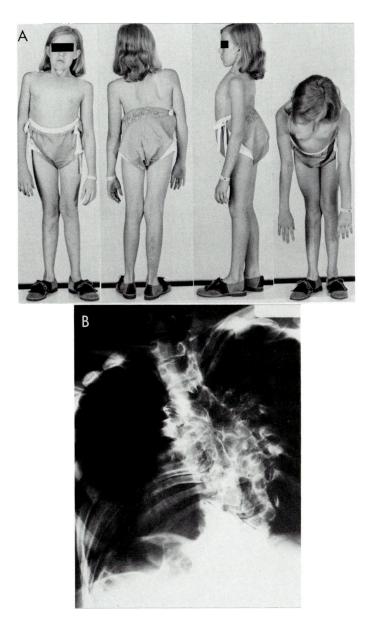

FIG 7–16.
Mixed congenital anomalies. A series of segmentation and formation abnormalities are present and have produced severe curvature. **A,** clinical photographs, age 10 years. **B,** radiologic appearance, age 17 years. At this time, lung vital capacity was 45% of predicted.

abnormalities. Unilateral renal agenesis is the most common genitourinary tract anomaly in patients with congenital scoliosis; duplication of the renal pelvis or ureters, renal ectopia, horseshoe kidney, and renal tubular ectasia have also been reported. Genital hypoplasia or absence on the affected side occurs on occasion. The incidence of obstructive uropathy in congenital scoliosis is about 2.5%. Because such patients may have no urinary tract symptoms at the time of discovery of congenital spine deformity, all should have a thorough urologic work-up as part of their initial evaluation.

Diastematomyelia, a longitudinal bifurcation in the spinal cord with an interposed bony, fibrous, or cartilaginous bar, occurs in about 5% of congenital scoliosis patients (Fig 7–17). Diastematomyelia is one of a group of associated congenital abnormalities of the spinal cord and vertebral column that includes myelomeningocele, dermal sinuses and dermoid cysts, neurenteric cysts, intradural lipomas, and diplomyelia. Patients with diastematomyelia often have skin abnormalities overlying the lesion; dimples, café au lait spots, and hairy patches are common.

Lower extremity weakness, reflex changes, and foot deformities such as pes cavus, equinovarus, and pes planus are frequent findings. Incontinence of urine or stool often occurs. Roentgenograms of patients with congenital scoliosis and diastematomyelia usually show widening of the interpeduncular distance in the region of the defect. Myelography and contrast-enhanced computed axial body tomography usually demonstrate the offending bar.

Diastematomyelia may cause tethering of the spinal cord during growth or during treatment of associated scoliosis, with resultant neurologic deficit. Previously asymptomatic children, with or without congenital scoliosis, who develop lower extremity weakness, progressive

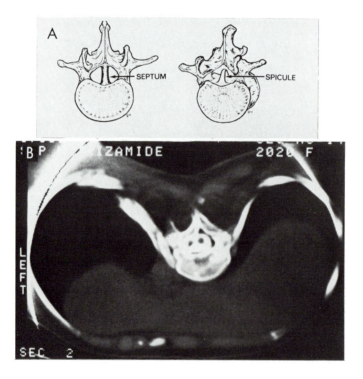

FIG 7–17.
Diastematomyelia. A longitudinal bar extends posteriorly from the vertebral body into the neural canal. It may be complete or incomplete and may be part bone and part fibrous tissue. **A,** diagrammatic representation. (From Hood RW, et al: Diastematomyelia and structural spinal deformities. *J Bone Joint Surg Am* 1980; 62:520. Reproduced by permission.) **B,** computed tomography combined with myelography in the patient illustrated in Figure 7–16 demonstrates bifurcation of the lower thoracic spinal cord.

foot deformity, or incontinence during growth must be carefully evaluated for spinal cord impingement. Exploration may be necessary in the presence of progressive neurologic impairment; it is essential if correction of coexistent congenital scoliosis is planned.

Congenital hip dysplasia, congenital heart disease, hearing impairments, and other musculoskeletal deformities such as clubfoot, metatarsus adductus, congenital elevation of the scapula (Sprengel's deformity), torticollis, and Klippel-Feil syndrome all have been reported in association with congenital scoliosis. Congenital scoliosis may be the least obvious of a number of congenital anomalies. The finding of one such anomaly in an infant signals the possibility of a significant embryonic insult and should lead to careful systemic evaluation.

Until recently, patients with congenital scoliosis were neglected, owing partly to lack of long-term follow-up information. Large-scale studies by MacEwen et al. and Winter et al. clearly show that all congenital curves are potentially progressive, and that once progression begins, it continues throughout growth. Compensatory curves develop above and below areas of vertebral deformity and become secondary structural deformities with time. When severe, these curves progress even after termination of growth and may themselves cause significant morbidity. Treatment of congenital scoliosis in almost all cases should begin as soon as progression is documented. Some curves, especially those produced by unilateral segmentation failures, are so likely to progress that treatment is justified as soon as the defect is demonstrated.

In most cases, treatment of congenital scoliosis is surgical. Spinal bracing rarely if ever prevents progression of congenital scoliosis. In some instances, bracing may be useful to encourage the development of compensatory curves necessary to maintain trunk balance or to prevent progression of compensatory curves after surgical stabilization of an area of congenital curvature. It is a grave mistake to delay referral of a patient with congenital scoliosis while awaiting further growth. When progression begins, it continues relentlessly. Patients do not get taller; they only become more deformed. Even though surgically fused segments do not grow, the functional and cosmetic results of a short, straight spine are far better than those of a short, deformed spine. In most cases of congenital spine deformity, short segmental fusions performed early in childhood prevent severe deformity and permit normal growth of unaffected segments.

Neuromuscular Scoliosis

A high percentage of children with paralytic diseases develop spine deformity. Scoliosis and kyphoscoliosis may complicate both progressive and nonprogressive neuromuscular conditions. Such patients are doubly at risk: postural difficulties and respiratory problems caused by the primary paralytic disorder are compounded by the development of spinal curvature. Neuromuscular curves do not behave like idiopathic or congenital curves; once curvature begins, it usually progresses even after termination of growth. Curves that begin early in life are especially likely to produce severe spinal deformity.

Collapse of the spine compounds the respiratory problems that many patients with neuromuscular diseases experience. Patients with static disorders often show decreasing pulmonary function directly related to increasing spine deformity (Fig 7–18); patients with progressive neuromuscular diseases are even more seriously affected. As curves progress, the ribs on the concave side of the curve impinge on the iliac crest, increasing respiratory compromise and causing pain and

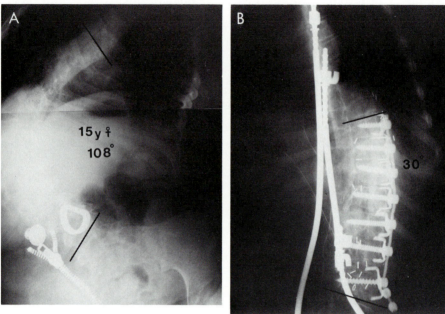

FIG 7–18.
Neuromuscular scoliosis. **A,** collapsing curves of large magnitude commonly develop in patients with paralytic disorders. This curve of greater than 100 degrees severely compromised respiratory function and made unsupported sitting impossible in this patient with fascioscapulohumeral dystrophy. **B,** anterior and posterior spinal instrumentation and fusion have improved pulmonary function and restored the ability to sit independently.

maceration of skin folds. Pelvic obliquity often develops, and the resultant uneven weight distribution may cause skin breakdown over the ischial tuberosities. As sitting balance deteriorates, patients are forced to use their arms for props, depriving themselves of much of their remaining independence. Eventually most patients become bedridden and completely dependent on others for care. Respiratory insufficiency and infection are the most frequent causes of death and are secondary to both the underlying disease and the resultant spine deformity.

Scoliosis and kyphoscoliosis occur in a wide variety of progressive and nonprogressive neurologic and muscle diseases. Paralytic curves can be divided into broad categories of primary neuropathic and primary myopathic disorders, although in some instances such as arthrogryposis multiplex congenita, the distinction is not clear. The nature of the primary neuromuscular disorder is important in planning treatment; progressive neurologic and myopathic diseases are far more difficult to manage than nonprogressive diseases. A partial listing of neuromuscular disorders associated with scoliosis is given in Table 7–1.

The goal of treatment in neuromuscular scoliosis is to prevent the complications of progressive spine deformity with minimum loss of function and minimum risk to the patient. Young patients with rapidly progressive neurologic or myopathic diseases present much more difficult management problems than older children or adolescents with static primary disorders.

In general, conventional bracing techniques are not as effective in children with neuromuscular disorders as in patients with idiopathic scoliosis. Children

TABLE 7–1.
Some Neuromuscular Disorders Associated With Scoliosis

Neuropathic disorders
  Progressive
    Spinal muscular atrophy
    Friedreich's ataxia
    Charcot-Marie-Tooth disease
    Syringomyelia
    Spinal cord tumors
  Nonprogressive
    Cerebral palsy
    Spinal cord trauma
    Poliomyelitis
    Arthrogryposis
    Reye's syndrome
Myopathic disorders
  Progressive
    Muscular dystrophies
    Duchenne type
    Fascioscapulohumeral
    Limb-girdle
  Nonprogressive
    Fiber-type disproportions
    Arthrogryposis

with paralytic diseases cannot participate in the exercise programs necessary for maximum benefit from bracing, and the dynamic effects of bracing are lost. Attempts to correct curvature passively with pressure pads often lead to skin breakdown and necrosis. Furthermore, bracing may prevent patients from achieving postures necessary for standing balance and may make a marginal walker a sitting patient. Finally, since neuromuscular curves may progress even after skeletal maturation, bracing may not be a practical alternative for patients with long life expectancies.

Custom-fabricated total contact braces are sometimes effective in controlling neuromuscular curves, especially in patients with progressive neurologic diseases who are not candidates for operative stabilization. These braces are manufactured around a plaster positive of the individual patient's trunk and distribute corrective forces over a wide area. In some designs, the posterior portion of the brace is incorporated into a custom-fabricated wheelchair insert that supports a patient comfortably while sitting. These devices are difficult to construct and require the best efforts of an experienced orthotist.

Surgical treatment of neuromuscular scoliosis is indicated in most patients with nonprogressive or slowly progressive primary disorders. Because bed rest is poorly tolerated and most patients have preexisting respiratory impairment, surgery must be preceded and followed by aggressive physical and respiratory therapy programs. Fusions often are extensive and often include the sacrum. Internal fixation with effective spine instrumentation is imperative to decrease the need for postoperative immobilization. Both anterior and posterior spine fusion may be necessary. The pseudarthrosis rate is higher than in other types of spinal fusion, and repeated grafting may be necessary. Nevertheless, surgical correction of neuromuscular scoliosis is presently the method of choice in patients who can safely tolerate the extensive procedures required.

Kyphosis and Lordosis

Unlike lateral deviation of the spine, which is always abnormal, anteroposterior curves are normal in the cervical, thoracic, and lumbar spine. The anteroposterior alignment of the spine changes with growth until, at maturity, lordotic configurations are present in the cervical and lumbar spine and a kyphotic curve is present in the thoracic region. The borderlines of normal for kyphotic and lordotic curves are not well defined, and the complications of progression are not as well documented as those of scoliotic progression. The normal range for thoracic kyphosis is usually said to be from 20 to 40 degrees. Lumbar and cervical lordosis standards are not as clear. Abnormal in-

creases in kyphosis and lordosis are un-
sightly and predispose to back pain in
adult life. In addition, severe kyphotic
curves may cause spinal cord impingement and paraplegia, although these complications are not seen consistently. Respiratory compromise may occur in some
patients with marked thoracic kyphosis,
although more moderate degrees of kyphosis are not associated with clinically
significant alterations in pulmonary function. Loss of thoracic kyphosis and thoracic lordosis interfere much more consistently with pulmonary function.

In some respects, kyphotic and lordotic curves are 90-degree rotational ana-
logues of scoliotic curves. Abnormal increases in curvature may be flexible or
structural, and they may be idiopathic,
congenital, or paralytic in origin. Minor
flexible increases in either thoracic kyphosis or lumbar lordosis produce a
round-shouldered or swaybacked appearance and are often caused by weak abdominal or trunk musculature. More severe curves may be associated with
anterior wedging of vertebral bodies,
sometimes called Scheuermann's disease,
or with congenital abnormalities of vertebral formation or segmentation. Paralytic
disorders, especially those associated with
congenital or surgical defects in the posterior elements of the vertebral column,
often produce extreme kyphosis.

Idiopathic Kyphosis

Roundback deformity is encountered
in 3% to 5% of otherwise healthy adolescents at the time of school screening examination for spine deformity (Fig 7–19).
The parents of such patients frequently
complain of their poor posture; prominent kyphosis is evident on forward
bending. Concomitant scoliotic deformities are sometimes present. Girls are affected slightly more often than boys. If repeated examination confirms initial
suspicions, then roentgenographic studies
are necessary.

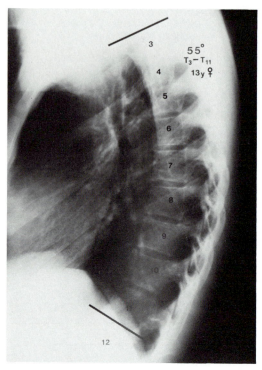

FIG 7–19.
Juvenile roundback. Kyphosis is present, but there
are no structural changes in the thoracic spine.

Initial roentgenograms should consist
of standing posteroanterior and lateral
views. Supine hyperextension films made
with a plastic bolster placed under the
apex of the deformity may be necessary if
initial roentgenograms are abnormal.
Careful shielding and collimation are essential, especially on lateral views, to
avoid excess radiation exposure. Kyphotic
and lordotic curves are measured in the
same manner as scoliotic curves, using
the Cobb-Lippman method. Maximally
tilted vertebral bodies are considered the
end points of curvature.

Two radiologic patterns are common
in children with roundback. Some children, especially preadolescents, have thoracic kyphotic curves of 40 to 60 degrees,
with no underlying structural vertebral
changes. Usually these curves are quite
flexible and readily correct on hyperextension. Compensatory increased lumbar lor-

dosis is often present, producing a sway-backed appearance. Thoracic kyphotic curves of this type are usually termed juvenile or adolescent postural roundback.

More rigid kyphotic deformities occur in some adolescents. Curves of greater than 60 degrees may be present, and little correction may be evident on hyperextension. Careful inspection of roentgenograms of these patients often shows endplate erosion and wedging of vertebral bodies at the apex of the curve. Such vertebral changes are sometimes called Scheuermann's disease, and affected patients are often said to have Scheuermann's kyphosis (Fig 7–20). The pathologic significance of vertebral body wedging and end-plate irregularity is not clear; it is not certain whether the radio-

logic changes of Scheuermann's disease are primary or secondary phenomena. They are significant in planning treatment, however, since patients with vertebral wedging are usually less flexible, and the curvature is more difficult to correct. Evidence indicates that these patients are more likely to have progression of curvature and back pain than patients with postural roundback.

Young patients with kyphotic curves of less than 60 degrees that are flexible and show no changes of Scheuermann's disease can often be successfully treated with a program of thoracic hyperextension exercises. These must be carefully supervised and faithfully performed to be effective, but in appropriately selected patients, they usually result in significant improvement in appearance. Patients must be carefully followed until the end of growth to guard against recurrence or progression of deformity.

Adolescents with kyphosis of greater than 60 degrees or with apical vertebral wedging do not respond well to exercise programs alone. Bracing is usually necessary to obtain correction. Modified Milwaukee or underarm braces are often quite effective in structural kyphotic curves of 50 to 70 degrees. Kyphosis brace programs differ slightly from scoliosis brace programs; often bracing may be started later in adolescence with success, and frequently full-time brace use is not required for as long as it is in patients with scoliosis. Night use, however, is often necessary until full spine growth is attained.

The indications for surgical treatment of idiopathic kyphosis are not well defined. It appears that patients with curves of greater than 70 degrees at skeletal maturity may have further progression in adult life and frequently have disabling back pain and fatigability. In addition, a small percentage of such patients may experience spinal cord compression later in life if curve progression occurs or if ar-

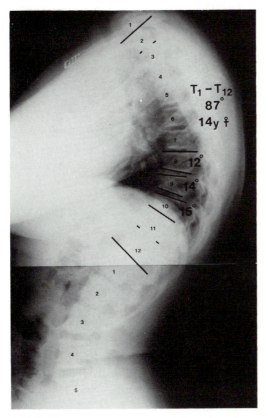

FIG 7–20.
Scheuermann's kyphosis. Severe roundback is present, associated with wedging of vertebral bodies at the apex of the curve.

thritic changes develop at the apex of curvature. At present, surgical correction of idiopathic kyphosis is reserved for adolescent patients with curves of greater than 70 degrees who are refractory to brace treatment and for older patients with pain and progression of deformity. Surgical correction is difficult and not without risk. Often both anterior and posterior spine fusion are necessary, and the risks of neurologic compromise are greater than in scoliosis surgery. Instrumentation failure is a well-documented problem, and pseudarthrosis occurs more often than in scoliosis surgery. When carefully performed, however, surgical correction of kyphosis can provide excellent functional and cosmetic results.

Congenital Kyphosis

Vertebral segmentation and formation errors located in the anterior or anterolateral portion of the spinal column consistently produce kyphotic and kyphoscoliotic deformities. In some patients, a gibbus located over the apex of deformity is present at birth. In other patients, kyphosis becomes evident later in infancy or childhood. Like congenital vertebral malformations that produce scoliosis, anterior and anterolateral spinal defects may be associated with other systemic anomalies. A careful search for renal, cardiac, auditory, and other skeletal abnormalities must be made.

Incomplete anterior segmentation of vertebrae into separate units produces kyphosis of varying severity. In some patients, incomplete segmentation is obvious on lateral roentgenograms made at birth. In other patients, incomplete segmentation may not become apparent until later in childhood when cartilaginous bridges between vertebral units ossify. Kyphotic curves produced by anterior segmentation errors tend to be less severe than scoliotic curves produced by lateral segmentation errors, but the prognosis in individual cases is unpredictable.

Congenital kyphosis caused by anterior vertebral formation failures is potentially much more severe. Hemivertebrae located in the posterior portion of the vertebral column serve as keystones around which severe kyphosis develops. Rapid progression is the rule, and a high incidence of associated neurologic impairment exists when uncontrolled progression occurs.

Patients with congenital kyphosis must be promptly referred for orthopedic evaluation and treatment. Careful observation is essential. Progression of congenital kyphosis cannot be tolerated. Brace treatment is usually ineffective, and spine fusion may be necessary early in life to prevent irreversible neurologic damage and vertebral column deformity.

Spondylolysis and Spondylolisthesis

Abnormal formation or traumatic disruption of the bony supporting elements of the lower lumbar and lumbosacral spine occur in about 6% of the North American population. The radiologic abnormalities may be incidental findings in entirely asymptomatic individuals, or lumbosacral dysplasia may be associated with back pain and progressive deformity. The theories about the etiology and natural history of these lesions and their classification and treatment are controversial.

Because of the normal lordotic tilt of the lumbar spine, the bodies of the fifth lumbar and first sacral vertebrae are not parallel to the transverse plane of the body. Shear forces are generated between the vertebrae in the seated and erect positions. Forward displacement of L-5 on S-1 is normally prevented by the stable articulation of the superior facets of S-1 and the inferior facets of L-5. Defective formation of the posterior elements of the lumbosacral joint or defects in the bony connection between the body and arch of the fifth lumbar vertebra render the anterior junction of L-5 and S-1 unstable and may lead to relative displacement.

Spondylolisthesis refers to forward displacement of one vertebral body upon another. Classic spondylolisthesis in children and adolescents almost always involves the fifth lumbar and first sacral units. Instability may be acute or chronic and may arise from a variety of traumatic or developmental lesions. Acute fracture dislocation of vertebral units resulting from violent trauma is, in a strict sense, one form of spondylolisthesis, but because it differs so greatly from other types of spondylolisthesis in etiology, presentation, and treatment, it is usually considered as a separate entity.

Defective formation of the posterior articular components of L-5 or S-1 decreases the stability of the lumbosacral joint (Fig 7–21,A). Forward displacement of L-5 may follow, especially if the anterior junction of L-5 and S-1 is quite oblique or if the S-1 body is defective. Such slips are termed *dysplastic* spondylolisthesis.

Defects in the bony connection of the posterior arch of L-5 with its body are called *spondylolysis* (Fig 7–21,B). Most patients with spondylolisthesis have spondylolytic defects. In such instances, the posterior articulation of L-5 and S-1 remains intact, but the body of L-5 slips forward, leaving a gap in the vertebral arch (Fig 7–22). The posterior elements of L-5 remain attached to the superior articular facets of S-1. The gap between the anterior and posterior elements of L-5 fills with cartilaginous tissue that may in time hypertrophy enough to cause nerve root impingement in later life.

The degree of displacement in both dysplastic and spondylolytic spondylolisthesis can be estimated by noting the position of the posterior border of the L-5 vertebral body with respect to the body of the first sacral vertebra. Slips less than 25% of the width of the first sacral body are considered mild; slips between 25% and 50% are considered moderate. Slips greater than 50% are considered severe. At times, slippage may be so severe that L-5 may be located in front of S-1. The angular relationship of the body of L-5 to the sacrum is often used in planning treatment of spondylolisthesis; a variety of measurement methods have been developed to aid in management, but they are complex and not necessary for diagnosis of spondylolysis or spondylolisthesis.

Etiology

The cause of spondylolysis is unclear. It appears to be multifactorial; both hereditary and mechanical factors have been implicated. Age, race, and sex appear to influence its occurrence. Spondylolysis is rare in children less than 5 years old, but by age 6 years, it is present in about 5% of white North American children. Another 1% develops defects later in childhood and adolescence. Spondylolysis appears to be less common in blacks and much more common in some North American Eskimo groups. The lowest incidence has been reported in black females and the highest in white males. Relatives of patients with spondylolisthesis are much more likely to be affected than individuals in the general population.

Fatigue fracture through the pars interarticularis or isthmus of L-5 is presently considered to be important in the development of spondylolysis and spondylolisthesis. In most patients with spondylolisthesis, this occurs through an area of congenital weakness or malformation that may be genetically determined as a result of the ordinary activities of childhood. Less commonly, fracture may occur in a previously normal vertebral isthmus as a result of strenuous, repetitive athletic activities. Activities that involve repeated trunk flexion and extension have been particularly implicated; adolescent divers and gymnasts are reported to be signifi-

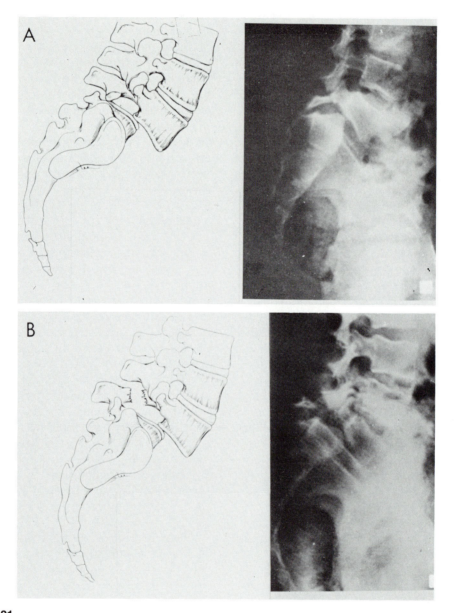

FIG 7–21.
Spondylolisthesis. **A,** forward displacement of L-5 on S-1 due to defective formation of the posterior L-5–S-1 joint. **B,** displacement associated with a spondylotic defect in the posterior elements of L-5 (see text). (From Hensinger RN, et al: Surgical management of spondylolisthesis in children and adolescents. *Spine* 1976; 1:207. Reproduced by permission.)

cantly more susceptible to spondylolysis and spondylolisthesis.

Spondylolysis differs from other fatigue fractures in a number of important respects. Spondylolytic defects develop much earlier than other fatigue fractures and usually without identifiable cause. In contrast to other fatigue fractures, healing of spondylolytic defects is the exception rather than the rule. Callus formation is

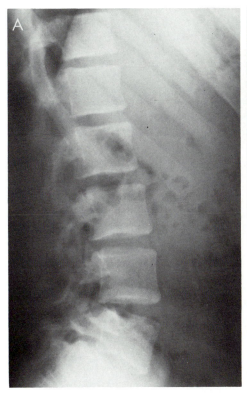

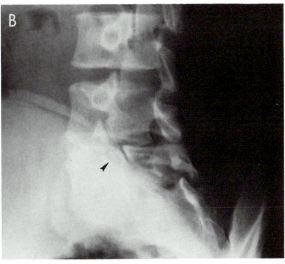

FIG 7–22.
A, moderate slip of L-5 on S-1 in a patient with spondylolysis. **B,** oblique roentgenogram demonstrates clearly the defect *(arrow)* in the posterior elements of L-5.

uncommon. Finally, in distinction to other fatigue fractures, patients with spondylolysis are usually asymptomatic at the time of presumed failure. Nevertheless, fatigue fracture seems at present to be the most likely cause of spondylolysis.

Presentation

Symptoms in patients with spondylolysis and spondylolisthesis are quite variable. Some patients with minimal slips have extreme pain, while others with moderate to severe slips have little or no discomfort. When present, pain is usually ill defined and poorly localized. Most patients complain of aching in the lumbar and lumbosacral regions. Buttock and posterior thigh pain may be present, but radicular symptoms of nerve root compression are usually absent. Discomfort is usually increased by exercise and relieved by rest.

Signs vary with the severity of spondylolisthesis. Asymptomatic patients with slips of mild severity may have no outward manifestations of vertebral abnormality. Patients with moderate to severe slips usually have tenderness on palpation of the lumbar spine and increased lumbar lordosis. Spasm of the hamstring muscles may extend the sacral spine, causing the buttocks to seem prominent and flattened or heart-shaped in appearance. In moderate and severe degrees of slip, the step-off of L-5 on S-1 can often be palpated. A flexible scoliotic deformity caused by paraspinal muscle spasm may be present. Lower extremity muscle strength, sensation, and reflexes are usually normal in children and adolescents except in the most severe slips. Bladder and bowel function are usually not affected. Symptoms and signs of nerve root compression and mechanical instability are much more common in the adult patient with progressive or severe untreated adolescent spondylolisthesis.

Hamstring muscle spasm is a common finding in patients with symptomatic spondylolisthesis and at times may be the chief presenting problem. Affected patients are unable to flex far enough forward to touch their toes without bending their knees. When severe, hamstring spasm causes a loss of normal lumbar lordosis and a flattened appearance of the low back. Hamstring muscle spasm also interferes with gait; stride length is shortened, and patients run with a peculiar stiff-legged posture. The cause of hamstring spasm in spondylolisthesis is unclear; it does not appear to be caused by compression of spinal nerves, and it is rarely accompanied by other signs of nerve root compromise. Most authorities feel it is a result of abnormal strain on the hamstring muscles caused by mechanical instability of the lumbosacral junction since surgical stabilization of the spine usually relieves hamstring spasm even without decompression of the neural elements.

Treatment

The management of patients with spondylolysis and spondylolisthesis is controversial. Treatment depends on the age of the patient, symptoms, degree of slip, and associated neurologic findings. Almost all authorities believe that asymptomatic children with minimal slips require no active treatment. Many of these children are discovered to have spondylolysis only as an incidental finding on roentgenograms made for other reasons. There is probably little reason to restrict activities when patients are asymptomatic and have only spondylolysis or mild spondylolisthesis. Since progression occurs in a small proportion of these patients, radiologic follow-up at 4- to 6-

month intervals from the time of discovery through adolescence is indicated.

Asymptomatic children and adolescents with moderate degrees of spondylolisthesis should be carefully followed. It is reasonable to restrict such patients from participation in contact sports and gymnastics. Radiologic signs of progression in these patients usually signal the need for surgical stabilization of the lumbosacral junction.

Symptomatic children with mild to moderate spondylolisthesis in most cases should be given a trial of nonoperative treatment. A period of bed rest, sometimes in a plaster body jacket, often relieves pain and associated muscle spasm. Gradual resumption of activities can be permitted after 4 to 8 weeks. A lumbosacral spine brace may be useful in older children after the initial period of immobilization. Those sports that require trunk flexion and extension may have to be restricted.

Surgical treatment is usually reserved for patients with severe or progressive slips or symptomatic patients with more mild slips who do not respond to nonoperative therapy. In most cases, fusion of L-5 to S-1 stops progression and eliminates pain. Fusion from L-4 to the sacrum may be necessary in more severe slips. Reduction of the deformity is rarely necessary in mild to moderate slips but is sometimes recommended in more severe slips. Nerve root decompression, often needed in adults with degenerative arthritis and spondylolisthesis, is rarely necessary in children.

Torticollis

Tilting of the head and neck, called *wryneck* or *torticollis*, may have a number of causes. Head and neck asymmetry may be present at birth, or torticollis may develop later in childhood or in adolescence.

Often torticollis is the principal manifestation of self-limiting muscular or inflammatory processes. In other cases, it may be the only outward sign of far more serious disease. A partial listing of the causes of torticollis is given in Table 7–2.

Torticollis in infants is most commonly associated with abnormalities of the sternocleidomastoid muscle (Fig 7–23). Birth trauma, intrauterine malposition, muscle fibrous "tumors," and venous abnormalities within the muscle have all been implicated, but no single cause has been identified. For whatever reason, shortening of the sternocleidomastoid muscle results in a tilt of the head toward the affected muscle and rotation of the chin toward the opposite side. A palpable lump is sometimes present within the affected muscle during the first few weeks of life, but it usually spontaneously disappears. Flattening of the head and slight facial asymmetry are usually present. If the deformity is not corrected, contractures of the soft tissues on the side of the affected sternocleidomastoid muscle occur, and pronounced facial asymmetry may develop.

TABLE 7–2.
Some Causes of Torticollis

Muscular
    Congenital sternocleidomastoid
       muscle abnormality
    Neck muscle stain
Skeletal
    Congenital cervical scoliosis
    Congenital abnormalities of the
       atlanto-occipital junction or C1–
       2 articulation
    Klippel-Feil syndrome
    Idiopathic cervicothoracic scoliosis
    Traumatic cervical subluxation
Inflammatory
    Cervical lymphadenitis
    Upper respiratory tract infection
    Intervertebral diskitis
Neoplastic
    Vertebral column tumors
    Spinal cord tumors

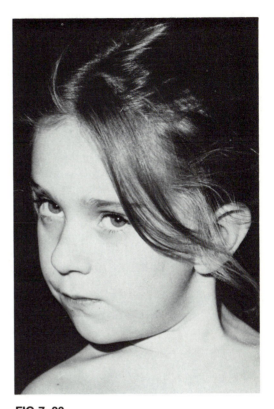

FIG 7–23.
Congenital muscular torticollis. Shortening of the sternocleidomastoid muscle tilts the head toward the affected muscle and rotates chin in the opposite direction. In this untreated 5-year-old girl, early facial asymmetry is present.

The first step in treatment of torticollis due to sternocleidomastoid contracture is confirmation of the diagnosis. Careful roentgenographic examination of the cervical spine is necessary. Anteroposterior and lateral views of the neck should be obtained initially; laminography may be necessary in some cases. Particular attention should be given to the atlanto-occipital and the atlantoaxial regions. Manipulative exercises in infants with upper cervical instability may have disastrous consequences.

If no underlying skeletal abnormalities are identified, a program of stretching exercises is indicated to lengthen the contracted sternocleidomastoid muscle. The head is first tilted toward the opposite shoulder, and the chin is then rotated toward the affected side. Exercises should be performed gently, and the corrected position should be maintained for 5 to 10 seconds on each repetition. A program of 10 to 15 repetitions 4 times daily is sufficient in most cases. Positioning the infant's crib with the normal side of the neck toward the wall will sometimes stimulate an infant who lies prone to turn his head and stretch the sternocleidomastoid muscle. It is not, however, a reliable method of treatment.

Surgical release of sternocleidomastoid contractures is necessary for the rare cases in which exercises do not achieve correction and for older children with untreated torticollis. Delay results in severe facial deformity that will not completely correct after release. Surgical results are mixed; younger children do best after sternocleidomastoid release. Recurrence of contracture is a problem in older children.

Neck muscle strain is a common cause of acute wryneck in older children who are active in contact sports. Injury produces muscle spasm and inflammation, which in turn produces torticollis. Treatment consists of excluding underlying cervical fracture or dislocation and then starting a program of warm soaks and mild anti-inflammatory medications. At times, a soft collar is useful in relieving pain.

Torticollis associated with congenital cervical vertebral anomalies is more serious (Fig 7–24). Because the primary cause of wryneck in these patients is skeletal,

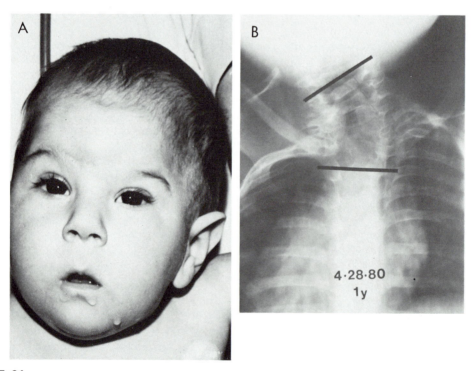

FIG 7–24.
Congenital cervical scoliosis may present as torticollis. **A,** the clinical appearance of a 1-year-old child with congenital cervical scoliosis. The chin is tilted toward the right, and the occiput is tilted toward the left. **B,** radiologic views of the cervical spine in this patient show multihemivertebra formation and an unsegmented congenital bar on the left side of the lower cervical spine. Note that by convention, scoliosis films are viewed as if the examiner were facing the patient's back.

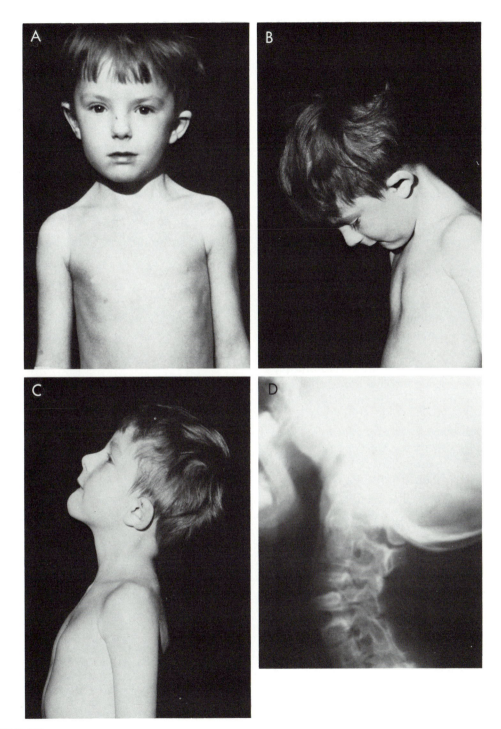

FIG 7–25.
Klippel-Feil syndrome. The clinical findings of a short neck, low hair line, and limited neck motion are often associated with congenital vertebral anomalies. **A–C,** clinical photographs of a 7-year-old boy with Klippel-Feil syndrome. **D,** roentgenograms showing congenital fusion of the posterior elements of C-1 and C-2 and fusion of the interspace between C-5, C-6, and C-7.

soft tissue stretching cannot provide lasting correction. The eventual severity of curvature and associated head deformity depends on the nature of the vertebral defect. Cervical hemivertebrae are sometimes less deforming than unsegmented unilateral cervical bars. As in other cases of congenital spine curvature, a careful search for other systemic anomalies must be made (Fig 7–25). Treatment of torticollis caused by congenital cervical scoliosis is difficult; surgical fusion of the affected area may be necessary to halt progression. It may be impossible to reverse facial asymmetry that has developed because of head tilt.

Acute torticollis in older children and adolescents may result from traumatic unilateral subluxation or dislocation of the facet joints of the atlantoaxial joint. The initial injury may be relatively minor, or it may be severe. Affected patients present with painful torticollis and cervical muscle spasm. The chin is rotated away from the side of subluxation, and the head is tilted toward the affected side. Active correction is not possible. Careful radiographic evaluation is essential. Anteroposterior, lateral, and open-mouth odontoid views should be obtained initially. Tomography may be necessary to rule out occult cervical fracture. Once the diagnosis is established, treatment may be started. Most acute cases subside with rest and cervical traction. A soft collar may provide pain relief after reduction. Surgical reduction has rarely been necessary for acute cases, but surgical fusion may be required when diagnosis has been delayed.

Occasionally children with acute bacterial or viral infections of the upper respiratory tract, middle ear, or cervical lymph nodes present with painful torticollis. Intervertebral diskitis may also cause torticollis. Treatment in these instances is directed toward the underlying disease. Associated torticollis usually subsides spontaneously.

Painful torticollis may be the presenting sign of vertebral or spinal cord tumors. Although such lesions are uncommon, they must be considered in the differential diagnosis of torticollis if no other cause is apparent. Neurologic abnormalities are uncommon in torticollis of nonneoplastic origin; their presence on initial examination makes the diagnosis of spinal cord tumor much more likely. Neurosurgical consultation should be obtained for children with torticollis and neurologic abnormalities and in cases where no other cause is found on initial physical and radiologic evaluation.

GLOSSARY*

Adolescent scoliosis: Lateral spine deviation developing after onset of puberty but before maturity.

Apex vertebra: Most rotated, least tilted vertebra in a curve; by convention, its location establishes the location of the curve in the spine, e.g., cervical, cervicothoracic, thoracic, thoracolumbar, lumbar.

Compensatory curve: A curve, most often initially nonstructural, that develops above or below a primary curve to maintain trunk alignment.

Congenital scoliosis: Lateral spine deviation that results from defective embryonic spinal formation.

Congenital kyphosis: Apex posterior spine deformity resulting from defective formation or segmentation of the embryonic spine.

End vertebra: Point of inflection of spinal curvature: most tilted, least rotated vertebral body at each end of a scoliotic curve; most tilted body at either end of a lordotic or kyphotic curve.

Idiopathic scoliosis: Most common type of structural scoliosis; spine deformity that develops for as yet unestablished reasons.

Infantile scoliosis: Lateral spine deformity present at birth or that develops during the first years of life.

Juvenile scoliosis: Spine deformity that develops after early childhood but before puberty.

Kyphosis: Apex posterior angulation of the spine.

Kyphoscoliosis: Combined kyphotic and scoliotic spine deformity.

Lordosis: Apex anterior angulation of the spine.

*Glossary adapted from Winter RB: The spine, in Lovell WW, Winter RB (eds): *Pediatric Orthopaedics.* Philadelphia, JB Lippincott Co, 1978, p 681.

Major curve: Largest magnitude curve; often but not always the first curve to develop and the most structural curve.

Minor curve: Curve of the lesser magnitude; often compensatory; may be structural or nonstructural.

Nonstructural curve: Spine deformity that corrects on supine lateral bending roentgenograms.

Primary curve: First curve to develop; often but not always the major curve.

Risser's sign: The extent of excursion of the iliac crest apophysis. An indicator of skeletal maturation.

Secondary curve: Curve that develops after primary curve to maintain compensation. When structural changes are present in all segments of a deformed spine at the time of first evaluation, it is not possible to distinguish primary from secondary curves.

Structural curve: Curve that does not fully straighten or derotate on supine lateral bending roentgenograms.

SUGGESTED READINGS

General

Moe JH, Winter RB, Bradford DS, et al: *Scoliosis and Other Spinal Deformities.* Philadelphia, WB Saunders Co, 1978.

Winter RB: The spine, in Lovell WB, Winter RB (eds): *Pediatric Orthopaedics.* Philadelphia, JB Lippincott Co, 1978, chapter 16.

Normal Growth: Embryology, Growth, and Development

Anderson M, Hwang SC, Green WT: Growth of the trunk in normal boys and girls during the second decade of life. *J Bone Joint Surg Am* 1965; 47:1554.

Parke WW: Development of the spine, in Rothman RH, Simeone FA (eds): *The Spine.* Philadelphia, WB Saunders Co, 1975.

Radiography

Gray JE, et al: Reduction of radiation exposure during radiography for scoliosis. *J Bone Joint Surg Am* 1983; 53:5.

Idiopathic Scoliosis

Collis DK, Ponseti IV: Long-term follow-up of patients with idiopathic scoliosis not treated surgically. *J Bone Joint Surg Am* 1969; 51:425.

Cowell HR, Hall JN, MacEwen GD: Genetic aspects of idiopathic scoliosis. *Clin Orthop* 1972; 86:121.

Ferriera JH, James JR: Progressive and resolving infantile idiopathic scoliosis: Differential diagnosis. *J Bone Joint Surg Br* 1972; 54:648.

Gore DR, Parsehl R, Sepic S, et al: Scoliosis screening: Results of a community project. *Pediatrics* 1981; 67:196.

James JIP: The management of infants with scoliosis. *J Bone Joint Surg Br* 1975; 57:422.

Mehta MH: The rib-vertebra angle in the early diagnosis between resolving and progressive infantile scoliosis. *J Bone Joint Surg Br* 1973; 54:230.

Nachemson A: A long-term follow-up study of nontreated scoliosis. *Acta Orthop Scand* 1968; 39:466.

Nilsonne V, Lundgren KD: Long-term prognosis in idiopathic scoliosis. *Acta Orthop Scand* 1968; 39:456.

Ponseti IV, Friedman B: Prognosis in idiopathic scoliosis. *J Bone Joint Surg Am* 1950; 32:381.

Riseborough EJ, Wynne-Davies R: A genetic survey of idiopathic scoliosis in Boston, Mass. *J Bone Joint Surg Am* 1973; 55:974.

Rogala EJ, Drummond DS, Gurr J: Scoliosis: Incidence and natural history, a prospective epidemiological study. *J Bone Joint Surg Am* 1978; 60:173.

Wynne-Davies R: Familial (idiopathic) scoliosis: A family survey. *J Bone Joint Surg Br* 1968; 50:24.

Congenital Scoliosis

MacEwen GD, Winter RB, Hardy JH: Evaluation of kidney anomalies in congenital scoliosis. *J Bone Joint Surg Am* 1972; 54:1451.

Winter RB, Moe JH, Eilers VE: Congenital scoliosis: A study of 234 patients treated and untreated. *J Bone Joint Surg Am* 1968; 50:1.

Winter RB, Haven JJ, Moe JH, et al: Diastematomyelia and congenital spine deformities. *J Bone Joint Surg Am* 1974; 56:27.

Neuromuscular Scoliosis

Bonnet C, Gibson DA: Thoracolumbar scoliosis in cerebral palsy. *J Bone Joint Surg Am* 1976; 58:328.

Hensinger RN, MacEwen GD: Spinal deformity associated with heritable neurologic conditions. *J Bone Joint Surg Am* 1976; 58:13.

Scheentker EP, Gibson DA: The orthopaedic aspects of spinal muscular atrophy. *J Bone Joint Surg Am* 1976; 58:32.

Wilkins KE, Gibson DA: The patterns of spinal deformity in Duchenne muscular dystrophy. *J Bone Joint Surg Am* 1976; 58:24.

Scoliosis—Treatment

Blount WP, Moe JH: *The Milwaukee Brace.* Baltimore, Williams & Wilkins Co, 1973.

Dickson JH, Harrington PR: The evolution of the Harrington instrumentation technique in scoliosis. *J Bone Joint Surg Am* 1973; 55:993.

MacEwen GD, Bunnell WP, Sriram K: Acute neurologic complications in the treatment of scoliosis. *J Bone Joint Surg Am* 1975; 57:404.

Kyphosis

Bradford DS, Moe JH, Montalvo FJ, et al: Scheuermann's kyphosis and roundback deformity—results of Milwaukee brace treatment. *J Bone Joint Surg Am* 1974; 56:740.

Bradford DS, Moe JH, Montalvo FJ, et al: Scheuermann's kyphosis—results of surgical treatment by posterior spine arthrodesis in twenty-two patients. *J Bone Joint Surg Am* 1975; 57:439.

Winter RB, Moe JH, Wong JF: Congenital kyphosis: Its natural history and treatment as observed in a study of 130 patients. *J Bone Joint Surg Am* 1973; 55:223.

Spondylolysis and Spondylolisthesis

Jackson DW, Wiltse LL, Cirincione RJ: Spondylolysis in the female gymnast. *Clin Orthop* 1976; 117:68.

Newman PH: The etiology of spondylolisthesis. *J Bone Joint Surg Br* 1963; 45:39.

Turner RH, Bianco AJ: Spondylolysis and spondylolisthesis in teenagers and children. *J Bone Joint Surg Am* 1971; 53:1298.

Wiltse LL, Widell EH, Jackson DW: Fatigue fracture: The basic lesion in isthmic spondylolisthesis. *J Bone Joint Surg Am* 1975; 57:17.

Wiltse LL, Jackson DW: The treatment of spondylolisthesis and spondylolysis in children. *Clin Orthop* 1976; 117:92.

Torticollis

Coventry MB, Harris LE: Congenital muscular torticollis in infancy: Some observations regarding treatment. *J Bone Joint Surg Am* 1959; 41:815.

Fielding JW: Selected observations on the cervical spine in childhood, in Ashtrom JP (ed): *Current Practices in Orthopaedic Surgery.* St Louis, CV Mosby Co, 1973, pp 31–55.

Hensinger RN, Long JR, MacEwen GD: The Klippel-Feil syndrome: A constellation of related anomalies. *J Bone Joint Surg Am* 1974; 56:1246.

MacDonald C: Sternomastoid tumor and muscular torticollus. *J Bone Joint Surg Br* 1969; 51:432.

Tachdjian MO, Matson DD: Orthopaedic aspects of intraspinal tumors in infants and children. *J Bone Joint Surg Am* 1965; 47:223.

8

Musculoskeletal Infection

Stephen C. Aronoff, M.D.
Peter V. Scoles, M.D.

Musculoskeletal infectious disease continues to present diagnostic and therapeutic problems 30 years after the introduction of effective antibiotic therapy. Mortality from bone and joint infection has fallen dramatically from about 25% in the preantibiotic era to about 1% to 2% at present, but morbidity from the diseases remains high. Extensive and often irreversible bone and joint damage predictably follow delayed diagnosis or inadequate treatment, and the consequent deformity and disability last a lifetime. Early diagnosis and prompt adequate therapy can greatly decrease the risks of long-term complications. A thorough understanding of the pathophysiology of bone and joint infection is an essential part of effective management of these patients.

OSTEOMYELITIS

Bacterial infection in bone can arise through several routes. Direct inoculation of bone often occurs at the time of open fracture or after penetration of skin and bone by a contaminated object such as a nail or fishhook. Unless prompt and thorough debridement is performed, bone infection may follow. Infection may also spread to bone from a contiguous site such as a septic joint or infected soft tissue wound. Osteomyelitis that arises from this contiguous spread is especially common in older patients with circulatory impairment, in patients with diabetic peripheral vascular disease, and in newborn infants.

Osteomyelitis may also begin after hematogenous seeding of bone during an episode of bacteremia. Hematogenous osteomyelitis occurs principally in two widely separated age groups. It is the most common type of osteomyelitis in children under age 15 years, ordinarily involving the metaphyseal area of long bones. Recently it has been reported with increasing frequency in the fifth, sixth, and seventh decades of life, usually involving the vertebral bodies or the sites of prosthetic implants. Hematogenous osteomyelitis is uncommon in otherwise healthy young adults.

The characteristics of infection vary within each age group. The pathophysiology and clinical manifestations of osteomyelitis in an individual patient depend on many factors, including age, precise site of infection, virulence of the offending organism, and host resistance.

Pathophysiology

The metaphyseal areas of long bones in the immature skeleton are particularly susceptible to blood-borne infection. The anatomical arrangement of the vascular supply of the metaphysis and the dynamic characteristics of fluid flow in the region are major factors in this predilection. The nutrient arterioles of the metaphysis terminate in sharp loops at the growth plate before emptying into tortuous and wide venous sinusoids. Blood flow in the sinusoids is slow and turbulent. Pressure in the system is low, and contaminants are not rapidly cleared. Bacteria may lodge in the metaphysis during episodes of systemic bacteremia and may not be mechanically flushed through the venous network.

In addition, evidence indicates that normal antibacterial responses within the metaphysis are impaired in the newborn. The afferent limbs of metaphyseal capillaries lack phagocytic lining cells, and the phagocytes of the venous sinusoids appear to be functionally inactive. In this en-

vironment of altered antibacterial response and limited blood flow, infection develops easily and spreads rapidly.

When bacterial proliferation occurs, pressure within the sinusoids is raised, and local circulation is compromised. As bacteria and leukocytes accumulate, pressure within the metaphysis increases and arteriolar thrombosis follows. Decompression of the metaphysis occurs by spread through the haversian canals of the metaphysis and rupture through the cortex to the subperiosteal space. Accumulations of pus strip the periosteum from the underlying bone and disrupt the periosteal contribution to bone blood supply. Areas of metaphyseal bone become sequestered and isolated from blood flow. New bone forms beneath the elevated periosteum in response to irritation, and the dead bone of the metaphysis may be completely encased by reactive bone. The necrotic underlying bone is known as a *sequestrum* and serves as a site of chronic infection.

The physis and epiphysis are particularly vulnerable in untreated or inadequately treated metaphyseal osteomyelitis. Lysosomal enzymes destroy the chondroid matrix of the growth plate and allow infection to spread to active proliferative regions of the physis. Septic thrombosis of vessels that supply epiphyseal and germinal layers of the physis may also occur. Permanent damage to the growth plate follows, and significant deformity will develop in an actively growing child.

Septic arthritis may be an early complication of metaphyseal osteomyelitis in several anatomical locations. Portions of metaphyseal bone lie within the capsules of the hip, shoulder, and elbow joints. If decompression of metaphyseal osteomyelitis occurs by rupture through cortex that lies within the joint capsule, septic arthritis will follow.

Osteomyelitis in the neonate and infant less than 1 year old has a different pathophysiology, clinical course, and morbidity from bone infection in older children. In most instances, osteomyelitis in the infant begins with hematogenous seeding of the metaphysis of a long bone, as in older children. Progression of infection occurs more rapidly in neonatal and infantile osteomyelitis. The cortex of infantile bone is quite thin, and there is early spread of infection through haversian canals to the subperiosteal space. The periosteum is easily elevated in infantile bone, resulting in circumferential stripping and subperiosteal spread along the shaft. Bacterial irritation usually invokes massive new periosteal bone formation, and the entire shaft may be encased in bone. In older infants or infants with less virulent infection, destruction of cortex may be limited to one side of the shaft. When this happens, sequestration is less severe.

Early spread of infection across the growth plate into the epiphysis is common in neonatal and infantile osteomyelitis. In the past, this was presumed to occur through vascular channels that crossed the physis from the metaphysis to the region of the secondary ossification center of the epiphysis. This may in fact occur in some cases. In other cases, spread probably occurs by destruction of chondroid matrix and contiguous spread from the infected metaphysis. In both cases, destruction of the germinal layer of the physis occurs, and growth disturbance follows.

Joint infection often complicates neonatal and infantile osteomyelitis. This may occur through several mechanisms: (1) direct spread across the articular surface from an infected epiphysis; (2) rupture through the cortex of an intra-articular metaphysis, usually in the hip, shoulder, or elbow; and (3) septic embolization and thrombosis of synovial and intra-articular vessels, with subsequent joint contamination.

Etiology and Incidence

Acute hematogenous osteomyelitis of infancy and childhood most often involves the long bones of the lower limb. The metaphyseal regions of the proximal and distal femur and tibia are the most common sites of infection; the humerus, fibula, calcaneus, radius, and ulna are less frequently but not uncommonly affected. Osteomyelitis has been reported in all components of the skeleton, including the bones of the skull, the chest, and the pelvis. In the hands and feet, infection secondary to contamination through puncture wounds or from contiguous spread from soft tissue infection occurs more often than hematogenous infection.

In many reported series, hematogenous osteomyelitis has been found to occur slightly more often in boys. Often there is a history of antecedent trauma, usually not severe enough to require medical attention. The relationship of trauma to osteomyelitis is unclear. It is possible that slight damage to metaphyseal bone may alter local blood flow slightly and provide a focus for subsequent incidental bacterial seeding. There is little experimental evidence to support this theory, and prior trauma may well be only incidental. Children are continually subject to minor injury, and the occurrence of an acute skeletal infection may simply bring to mind an otherwise forgotten mishap.

Some patients have a history of antecedent systemic or soft tissue infection. Otitis media, urinary tract infection, tonsillitis, pneumonia, and skin abscesses have all been implicated as possible sources of transient bacteremia. Two to three weeks may pass between the primary infection and the onset of clinically evident bone infection. Prodromal infection is particularly important in patients with altered immunity secondary to blood dyscrasias, renal disease, malabsorption syndromes, or other chronic illnesses.

High-risk infants are especially susceptible to hematogenous osteomyelitis. Bleeding during pregnancy, preeclampsia, premature rupture of membranes, prolonged labor, cesarean section, traumatic delivery, and prematurity all predispose an infant to infection. Pustules, furuncles, infected cutdown sites, and infected umbilical catheters may initiate bacteremia with subsequent metaphyseal seeding. Multifocal bone involvement is common in these patients and is probably a manifestation of poor host response. As many as 50% of patients have more than one bone involved.

In summary, the factors that predispose an infant or child to hematogenous osteomyelitis are incompletely understood. In some instances, prodromal illness or antecedent trauma can be implicated with reasonable certainty. Most often, however, the disease occurs spontaneously in previously healthy patients with no known metabolic or immunologic deficiencies.

Bacteriology

Staphylococcus is the most common bacterium responsible for acute hematogenous osteomyelitis in otherwise healthy children. In most series, more than 60% of organisms identified from blood or bone cultures are *S. aureus* or, less commonly, *S. epidermidis*. Other organisms may cause bone infection as well, especially in very young patients. Group B *Streptococcus* (*S. agalactiae*) has been isolated with increasing frequency from neonates and infants with osteomyelitis. *Escherichia coli* and *Hemophilus influenzae* type B have also been implicated in neonatal and infantile bone infection.

Patients with preexistent diseases or unusual histories may develop osteomyelitis from uncommon organisms. Osteomyelitis caused by *Salmonella* species is frequently associated with sickle-cell disease and the sickle cell trait. It may occur following *Salmonella*-related gastroenteritis in otherwise healthy children. Osteomyelitis caused by *Pseudomonas aeruginosa* is a frequent and troublesome complication of puncture wounds of the foot; osteomyelitis caused by hematogenous *Pseudomonas* is a recognized complication of drug addiction.

Effective therapy requires isolation of the responsible organism as early as possible. Blood cultures obtained at the time of initial evaluation yield positive results in about 50% of patients. Cultures of metaphyseal pus obtained by needle aspiration of the affected area have been reported to be positive in approximately 40% of patients. Cultures of bone obtained at surgical drainage are positive slightly more often. The highest rate of identification of the offending organism can be obtained by culture of multiple sources. Cultures of blood, pus, bone, and, where applicable, joint fluid yield results in over 90% of cases.

Often, culture results may be obscured by previous antimicrobial therapy. In cases such as this or when cultures are negative, detection of bacterial antigen in the blood, urine, or bone aspirate may aid in etiologic diagnosis.

Counterimmunoelectrophoresis (CIE), a technique available in many hospitals, can detect small amounts of bacterial cell wall antigen by electrophoretic precipitation with specific antibodies. Currently, it is available for group B *Streptococcus*, *H. influenzae* type B, and *S. pneumoniae*. Any body fluid may be evaluated by CIE.

Latex agglutination is a rapid test for evaluation of bacterial antigen. Latex particles are coated with antibody to specific bacterial cell wall antigen. The fluid to be examined is added to a solution of the latex particles; agglutination indicates a positive reaction. This test is available for *H. influenzae* type B, group B *Streptococcus*, and *S. pneumoniae.* Although it is more rapid than CIE, it is no more accurate and is available in only a few institutions.

Unfortunately, neither CIE nor latex agglutination can detect staphylococcal cell wall antigens. Teichoic acid antibodies have been shown to correlate with recent staphylococcal infection, but this examination is available only as a research tool.

Clinical Findings

The clinical manifestations of hematogenous osteomyelitis in the infant and child are reflections of the severity of infection and the individual patient's inflammatory response. The usual findings in neonatal osteomyelitis are different from those of osteomyelitis later in childhood. In older children, symptoms and signs vary with the site of infection and virulence of the responsible organism.

In the early stages of infection, differentiation of acute hematogenous osteomyelitis from cellulitis, septic arthritis, and recent fracture may be difficult. In most instances, however, careful evaluation of the patient's history, thorough examination, and appropriate laboratory studies permit early diagnosis and treatment.

There is often a striking lack of symptoms and signs in neonatal osteomyelitis. The paucity of physical findings in neonatal osteomyelitis often is responsible for prolonged delay in diagnosis and treatment. Local inflammatory reaction may be minimal, and swelling and redness of the involved area may or may not be present. When extremities are involved, lack of active motion is the most consistent finding. Irritability and fussiness are common, especially when the infant is moved. These may be the earliest findings in infection of the bones of the trunk. Pain on attempts at passive motion of an involved limb and localized tenderness at the site of infection are usually present in otherwise

healthy neonates and older infants. Unfortunately, many of these patients are seriously ill and may respond minimally to such stimuli. Effusion in a superficial joint such as the knee, ankle, or wrist may indicate osteomyelitis of adjacent long bones, but effusion in the hip and shoulder is difficult to detect. White blood cell counts are often normal or depressed in affected neonates with serious infection. Erythrocyte sedimentation rates are usually elevated. Apparent limb paralysis, irritability, and temperature instability are cardinal indications of osteomyelitis in a high-risk neonate.

Two presentation patterns are common in older children with hematogenous osteomyelitis. Most patients with the first pattern of presentation experience the acute onset of pain as pressure builds in the affected bone. Inflammation in the soft tissues of the involved limb develops rapidly and may be confused with cellulitis. Exquisite focal tenderness on palpation over the involved area of the metaphysis is characteristic. Temperatures above 39.5°C are common, and often affected children appear systemically quite ill. White blood cell counts greater than 15,000/cu mm and erythrocyte sedimentation rates greater than 50 mm/hour are usually found. The interval between onset of symptoms and presentation in such patients is usually short.

Systemic signs of infection appear to be less severe in children with the second pattern of presentation of hematogenous osteomyelitis. In this group of patients, pain is less intense, and inflammation is more localized. Tenderness on palpation over the involved area is always present. Temperatures are often below 39.5°C. White blood cell counts are often between 10,000 and 15,000/cu mm, and sedimentation rates are often below 50 mm/hour. The interval between onset of symptoms and first examination may be 5 days or more. In such patients, the offending organism may be less virulent or host response more effective. Rupture through the cortex with metaphyseal decompression may occur before significant sequestration occurs. In either group of patients, subperiosteal spread of the infection worsens prognosis. Serial physical examination will show diffusion of tenderness along the shaft of the involved bone when extension of periosteal elevation occurs.

Radiologic Findings

Radiologic and radioisotopic signs of osteomyelitis are manifestations of response to disease rather than specific demonstrations of infection. They lag behind clinical signs and are rarely pathognomonic. Many of the bone changes in patients with osteomyelitis also occur during fracture healing, in metabolic bone disease, and in certain bone tumors. No currently available radiologic or radioisotope technique directly demonstrates the presence of an offending organism. Roentgenograms and bone scans are best interpreted along with clinical findings in patients with suspected osteomyelitis.

Changes in the soft tissues around the infected bone in response to inflammation are the earliest radiologic signs of osteomyelitis (Fig 8–1). Deep soft tissue swelling, manifested by displacement or obliteration of normal muscle planes, often occurs within the first week of infection. These findings are subtle and easily overlooked if films are of poor quality or if the index of suspicion is low. Often soft tissue changes are evident only in retrospect.

Bone changes in response to infection usually do not occur until 10 to 14 days after the onset of disease. Rarefaction of the involved metaphysis is the first change to occur; cortical erosion follows soon afterward (Fig 8–2). Periosteal elevation and new bone formation usually begin within 2 weeks of the onset of disease. If infection continues untreated, pus may permeate the new subperiosteal bone and again elevate the periosteum. A lamellar pattern of bone formation develops that can be difficult to distinguish from rapidly progressive osteogenic sarcoma or round cell tumor.

Sequestration and involucrum formation are indicated by development of radiodense areas within the affected bone. The increased density is both relative and absolute. Sequestered bone is avascular; the disuse osteoporosis usually evident in surrounding bone does not affect the sequestrum. In addition, calcium salts often precipitate within the empty marrow spaces of the necrotic bone. The pathologic process resembles the changes seen within the femoral head in patients with Legg-Calvé-Perthes disease.

Radioisotope scans show abnormalities earlier in the course of osteomyelitis than do routine roentgenograms. Like radiographic changes, scans are evidence of response to injury, and often are not specific. Correct bone scan interpretation requires full knowledge of the clinical setting and a thorough understanding of bone physiology radioisotope physics. Two radioisotope compounds are in common use for early evaluation of suspected infection. Technetium 99m polyphosphate localizes at sites of rapid bone turnover (Fig 8–3). Gallium 67 localizes in white blood cells, which later accumulate at a site of infection.

Technetium 99m polyphosphate scans often remain abnormal long after successful treatment of acute osteomyelitis. Like roentgenograms, scans reflect the extent of initial damage and subsequent reconstruction of involved bone. They cannot normally be used to monitor the efficacy or duration of treatment.

Gallium 67 is a cyclotron-produced radioisotope with a half-life of 78 hours. When complexed with citrate, it binds to

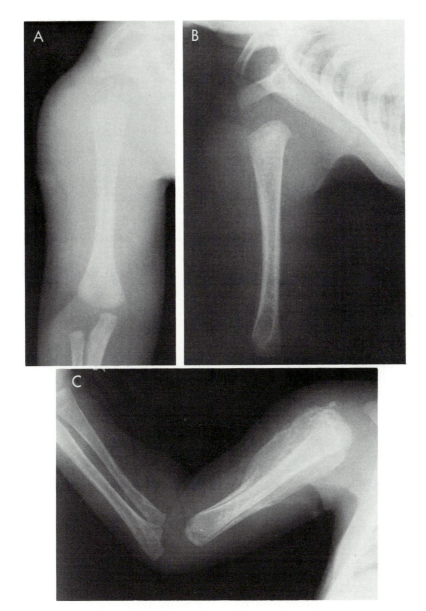

FIG 8–1.
Radiologic changes in neonatal osteomyelitis. **A,** early proximal humeral osteomyelitis. Soft tissue swelling around the affected bone is present. **B,** periosteal elevation is manifested by subperiosteal bone formation. **C,** massive subperiosteal new bone formation. The humeral shaft has become surrounded by new bone.

plasma proteins and accumulates within lysozomes of white blood cells. Non-bound gallium is slowly excreted through the kidneys and colon. Scanning is usually performed 1 to 3 days after the intra-venous administration of 5 mCi to allow time for localization. The estimated radiation absorbed dose is about 0.25 rad/mCi.

Tagged leukocytes tend to localize in abscesses present at the time of injection.

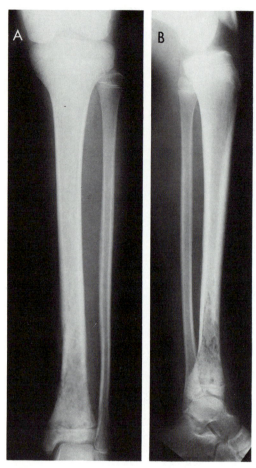

FIG 8–2.
Radiologic changes in adolescent hematogenous osteomyelitis. Rarefaction, bone destruction, and new
subperiosteal bone formation are present in this
case, in which the diagnosis was not suspected for 3
weeks after the onset of infection.

Since isotope accumulation does not depend on bone reaction, ^{67}Ga scans may
show increased uptake slightly earlier
than ^{99m}Tc scans. Penetration still depends on blood flow, and bone infarction
may interfere with leukocyte accumulation. In addition, the necessary delay between injection and scanning limits the
usefulness of gallium scanning for early
diagnosis.

Abnormal bone scans are sometimes
seen in patients with septic arthritis and
cellulitis. Uptake in the affected area is
diffuse, rather than focal with bone, and
usually returns to normal as infection
clears and synovitis resolves. The radioisotope scan pattern seen in these instances
is probably a result of increased blood
flow in the involved limb.

In most cases, the diagnosis of acute
osteomyelitis should be based on clinical
observations and laboratory findings. Although roentgenograms and radioisotope
scans frequently become abnormal in patients with osteomyelitis, they are often
normal early in the course of the disease.
In no instance should treatment be delayed in patients with symptoms and
signs of bone infection until bone scan or
radiologic findings develop.

Treatment

Successful treatment of osteomyelitis
with minimal morbidity and mortality requires accurate diagnosis and prompt and
adequate therapy. The principles of effective care include:

1. Early diagnosis.
2. Identification of the responsible organism.
3. Specific antibiotic therapy.
4. Attainment of bactericidal drug
levels throughout infected bone.
5. Drainage of abscesses and removal
of large sequestra.
6. Maintenance of adequate drug levels for a period of time sufficient to eradi-
cate the infection.

A high index of suspicion is necessary
for early identification of hematogenous
osteomyelitis. Diagnosis is simple when
the classic findings of fever, extremity
pain, and discrete intense tenderness in
bone are present. Frequently symptoms
and signs are not so pronounced early in
the course of infection, and osteomyelitis
may be confused with cellulitis, traumatic

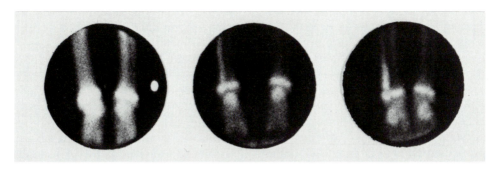

FIG 8–3.
Technetium bone scan patterns in acute fibular osteomyelitis. **Left,** diffuse hyperactivity is seen within both bones of the affected extremity. **Center,** 10 days later focal hyperactivity is present within the affected fibula. **Right,** 2 weeks later focal hyperactivity persists despite clinically adequate treatment. (From Scoles PV, et al: Bone scan patterns in acute osteomyelitis. *Clin Orthop* 1980; 153:210. Reproduced by permission.)

inflammation, rheumatic fever, and juvenile rheumatoid arthritis. Diagnosis may be especially difficult in the neonate.

Aspiration of bone at the site of maximum tenderness is the most important diagnostic study in patients with suspected osteomyelitis. It should be part of the initial evaluation in all patients and should not be delayed pending results of blood cultures or bone scans. Needle aspiration will not alter the results of radioisotope scanning. Under sterile conditions, with mild sedation and local anesthesia, an 18-gauge spinal needle is inserted through the skin and advanced to bone. The periosteal region is aspirated first. If no fluid is obtained, the needle may be drilled by hand through the cortex into the medullary cavity. Specimens from both aspirates should be sent immediately for Gram stain, aerobic and anaerobic bacterial cultures, fungal cultures, and, if indicated, cultures for tuberculosis.

If pus is obtained either from the subperiosteal area or medullary cavity, a significant amount of metaphyseal bone is likely to have been deprived of blood flow by increased pressure. Surgical drainage is necessary for decompression.

Staphylococcus aureus is the most common cause of hematogenous osteomyelitis

in infants and children. Initial therapy should consist of an antistaphylococcal agent such as nafcillin, oxacillin, or a cephalosporin. Aminoglycoside derivatives should be added if gram-negative organisms are identified on stained specimens and in cases of osteomyelitis secondary to puncture wounds of the foot. In cases where *H. influenzae* type B is suspected, chloramphenicol should be included in the initial treatment regimen. The incidence of ampicillin resistance in *Hemophilus* infection is increasing; ampicillin should be substituted for chloramphenicol only if the organism isolated does not produce β-lactamase.

Neonates present a slightly different problem. Group B *Streptococcus* and Enterobacteriaceae, in addition to *S. aureus*, are frequent offenders. Optimal primary coverage can be provided with a semisynthetic penicillin such as oxacillin or nafcillin and an aminoglycoside such as gentamicin or kanamycin. Antibiotics can be altered appropriately when culture and sensitivity results are available. Group B *Streptococcus*, when present, is best treated with high doses of penicillin.

The early response of patients who are not treated by primary surgical decompression is critical. Improvement, manifested by reduced fever, decreased local pain, and lowered white blood cell count should occur within 24 to 36 hours of the start of treatment. If little or no improvement occurs or if tenderness spreads along the shaft of the bone, surgical decompression is indicated. In most instances, if surgery is performed early, before extensive sequestration has occurred, simple windowing of the metaphysis provides adequate drainage. Removal of extensive amounts of necrotic sequestrum may be necessary if surgery is inappropriately delayed. Whether or not surgery is necessary, immobilization of the affected limb in splints or balanced traction decreases pain and facilitates nursing care.

High antibiotic levels in serum and bone can be reliably achieved by intravenous administration. Patient compliance and drug absorption are rarely problems. It is the primary treatment of choice of acute osteomyelitis. Long-term intravenous therapy is often inconvenient and uncomfortable and carries the risks of phlebitis and secondary infection. It has been demonstrated that bactericidal levels of antibiotics can be achieved in blood, joint fluid, and bone by oral administration, and in some instances, oral antibiotics may provide an alternative to intravenous drugs after the acute phase of infection has passed.

There are a number of critical requirements for safe oral antimicrobial therapy of osteomyelitis. In most cases, the offending organism must be isolated. Adequate laboratory facilities for the dilution studies necessary for drug titration must be available. An oral antibiotic must be available that is effective against the organism in vivo, well absorbed, nontoxic, and palatable. The half-life of the drug should be long enough to permit dosing at convenient intervals. In almost all cases, oral antibiotic therapy should be administered initially on an inpatient basis to permit adequate monitoring and to ensure compliance.

Oral therapy should not begin until the patient has received 7 to 10 days of parenteral therapy and has stabilized. The offending organism must be isolated, and the mean inhibitory concentrations (MIC) of potential oral agents must be determined. Laboratory facilities capable of determining serum inhibitory concentrations (SIC) or serum bactericidal concentrations (SBC) must be available.

Serum inhibitory concentrations are obtained by serially diluting the patient's serum with broth and adding known concentrations of the infecting organism to each tube. The largest dilution that remains clear after 18 hours of incubation is the SIC. If, after 18 hours of incubation, the SIC tubes are subcultured onto agar mediums, in 24 hours the SBC may be determined. The SBC is the largest dilution of serum that has no growth on agar. In most cases, the SIC and SBC differ by one tube.

The timing of blood drawing for SIC or SBC determination is critical. Most authors use peak and trough SIC and SBC values to determine efficacy of treatment.

After 4 to 6 doses of antibiotic, efficacy of treatment must be tested by SIC or SBC determinations. Peak values are obtained 1 hour after oral administration on an empty stomach; trough values should be obtained immediately prior to dosage. If the SIC is used to monitor treatment, peak SIC values should be equal to or greater than 1 to 16, and trough values should be equal to or greater than 1 to 4. If the SBC is used to follow treatment, peak values should be equal to or greater than 1 to 8, and trough values equal to or greater than 1 to 2. Peak SIC and SBC values can be raised by increasing total drug dose; trough values can be improved by shortening the interval between drug doses.

Three to 4 weeks appears to be the optimal duration of treatment in most cases of acute hematogenous osteomyelitis. Successful treatment is marked by falling fever, decreased symptoms, and return of white blood cell counts and sedimentation rates to normal. There is a significant risk of recurrent infection if treatment is halted before 3 weeks, even in the presence of a rapid response to antibiotics. On the other hand, there does not seem to be an advantage to continuing treatment past 4 weeks in uncomplicated disease. Antibiotics can be safely stopped at the time of discharge from the hospital. Close outpatient follow-up is necessary to guard against recurrent infection and to detect possible orthopedic complications.

Chronic osteomyelitis may develop if early medical or surgical therapy has been inadequate. Sequestra serve as foci of chronic infection; repeated episodes of spontaneous drainage from sinus tracts and abscess cavities will occur until all dead bone is removed surgically. Radical debridement, bone grafting, and long-term antibiotic administration are usually required. One to 2 years of high-dose antibiotic therapy may be necessary. Squamous cell carcinoma of sinus tracts is a frequent long-term complication of chronic osteomyelitis. Amputation is required, and death from metastatic disease may result.

INFECTIOUS ARTHRITIS

Morbidity and mortality from acute infectious arthritis were high in the preantibiotic era. Suppurative arthritis often led to severe and permanent loss of motion and limb deformity; complications from systemic seeding were frequent. Effective medical and surgical management has lessened the risks of irreversible joint damage, but successful therapy depends primarily on prompt diagnosis.

Pathophysiology

The details of joint infection vary in different age groups and with different organisms, but the natural history of untreated infection is similar in infants, children, and adolescents. Bacterial contamination of a joint may occur by hematogenous seeding of synovium, through spread from an adjacent site of bone infection, or by direct inoculation through a penetrating wound or foreign body. Once bacteria are introduced into the joint space, an inflammatory reaction ensues. The synovial membrane thickens, and synovial capillary permeability increases. Fluid accumulates in the joint, and an effusion may be noted on examination. Large numbers of leukocytes enter the joint, and the synovial fluid becomes purulent. Degranulation of neutrophils releases lysozymes and trypsin-like enzymes into the effusion; these in turn degrade hydroxyproline, a major constituent of the ground substance of articular cartilage.

Increasing intra-articular pressure interferes with joint nutrition. Tissue pressure around the joint rises, and blood flow is shunted away from the synovium. Accumulations of pus and fibrin clots on the joint surfaces block diffusion of substrates necessary for chondrocyte metabolism. The articular surfaces become pitted and fibrillated. Infected pannus may completely cover joint surfaces, and extension of infection to subchondral bone is possible. Fibrocartilaginous scar tissue replaces articular cartilage, and restriction of joint motion follows. Eventually, bony ankylosis of opposing joint surfaces may develop.

Rupture of pus through the synovial membrane into surrounding tissues may occur if intra-articular pressures continue to rise. Cellulitis, soft tissue abscesses, and external draining sinuses may develop. Chronic drainage may persist indefinitely. Permanent loss of function can be expected.

The clinical presentation, bacterial etiology, and prognosis in septic arthritis vary with age. Most cases of hematogenous joint infection occur in children between the ages of 6 months and 12 years. Joint infection in early infancy is less common but often occurs in systemically ill, high-risk babies. In adolescence and young adult life, venereal arthritis is the most common form of joint infection.

Infectious Arthritis in Childhood

Septic arthritis in childhood is an uncommon disease. In one review of the subject, it accounted for less than 10 admissions per year to a major university center. In children between ages 6 months and 12 years, the most common cause of joint infection is hematogenous seeding. After the neonatal period, joint infection caused by direct spread from an area of adjacent osteomyelitis accounts for only about 10% of all cases. Penetration of the joint space by a foreign body such as a needle, splinter, glass fragment, or thorn may directly contaminate the joint and initiate infection; this is the least common etiology of septic arthritis in children.

Preexisting infection is an important predisposing factor in septic arthritis. Bacteremia has been documented in children with otitis media, pneumonia, upper respiratory tract infection, urinary tract infection, and cellulitis; it is not surprising that more than half of the children with septic arthritis have a history of antecedent infection. Patients with meningitis, septicemia, epiglottitis, and distant osteomyelitis may also develop hematogenous septic arthritis. The organism that is iso-lated from the extra-articular source is usually the organism responsible for joint infection.

Chronic illness seems to predispose to joint infection. Lymphoproliferative diseases, sickle cell anemia, congenital immunoglobulin deficits, leukocyte chemotactic defects, asplenia, chronic renal failure, and immunosuppressive therapy all have been associated with an increased risk of pyogenic arthritis.

The relationship of trauma to joint infection is not clear. A history of minor recent injury in septic arthritis patients is common. Synovial injury has been proposed as a cause of local stasis and a possible focus for bacterial seeding, but this has not been well documented. It may well be that trauma is only incidental in children with joint infection.

Etiology

The organisms responsible for septic arthritis of childhood vary with the source of infection and the age of the child. There is also evidence that indicates the prevalence of infection caused by particular bacteria is changing with time. In most reports, *S. aureus* and group A *Streptococcus* are responsible for the majority of cases of septic arthritis. *Hemophilus influenzae* type B accounts for one third to one half of cases of septic arthritis in patients less than 2 years old. Recently, this organism has been isolated with increasing frequency in patients over age 2 years, but it remains uncommon in patients over 6 years old. *Staphylococcus aureus* is the most common organism isolated from patients between the ages of 6 and 14 years; group A *Streptococcus*, Enterobacteriaceae, and *S. pneumoniae* follow.

Other agents have been occasionally reported to cause septic arthritis in childhood. *Aerobacter* sp, *Neisseria meningitidis*, and *Salmonella* species may cause arthritis in otherwise healthy children. Pseudomonas species have been isolated from infected joints in habitual drug abusers and following puncture wounds of the foot. Viral agents such as varicella, rubella, and hepatitis B may cause arthralgia or tenosynovitis but rarely cause septic arthritis.

Tuberculous arthritis was common in North America in the 19th and early 20th centuries. It remains common in underdeveloped countries but is now rare in America and northern Europe.

Penetrating wounds may inoculate a joint with unusual organisms. Human bite wounds are often contaminated with anaerobic oral flora, and animal bites may be infected with *Pasteurella multocida*. Secondary *Staphylococcus* infections occasionally occur. Thorn puncture may result in a sterile inflammatory process or may contaminate a joint with uncommon bacterial or fungal organisms.

Presentation

The principal symptoms and signs of childhood infectious arthritis are pain, fever, limitation of motion, and joint swelling. Fever may antedate joint symptoms by several days; prodromal infection may be present elsewhere. The onset of joint symptoms is most often acute and limited to one joint. The involved joint is usually tender, and the surrounding area is often warm and reddened. Active motion is limited, and attempts at passive motion are vigorously resisted.

The knee is the most common site of infection, followed by the hip, ankle, elbow, and wrist. The shoulder and sacroiliac joints are involved less often. The small joints of the hands and feet are rarely involved in hematogenous infection but may be the sites of infection from puncture wounds. When the joints of the pelvis or lower extremity are involved, the child may refuse to walk. When the hip joint is infected, the extremity is most often held in a position of hip flexion, abduction, and external rotation. The knee is usually slightly flexed when infected.

Obliteration of the recesses on either side of the patella is an early sign of knee effusion. As fluid accumulates, the patella may seem to ''float'' over the knee joint. Fullness around the elbow, ankle, and wrist is usually present as effusion collects within the joint.

Most children with septic arthritis have white blood cell counts greater than 10,000 cells/cu mm. White blood cell counts of 20,000 to 30,000 cell/cu mm are not uncommon. The erythrocyte sedimentation rate is almost always greater than 20 mm/hour. In the absence of other systemic diseases, other common blood chemistry studies are usually normal.

Radiologic findings are variable. Early in the course of the disease, roentgenograms may be normal or show only deep soft tissue swelling. Occasionally joint-space widening caused by intracapsular effusion may be present. Disuse osteoporosis may be present in septic arthritis of longer standing. Joint-space narrowing and subchondral bone destruction may be present in chronic or late cases.

Technetium 99m polyphosphate bone scanning is most often not helpful in the early diagnosis of septic arthritis. Bone scans may show normal uptake or diffusely increased uptake in the region of the suspect joint (Fig 8–4). Diffuse hyperactivity may persist for long periods. Gallium 67 scanning may be more valuable, since gallium localizes in the granules of neutrophils. However, the 24- to 48-hour localization time limits the value of gallium scans in early diagnosis.

Evaluation

Joint aspiration and synovial fluid analysis are the most important steps in the management of the child with suspected septic arthritis. Arthrocentesis should be promptly and carefully performed under sterile conditions by an experienced physician. In most cases, the child should be sedated and the involved

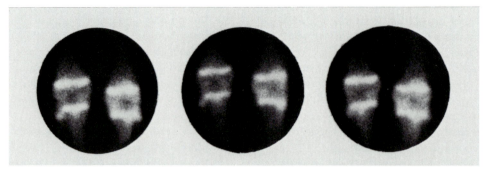

FIG 8–4.
Bone scan patterns in septic arthritis. Persistent, diffuse hyperactivity is present around the left knee, despite clinically adequate treatment. Normal increased uptake is present in the epiphyseal centers around the knee. Scans were taken at 1-week intervals, **left to right.** (From Scoles PV, et al: Bone scan patterns in acute osteomyelitis. *Clin Orthop* 1980; 153:210. Reproduced by permission.)

joint carefully prepared and draped. Local anesthetic infiltration should be used. A large-bore spinal needle should be passed into the involved joint and suction created with a large-volume syringe. Repeated attempts to penetrate a joint may damage the joint surface and inoculate underlying bone. Fluoroscopy and contrast injection should be employed when necessary to ensure proper needle placement.

The gross appearance of joint fluid gives important information about the cause of effusion. Normal joint fluid is clear to slightly yellow. Infected joint fluid is cloudy or purulent. Grossly bloody fluid usually indicates traumatic effusion. A drop of normal fluid placed between the thumb and index finger will stretch 1 to 2 cm as the fingers are drawn apart. Infected fluid is considerably less tenacious.

Joint fluid obtained by aspiration must be promptly and carefully handled. Samples should be processed to determine cell counts and glucose, protein, and lactic dehydrogenase levels; culture and microscopic examination should also be undertaken. Counterimmunoelectrophoretic studies of likely bacterial agents, when available, are valuable aids in diagnosis.

One milliliter of heparinized joint fluid should be examined microscopically for cell counts and differentials. Normal synovial fluid contains less than 400 white blood cells per cubic milliliter, with a preponderance of mononuclear cells. In septic arthritis, white counts of 80,000 to 1 million cells/cu mm are often found. Polymorphonuclear leukocytes predominate.

Carefully planned and performed bacteriologic studies are critical. If only a small amount of joint fluid is obtained on aspiration, it should be reserved for Gram stains and cultures; fluid chemistry determinations are less important. If only one to two drops of joint fluid can be aspirated, the joint should be irrigated with several milliliters of nonbacteriostatic sterile saline. This fluid should then be withdrawn and sent for cultures.

A Gram stain should be promptly performed on a drop of joint fluid streaked onto a clean slide. Bacterial morphology and staining characteristics are important aids in selection of initial antibiotic therapy. Unfortunately, bacteria are often not isolated by Gram staining, even in cases of obvious joint infection.

Blood, chocolate, and MacConkey's and Sabouraud's agar plates should be inoculated with 0.1 ml of joint fluid and promptly incubated. Synovial fluid cultures are positive in about two thirds of patients with joint infections. The high rate of negative cultures is probably the result of several factors. Delay in processing joint fluid and improper culture techniques account for some false negative cultures. In addition, there is evidence that purulent joint fluid is bacteriostatic. Large concentrations of neutrophils inhibit bacterial growth. Transfer of 0.1 to 0.2 ml of joint fluid to 10 ml of thioglycolate broth or tryptocase soy broth lessens the possibility of bacterial inhibition. Diluted fluid can be held for subculture if initial cultures are negative.

About 40% of children with septic arthritis have positive blood cultures. Occasionally, grossly purulent joint fluid will not yield an organism in patients with positive blood cultures. For that reason, blood cultures should be obtained in all patients with suspected septic arthritis before antimicrobial therapy is started.

If enough fluid is available, 3 to 4 ml should be placed in a clean test tube that has been anticoagulated with 0.1 ml of 1,000 units/ml of sodium heparin solution and sent for glucose, protein, and lactic dehydrogenase (LDH) determinations. Normally synovial fluid glucose, protein, and LDH levels approximate plasma levels. In infected joint fluid, glucose concentration is often below 40 mg/dl, protein is elevated above 3 gm/dl, and the LDH is markedly increased above levels in simultaneously obtained serum samples.

Counterimmunoelectrophoresis is a useful adjunct to bacterial cultures in identification of the organism responsible for joint infection. The yield of CIE is highest when fluid from several sources is tested. Joint fluid, blood, and urine specimens should all be analyzed. Antimicrobial therapy has no immediate effect on electrophoresis, and fluids may remain positive for several days after the start of antibiotic treatment.

Treatment

If the permanent complications of infectious arthritis are to be avoided, effective treatment must be started immediately. Management depends on the age of the patient, the site of infection, and the most likely organism responsible for infection. Since adequate antimicrobial therapy is urgent in all suspected cases of septic arthritis, often it must be started before the responsible organism can be identified. Surgical drainage and debridement are often necessary to decompress an infected joint and evacuate abscesses.

Initial antibiotic selection must often be made on a "best guess" basis (Table 8–1). After cultures are available, treatment can be altered if necessary. *Hemophilus influenzae* type B, *S. aureus*, and group A *Streptococcus* are the major pathogens in children between ages 1 month and 6 years; a combination of a penicillinase-resistant penicillin such as oxacillin or nafcillin and anti-*Hemophilus* agent should be used in primary treatment. Ampicillin has been used against *Hemophilus* in the past, but increasing resistance rates have been recently reported. Chloramphenicol should be considered in the primary treatment of septic arthritis in this age group.

Cefamandole, a broad-spectrum cephalosporin, is effective against both penicillin-resistant *Staphylococcus* and β-lactamase-producing *Hemophilus* and can be used as a single agent in primary treatment of septic arthritis. Like most cephalosporins, cefamandole penetrates the blood-brain barrier erratically and will not reliably prevent secondary *Hemophilus* meningitis in patients with *Hemophilus* arthritis. Persistent fever, headache, meningeal irritation signs, and changes in mental status should be carefully evaluated in septic arthritis patients. Spinal tap cerebrospinal fluid analysis is mandatory if manifestations of CNS infection develop. Newer third-generation cefamycins currently under investigation may be use-

TABLE 8–1.
Initial Therapy in Septic Arthritis

	PATIENT AGE			
	NEWBORN–1 MO	1 MO–6 YR	6–10 YR	> 10 YR
Most likely organism	Group B *Streptococcus* *Sta. aureus* Enterobacteriaceae	*Hemophilus influenzae* type B *Sta. aureus* Group A *Streptococcus*	*Staphylococcus aureus* Group A *Streptococcus* Enterobacteriaceae *Str. pneumoniae*	*Neisseria gonorrhoeae* *Sta. aureus* Group A *Streptococcus* Enterobacteriaceae
Antibiotics for primary use	Oxacillin or nafcillin, plus gentamicin or tobramycin	Oxacillin or nafcillin plus chloramphenicol	Oxacillin or nafcillin alone; if gram-negative bacilli on arthrocentesis, ampicillin plus gentamicin or tobramycin	Oxacillin or nafcillin; if gram-negative bacilli on arthrocentesis, ampicillin plus gentamicin or tobramycin

ful in the management of both *Hemophilus* arthritis and meningitis.

Staphylococcus aureus and group A *Streptococcus* are most often responsible for septic arthritis between age 6 years and adolescence. Penicillinase-resistant penicillins or cephalosporins may be employed safely in primary treatment in this age group. Anti-*Hemophilus* therapy is not necessary.

In cases where *Pseudomonas* species or other Enterobacteriaceae are suspected, initial therapy should include an aminoglycoside such as gentamicin or kanamycin and a broad-spectrum penicillin such as carbenicillin or ticarcillin. If *Salmonella* species are suspected, ampicillin or chloramphenicol should be used. Antimicrobial therapy can be adjusted once sensitivities are known (Table 8–2).

Surgical drainage of infected joints is a controversial treatment. It has been established that pus under pressure is detrimental to articular cartilage and that lysozomal enzymes in purulent joint fluid degrade cartilage ground substance. Accumulations of pannus on joint surfaces block diffusion of necessary chondrocyte nutrients. In addition, in areas where secondary ossification centers lie within joint capsules, increased intra-articular pressure may occlude blood flow to the epiph-

TABLE 8–2.
Antibiotics in Special Conditions

Condition	Open wound of joint	Puncture wound of foot	Animal bite of joint	Adjacent osteomyelitis	Fungal arthritis
Probable agents	*Staphylococcus aureus* Group A *Streptococcus*	*Pseudomonas* sp.	*Pasteurella multocida*	*Sta. aureus*	*Candida albicans*
Initial therapy	Oxacillin or nafcillin; if allergic, vancomycin, or cephalosporin	Ticarcillin or carbenecillin plus gentamicin or tobramycin	Penicillin or chloramphenicol	Nafcillin, oxacillin, or vancomycin	Amphotericin B plus 5-fluorocytosine

ysis. This is particularly important in the hip and shoulder.

Most investigators agree that evacuation of large volumes of purulent joint fluid is beneficial in primary treatment of septic arthritis. Intra-articular instillation of antibiotics is not necessary, however, since systemic antibiotics penetrate the synovial membrane well and high intra-articular antibiotic concentrations can be achieved without direct injection. In some instances, careful joint aspiration and irrigation through a large-bore needle or arthroscope can adequately decompress and debride an infected joint. The knee, elbow, and ankle joints can at times be adequately treated by aspiration and systemic antibiotic treatment. Repeated joint aspiration may be appropriate if initial systemic response to antibiotics is good yet joint effusion reaccumulates after one aspiration. Persistent systemic signs, rapid reaccumulation of effusion, and increased local signs of infection mandate surgical drainage.

There are few random comparisons of repeated aspiration and open surgical drainage. The morbidity from one or two careful aspirations is certainly less than that from arthrotomy in the knee, ankle, and elbow, but persistent infection after two attempts at aspiration is probably more harmful than primary arthrotomy. Aspiration is not indicated for treatment of septic arthritis of the hip joint or the shoulder. The dangers of damage to the growth plates and secondary ossification centers of the proximal humerus and proximal femur from increased intracapsular pressure are greater than the potential risks of surgery. In addition, repeated, poorly executed needle aspirations of other joints may permanently damage articular surfaces and inoculate underlying bone.

Arthrotomy and debridement are mandatory when septic arthritis results from direct joint puncture. The joint must be carefully inspected for foreign materials. Small pieces of glass, metal fragments, splinters, or plant thorns may induce persistent infection unless removed. In some cases, a sterile, foreign body inflammatory response is present within the joint. In others, bacterial infection is present as a result of puncture with a contaminated object. The decision to use antibiotics must be made individually, based on signs of infection and joint cultures.

Duration and route of antimicrobial therapy depend on the location and agent of infection. Septic arthritis of superficial joints such as the knee, ankle, or wrist caused by *Hemophilus* or *Streptococcus* can be treated by 2 to 3 weeks of antibiotic therapy if a prompt response to initial therapy occurs. Staphylococcal infections, particularly in the hip and shoulder, require longer treatment. Three to 4 weeks of antibiotic treatment is recommended. Longer treatment may be necessary if a prompt response does not ensue.

Oral antibiotic therapy may be appropriate for patients with septic arthritis in some circumstances. Before oral therapy is initiated, the following criteria must be fulfilled:

1. The responsible agent must be isolated from synovial fluid or blood cultures.
2. An appropriate oral agent must be available.
3. Synovial fluid penetration must be good.
4. Facilities to monitor and adjust serum bactericidal antibiotic levels must be available.
5. Patient compliance must be assured.

When appropriate, oral antibiotic therapy should be started 5 to 7 days after the start of parenteral therapy. Serum bactericidal levels should be monitored and adjusted as in oral antibiotic treatment of osteomyelitis. Oral therapy is not appropriate if no organism has been isolated, or if a palatable form of antibiotic is not available. Because of the need for strict compliance, outpatient therapy is difficult.

Results

Long-term complications of septic arthritis in children have been reduced with effective medical and surgical care. Nevertheless, joint stiffness, restriction of motion, and permanent deformity remain common. Residual disability has been estimated to occur in 10% to 20% of children with septic arthritis; limitation of motion is the most frequent sequela.

Pyogenic arthritis of the hip is especially likely to produce late complications. Destruction of the hip joint by pus occurs rapidly, and tamponade of the vessels that supply the secondary ossification center of the femoral head is common. Loss of articular surfaces is usually followed by fibrous ankylosis, often in a disabling amount of flexion. Significant shortening follows destruction of the growth plate by infection or secondary ischemic necrosis. Premature painful degenerative arthritis is common. Many children with septic arthritis of the hip in childhood reach maturity with several inches of shortening and stiff, painful hips. They are poor candidates for reconstructive surgery because of the high risk of secondary infection around a prosthetic implant. Septic arthritis of the hip is an absolute surgical emergency; prompt drainage is mandatory to minimize late sequelae.

Careful attention to joint position during treatment can minimize disabling contracture. During the acute phases of infection, affected limbs should be splinted in plaster in positions of comfort. Active-assisted range-of-motion exercises should be started by trained therapists as soon as local symptoms begin to subside. Isomet-

ric exercise programs are valuable in preventing quadriceps atrophy following knee joint infections. Protected weight bearing may be helpful in preventing further damage to articular surfaces weakened by proteolytic enzymes; this, however, has not been clearly established. Cast immobilization may be necessary if extensive capsular incisions in the hip are required for adequate drainage.

Long-term clinical and radiologic follow-up is advisable. Signs of growth plate damage and avascular necrosis may not appear for 6 months to a year after joint infection. It may become necessary to protect an involved hip by bracing or to compensate surgically for increasing limb-length inequality.

Neonatal Infectious Arthritis

Joint infection in infants less than 6 months old may arise from hematogenous seeding or by spread from an adjacent focus of osteomyelitis. Inadvertent inoculation of the hip joint sometimes complicates femoral venipuncture in septic infants. Primary joint infection is less common than septic arthritis associated with osteomyelitis; although the mechanisms of infection are different, the clinical characteristics of both processes are similar. Treatment methods and outcome depend on the nature of infection, rapidity of diagnosis, and associated illnesses.

Predisposing Factors

Almost all infants with septic arthritis have serious systemic illnesses or preexistent infections. Prematurity, low birth weight, maternal toxemia, bleeding during pregnancy, respiratory distress syndrome, meconium aspiration, asphyxia, erythroblastosis fetalis, and multiple anomalies all appear to be predisposing factors. Umbilical or central indwelling catheters increase risk. Meningitis, septicemia, and remote or adjacent osteomyelitis are common associated infections. Contamination of synovium may occur during episodes of bacteremia; bacterial proliferation and joint infection follow in neonates with lowered resistance.

Joint infection frequently complicates osteomyelitis of the long bones in infants. Direct spread across the growth plate into the intra-articular portion of a bone occurs rapidly in neonates with metaphyseal osteomyelitis. In some anatomical locations, portions of the metaphysis of adjacent bones are intracapsular, and rupture of pus through the metaphyseal cortex into the joint may occur. The hip, shoulder, and elbow are often infected in this manner. In many instances, both bone and joint infection are present at the time of initial evaluation.

Etiology

In the past, most cases of neonatal septic arthritis, with or without associated osteomyelitis, were caused by *S. aureus*. In recent years, the incidence of group B streptococcal infection has increased; in some series, group B *Streptococcus* accounts for more than 60% of cases. Group A *Streptococcus*, *Klebsiella pneumoniae*, *E. coli*, *Pseudomonas* sp., and other Enterobacteriaceae occasionally are isolated from infected joint fluid. *Hemophilus influenzae* is uncommon in infants less than 1 month old but rapidly increases in incidence in older infants.

Candida albicans arthritis is an unusual complication of systemic neonatal candidal infection. Most affected patients have associated candidemia, meningitis, or nephritis.

Presentation

The paucity of local symptoms and signs belies the serious nature of neonatal joint infection. Fever is often absent in neonates with isolated septic arthritis or septic arthritis and osteomyelitis. When present, it may be attributed to preexisting systemic illness. Listlessness, poor feeding, fussiness, and irritability usually accompany neonatal bone and joint infection but are nonspecific signs of illness.

White blood cell counts and erythrocyte sedimentation rates may be normal or only minimally elevated. Abnormalities, when present, may be attributed to other causes. Roentgenograms made early in the evolution of septic arthritis or septic arthritis with osteomyelitis may show obliteration of deep soft tissue planes or may be entirely normal.

Swelling and tenderness around an involved joint are often not dramatic early in the course of infection. Local signs are easily overlooked in the treatment of serious systemic illness. Later, induration and edema become much more obvious, but permanent joint destruction may have already occurred.

Pseudoparalysis is the most consistent finding in infants with septic arthritis with or without associated osteomyelitis. Active motion may be absent or markedly decreased, and passive motion produces pain. Pseudoparalysis is not pathognomonic of infection—it is also found in limb fractures in infants—but it is always abnormal. Decreased or absent voluntary motion indicates the need for careful clinical and radiologic evaluation. In the absence of radiologic evidence of fracture, bone or joint infection should be assumed to be present in infants with pseudoparalysis.

Evaluation

Arthrocentesis is the single most important diagnostic study in infants with suspected joint infection. Because of the high association of osteomyelitis and septic arthritis in the hip, shoulder, and elbow, and the similarity of symptoms of septic arthritis and osteomyelitis, aspiration of the metaphysis of the proximal humerus, proximal femur, and distal humerus should be performed as well.

Aspirated fluids should be promptly and carefully processed. Bacterial studies take precedence over chemistry determinations if only a small amount of fluid is obtained.

Blood cultures are vital; cerebrospinal fluid analysis and cultures are recommended in septic neonates as well. Urine cultures and CIE of joint fluid, blood, and urine increase the rate of identification of the responsible organism.

Roentgenograms of the suspect extremity should be obtained before starting treatment. Some of the signs and symptoms of neonatal fractures mimic those of infection. Later in the course of disease, it may be impossible to differentiate fracture callus from new bone formation in osteomyelitis.

Radioisotope scans can be helpful in determining if osteomyelitis and septic arthritis are both present in infants with signs of several days' duration. Technetium 99m scans may be normal early in the course of osteomyelitis and may never be abnormal in septic arthritis. Gallium 67 scanning may be of greater theoretical value, but treatment should not be delayed while awaiting radioisotope studies.

Treatment

The basic principles of treatment of neonatal septic arthritis are similar to those in older infants and children. Effective antimicrobial therapy and prompt joint decompression are essential. The choice of antibiotics and methods of joint debridement differ slightly from those used in older children.

The Gram stain is a valuable aid in the selection of initial antibiotic therapy. If gram-positive cocci are seen on examination of joint fluid, intravenous oxacillin or nafcillin should be started. Intravenous gentamicin, kanamycin, or tobramycin should be started if gram-negative rods are present. When no organisms are iden-

tified, combination therapy must be used. Antibiotics can be adjusted appropriately when culture results are available.

At present, *H. influenzae* type B is uncommon in infants less than 1 month old. However, it is being isolated with increasing frequency in older infants and young children. Ampicillin or chloramphenicol may become necessary additions to antibiotic coverage in neonates if *Hemophilus* infection rates continue to rise.

If a diagnosis of *Candida* arthritis is established by Gram stain or culture of joint fluid, blood, or cerebrospinal fluid, therapy should be started with amphotericin B and 5-fluorocytosine. Renal function must be carefully monitored. Because of the toxicity of antifungal agents, treatment should not be started until the diagnosis of candidal infection is definitely established.

Oral antibiotic therapy in neonates is not advisable. Drug administration is difficult, and absorption is unreliable. Vomiting and diarrhea interfere with attempts at oral therapy.

Joint decompression and debridement are as important in neonates as in older children. Emergency drainage of infected hips is especially important; the danger of permanent damage to the hip from septic arthritis is very high. Needle aspiration is an unreliable means of joint decompression; it may be attempted in other locations if an infant's medical condition is unstable. Aspiration of small joints is difficult, and the potential for damage to joint surfaces is high. Open drainage can often be safely and quickly performed under local anesthesia.

When septic arthritis complicates osteomyelitis, decompression of both the involved bone and joint may be necessary. This is especially important in the hip joint and proximal femur. Reaccumulation of fluid or lack of clinical response to antibiotic therapy in other areas indicates the need for open drainage.

Results

The prognosis in neonatal septic arthritis depends on the site of involvement, offending organism, duration of infection before treatment is begun, and response to therapy. The incidence of permanent joint damage in staphylococcal infection of the hip joint approaches 90%. *Hemophilus* infections and streptococcal infections seem less likely to result in permanent damage, especially if promptly and adequately treated. Long-term follow-up is essential to minimize the complications of hip subluxation and avascular necrosis. Splintage in flexion and abduction for prolonged periods may be necessary to permit normal acetabular and femoral head development to resume.

Gonococcal Arthritis

In adolescents and young adults, *N. gonorrhoeae* is the most common cause of acute suppurative arthritis. Since the advent of modern antimicrobial therapy, the features of gonococcal arthritis have changed. Originally gonococcal arthritis afflicted men primarily, and a majority of patients had permanent joint damage. Today the illness primarily affects women; with effective antibiotic therapy almost all patients recover fully.

Approximately 1% of patients with documented gonorrheal genitourinary disease develop arthritis. Meningitis, myocarditis, pericarditis, and perihepatitis have all been described in association with gonorrheal infection, but arthritis is by far the most common complication.

Presentation

Gonococcal arthritis begins as a venereally acquired infection of the genitourinary tract, rectum, or pharynx. In patients who subsequently develop gonococcal arthritis, the initial infection is asymptomatic and not treated prior to the onset of arthritis. After an uncertain incubation period, genitourinary infection produces a bacteremia. Tenosynovitis and periarthritis develop and may progress to frank arthritis. Two gonococcal arthritis syndromes have been described: a predominantly septicemic syndrome and a predominantly arthritic syndrome. The distinctions are sometimes not clear, and many patients have features of both syndromes.

The septicemic form of gonococcal arthritis is characterized by a 2- to 4-day prodrome of fever, stiffness, and joint pain. Many patients have vesicular skin lesions. Joint symptoms are migratory, and multiple joints may be involved. The knee, ankle, wrist, elbow, and small joints of the hand are most frequently involved. Effusions may be minimal and difficult to aspirate. Radiologic examination of affected joints is normal.

Most patients have a significant peripheral leukocytosis, and most have positive cervical or urethral cultures for *N. gonorrhoeae*. Gram stains of pustular contents of skin lesions may show gram-negative cocci, but cultures of skin lesions are rarely positive. Blood cultures are routinely positive in the septicemic form of gonococcal arthritis; synovial fluid cultures usually are not positive.

The arthritic form of gonococcal arthritis is characterized by a 5- to 10-day prodrome of joint pain. Fever is present in about 30% of patients, and about half have migratory polyarthralgia. Skin lesions occur in about 10% of cases. Leukocytosis is common, but peripheral white blood cell counts are not as high as those in septicemic gonococcal arthritis. Most such patients have only one or two joints involved. Marked effusion is usually present, and the joints are tender, painful, and erythematous. Roentgenograms often show surrounding soft tissue edema. Synovial fluid cultures are positive, and blood cultures are negative. Genitourinary cultures are positive in slightly more than half of affected patients.

Evaluation

Because of the high incidence of gonococcal arthritis in adolescents and young adults, genitourinary, pharyngeal, and rectal cultures, in addition to blood and joint fluid cultures, are recommended in the initial workup of patients with acute suppurative arthritis. Skin lesions should be carefully sought out, stained, and cultured. Management of gonococcal arthritis is quite different from management of other forms of septic arthritis, and every attempt must be made to identify the organism early in the course of infection.

Treatment

Gonococcal arthritis is exquisitely sensitive to penicillin; cessation of symptoms within 72 hours of the start of therapy is supportive evidence of gonococcal infection.

Gonococcal infections respond well to tetracyclines; oral tetracycline may be used in documented gonococcal disease in patients with penicillin allergies. Ten days to 2 weeks of treatment with either penicillin or tetracycline usually suffices; oral penicillin may be used after 2 or 3 days of parenteral therapy. Since *S. aureus* is the other major cause of septic arthritis in adolescents, oxacillin or nafcillin should be used if a clear diagnosis of gonococcal disease cannot be established.

Surgical drainage is rarely necessary but should be considered in hip joint disease in young adolescents to decompress articular vessels. Late complications are uncommon.

SPINAL INFLAMMATORY DISORDERS

Inflammatory lesions of the spine produce a wide variety of clinical syndromes in infants and children. Some affected patients are acutely ill, with severe back pain and signs of systemic sepsis. Others have few signs of serious illness and may be irritable or refuse to stand or walk. The etiology and nature of inflammatory spine disease in children are controversial. Delay in diagnosis is common, and approaches to treatment vary widely. Regardless of etiology, prompt recognition and adequate management can significantly decrease the severity and duration of symptoms in inflammatory diseases of the immature spine.

Pathophysiology

Primary vertebral body osteomyelitis, common in adults, is rare in children. Instead, spine inflammation before skeletal maturity begins most often in the intervertebral disk space. The signs, symptoms, and late radiologic findings in both processes are similar, however, and it may be impossible to differentiate vertebral osteomyelitis from intervertebral diskitis when diagnosis has been delayed. In most cases where spinal inflammatory disease has been suspected early, serial roentgenograms show first loss of disk-space height and later erosion of vertebral end-plates, suggesting primary intervertebral disk involvement.

Intervertebral diskitis is probably the common clinical and radiologic result of a number of pathologic processes. Bacterial infection is responsible for many cases. Cultures of intervertebral disk-space material obtained by needle aspiration or open biopsy are positive in about half of the instances in which they are performed; *S. aureus* is most often isolated. Contamination of the disk space in children could occur by contiguous spread from the metaphyseal vessels of adjacent vertebral bodies or by hematogenous seeding of the intervertebral space through persistent embryonic capillaries within the disk itself.

The benign course of many patients with intervertebral diskitis suggests that at times other inflammatory processes may be responsible for the clinical and radiologic findings. Often patients obtain dramatic relief with immobilization alone; this is not consistent with the course of musculoskeletal infections in other parts of the body. Viral infection and trauma have been implicated in some instances of diskitis. Herniation of the nucleus pulposis through the vertebral end-plate as a result of trauma may initiate an inflammatory response that produces findings similar to diskitis of infectious origin.

Regardless of etiology, inflammation within the intervertebral space results in destruction of the nucleus pulposis. Loss of disk-space height follows. If the inflammatory process continues, erosion of adjacent vertebral end-plates may occur, mimicking vertebral osteomyelitis. These changes persist after clinical and laboratory evidence of inflammation has disappeared. Although restoration of disk height may occur during the first few years after infection, narrowing and end-plate changes are usually permanent. Intervertebral calcification is common, and spontaneous interbody fusion may occur. Mild scoliosis has been reported in some patients, but late symptoms are uncommon, and acute inflammation rarely occurs.

Presentation

The clinical manifestations of diskitis vary with the age of the patient and the nature of the inflammatory lesion. Staphylococcal disk-space infection may be associated with acute back pain and systemic signs of septicemia. Symptoms in patients with less virulent infections and post-traumatic inflammatory lesions are not as severe. Fever is often present at the time of initial evaluation in acutely ill patients. Less symptomatic patients may have normal temperatures.

Symptoms in the early phases of diskitis may be the result of irritation of the nerve fibers that supply the annulus fibrosis and spinal ligaments, or of edema and compression of spinal nerve roots. Inflammation may produce irritation of the anterior paraspinal muscles and splanchnic nerves. A variety of clinical syndromes may result.

In infants, fussiness, irritability, and refusal to stand when supported are common signs of diskitis. Affected toddlers become cranky and cease walking. Tenderness may be present on palpation of the spine, but the site of maximum discomfort may be impossible to localize. Loss of normal lumbar or cervical lordosis is common when those spinal segments are involved. Acute torticollis and restriction of passive neck motion may be present in infants and children with cervical diskitis.

Back pain is a common complaint in older children and adolescents with diskitis. The patient can often localize the site of maximum discomfort to the affected area of the spine. Coughing and straining usually increase back pain. Leg pain may be present if inflammation involves the spinal nerves to the lower extremities. Irritation of the psoas muscles produces painful hip flexion contractures and loss of lumbar lordosis.

Abdominal symptoms predominate in some patients with diskitis involving the splanchnic nerves. Nausea, vomiting, and abdominal tenderness may be mistaken for signs of acute abdominal disease.

Erythrocyte sedimentation rates are almost always abnormal in patients with intervertebral diskitis, regardless of etiology. Rates greater than 50 mm/hour are not uncommon. White blood cell counts are elevated in about half of patients with diskitis. Blood cultures are positive on occasion in some patients with fever and signs of systemic sepsis.

Radiologic findings depend on the severity and duration of the inflammatory process. Loss of intervertebral disk height is the earliest radiologic manifestion of diskitis and may occur within 1 week to 10 days of the onset of symptoms. Erosion of vertebral end-plates occurs later; 2 to 3 weeks may be required for bony changes to develop (Fig 8–5). Signs of disk destruction and end-plate reaction persist long after all clinical and laboratory signs of inflammation have subsided.

Radioisotope bone scans become abnormal earlier in the evolution of intervertebral diskitis than do routine roentgenograms. Increased radioisotope turnover in adjacent vertebrae may be manifested within 10 days when ^{99m}Tc scans are employed. Gallium 67 scans reportedly become abnormal even earlier. Both technetium and gallium scanning techniques depend on reaction to inflammation, and both scans may be normal in the early phases of intervertebral diskitis. Because isotope uptake is a nonspecific reflection

of bone turnover, bone scans may remain abnormal after other signs of inflammation have subsided.

Treatment

A high index of suspicion is required for the early diagnosis of diskitis. Symptoms are often vague, and signs are frequently not specific. Back pain, muscle spasm, and tenderness along the spine are significant abnormalities in children with no history of trauma. They are often the earliest findings in patients with inflammatory or neoplastic lesions of the spine. Diskitis must be considered as well in the differential diagnosis of infants who are irritable when turned, refuse to stand, or cease walking. Unexplained abdominal pain or lower extremity pain may also be symptoms of intervertebral diskspace inflammation.

Children with symptoms and signs of

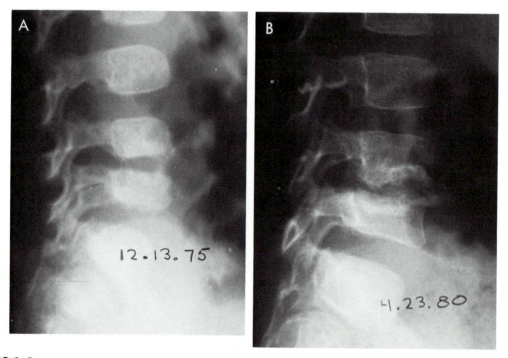

FIG 8–5.
A, loss of intervertebral disk height is the earliest radiologic manifestation of diskitis. **B,** progressive end-plate erosion and vertebral body sclerosis may reflect either ongoing disease or the severity of the initial insult.

diskitis should be hospitalized for evaluation. Careful examination of the musculoskeletal and neurologic systems is essential. Initial laboratory studies should include complete blood cell counts, sedimentation rates, and urinalysis. Tuberculin skin tests should be performed, and blood, urine, throat, and sputum cultures collected. Anteroposterior and lateral spine roentgenograms and bone scans with either or both gallium and technetium should be obtained on admission. Spinal tap is not indicated in the absence of signs of meningeal irritation or neurologic deficit.

New radioisotope techniques have decreased the delay and increased the accuracy of diagnosis of diskitis. Unfortunately, isolation of an organism even in cases where infection seems likely remains difficult. Biopsy of the intervertebral space is difficult, and the yield of cultures obtained by needle aspiration or open biopsy is low. The magnitude of the procedure is greater than the disease usually warrants.

Antibiotic therapy should be reserved for patients with fever and leukocytosis. If an organism is isolated from routine cultures, appropriate antibiotics should be started parenterally and continued for 7 to 10 days. Oral antibiotic therapy can then be employed, as in osteomyelitis and septic arthritis. If no organism is isolated, then "best guess" antibiotic therapy should be started with a semisynthetic penicillin or cephalosporin. A total of 4 weeks of antibiotic therapy should be used in patients with infectious diskitis. Cast immobilization during this period relieves symptoms and facilitates nursing care.

The often benign course in patients with diskitis despite long delays in diagnosis and little or no antibiotic therapy suggests that, at times, diskitis must be the result of either very low-grade infec-

tion or other noninfectious inflammatory processes. Antibiotic therapy is not indicated for patients without fever or leukocytosis. Such patients can be managed by immobilization alone. Most respond rapidly, with dramatic relief of symptoms. Four to 6 weeks of cast immobilization is ordinarily sufficient.

Surgical drainage, a critical component of effective treatment of other musculoskeletal infections, is rarely required in diskitis. Biopsy should be reserved for patients in whom tuberculosis is suspected on the basis of history and skin testing, for patients in whom diagnosis is in doubt, and for patients who do not respond to antibiotics and/or cast immobilization within 1 week.

Recurrent disk-space infection is uncommon, and most patients have no symptoms of back pain in later life despite persistent radiologic changes. Progressive spine deformity rarely if ever complicates diskitis.

SUGGESTED READINGS

Osteomyelitis

Curtiss PH Jr: *Bone and Joint Infection in Childhood*, American Academy of Orthopaedic Surgeons: Instructional Course Lectures. St Louis, CV Mosby Co, 1977, vol 26, pp 14–19.

Dich VQ, Nelson JD, Haltalin DC: Osteomyelitis in infants and children: A review of 163 cases. *Am J Dis Child* 1975; 129:1273–1278.

Fox L, Sprunt K: Neonatal osteomyelitis. *Pediatrics* 1978; 62:535–542.

Scoles PV, Sfakianakis GN, Hilty M: Bone scan patterns in osteomyelitis *Clin Orthop* 1980; 152:210–217.

Tetzlaff TR, McCracken GH, Nelson JD: Oral antibiotic therapy for skeletal infections in children. *J Pediatr* 1978; 92:485–490.

Trueta J: The three types of acute haematogenous osteomyelitis. *J Bone Joint Surg Br* 1959; 41:671–680.

Waldvogel FA, Medoff G, Swartz MN: Osteomyelitis: A review of clinical features, therapeutic considerations, and unusual aspects. *N Engl J Med* 1970; 282:198–206, 260–266, 316–322.

Waldvogel FA, Vasey H: Osteomyelitis: The past decade. *N Engl J Med* 1980; 303:360–370.

Infectious Arthritis

Pittard WB, Thullen JD, Fanaroff AA: Neonatal septic arthritis. *J Pediatr* 1976; 88:621–624.

Nelson JD, Koontz WC: Septic arthritis in infants and children: A review of 117 cases. *Pediatrics* 1966; 38:966–971.

Nelson JD: The bacterial etiology and antibiotic management of septic arthritis in infants and children. *Pediatrics* 1972; 50:437–440.

Goldenberg DH, Cohen AS: Acute infectious arthritis. *Am J Med* 1976; 60:369–373.

Brogadir SP, Schimmer BM, Myers AR: Spectrum of the gonococcal arthritis–dermatitis syndrome. *Semin Arthritis Rheum* 1979; 8:177–183.

Diskitis

Fischer GW, Popich GA, Sullivan DE, et al: Discitis: A prospective diagnostic analysis. *Pediatrics* 1978; 62:543.

Spiegel PG, Kengla K, Isaacson A, et al: Intervertebral disc space inflammation in children. *J Bone Joint Surg Am* 1972; 54:284.

Wenger DB, Bobechko WP, Gilday DJ: The spectrum of intervertebral disc space infection in children. *J Bone Joint Surg Am* 1978; 60:100.

9

Neuromuscular Diseases

Cerebral Palsy
Myopathic and Neuropathic Diseases
  Muscular Dystrophies
  Neuropathic Diseases
  Inherited Disorders of Motor, Sensory,
    and Autonomic Neurons

Arthrogryposis Multiplex Congenita
Brachial Plexus Injuries
Spinal Dysraphism

A number of disorders of the central nervous system, peripheral nerves, and skeletal muscle affect the developing musculoskeletal system. In some syndromes, such as cerebral palsy, the pathologic process is static, although its outward manifestations may change with growth and development. In other conditions, such as Duchenne type muscular dystrophy, disease progression and declining functional ability coincide.

Although intellectual and perceptual deficits accompany many neuromuscular disorders of childhood, the earliest manifestations are often abnormalities of motor function. Developmental delay, persistence of infantile reflex patterns, or decreasing function must be viewed with concern. The unfortunate tendency to dismiss subtle abnormalities as normal variations delays diagnosis, confuses parents, and generates considerable hostility. Early recognition permits a coordinated approach to the long-term care necessary for these children.

CEREBRAL PALSY

Cerebral palsy is the term applied to a number of clinical syndromes resulting from static lesions of the immature central nervous system. The nature and location of brain damage is variable, but by definition it must be fixed and nonprogressive. Delayed motor development and abnormalities of motor function are often the most obvious signs in affected children, but sensory and intellectual impairment are frequently present as well. Proprioception, stereognosis, and tactile discrimination are often compromised, and intellectual deficits ranging in severity from profound retardation to minor learning disorders are present in approximately half of involved patients. Often the degree of retardation corresponds to the severity of the motor involvement.

Cerebral palsy is one of the most common handicapping conditions of childhood. There has been no evidence of a decline in overall incidence over the past two decades despite improvements in obstetric and neonatal care. It has been estimated that as many as 1 in 500 school-age children are affected and that a number of more severely involved infants die before reaching school age. The spectrum of involvement is wide. Some patients have such profound motor and intellectual retardation that they require full-time nursing care and frequently must be institutionalized. Others are so minimally involved that they function independently at normal or near-normal levels in all activities of daily life. The majority of patients fall between these extremes and require varying amounts of pediatric, neurologic, and orthopedic care to maximize function.

The central nervous system (CNS) lesions that produce the clinical syndromes of cerebral palsy may arise during fetal development, at birth, or in the neonatal period. In his original descriptions of cerebral palsy, William Little concluded that abnormalities of birth were the principal etiologic factors. Recent large incidence studies support the later views of Freud, that, in many cases, problems at birth were the incidental consequences of prenatal abnormalities that produced the central nervous system lesion. Prematurity, low birth weight, and birth asphyxia have been clearly documented to greatly increase the risk to an infant of cerebral palsy, but the majority of children with cerebral palsy have no such history. Many times the etiology of developmental delay and cerebral palsy cannot be accurately established, and at times, multiple factors are involved. Trauma, asphyxia in the perinatal period, multiple births, neonatal or maternal infection, vascular anomalies, seizure disorders, and brain malformations all may produce nonprogressive brain damage with musculoskeletal manifestations. Maternal mental retardation, maternal illness, and fetal malformation have been recently reported to be the most significant predictors of cerebral palsy in term or near term infants.

Cerebral palsy is common in extremely low-weight and markedly premature infants. Intraventricular hemorrhage with focal brain damage and secondary hydrocephalus has been demonstrated on postmortem studies and by computed tomography in a significant percentage of infants with gestational age less than 32 weeks or birth weight less than 1,500 gm. Although not all affected infants show clinical symptoms, many later manifest developmental delay and neurologic impairment.

The motor deficits in cerebral palsy syndromes have been used to classify patients into a number of groups. Hoffer has proposed a simple scheme based on functional goals that may be summarized as follows:

Spasticity.—Syndromes characterized by increased activity of muscle stretch reflexes, resulting in exaggerated tendon jerks and clonus. Because control of deep tendon reflexes involves several levels of neural function, spasticity is no longer considered a purely pyramidal tract syndrome. Spasticity is the most common form of cerebral palsy and the form with the best prognosis.

Motion and Balance Disorders.—Syndromes characterized by involuntary movements such as athetosis and tremor, rigidity, or ataxia. These syndromes indicate more diffuse brain damage and present much more complicated treatment problems than pure spasticity.

Mixed Disorders.—Combinations of spasticity and dyskinesia are common and may be second to pure spasticity as the most frequent type of cerebral palsy.

Cerebral palsy patients, especially spastics, are usually classified by distribution of paresis as well as by type. *Monoplegia* refers to single limb involvement. *Hemiplegia* involves upper and lower limbs on the same side of the body. Patients with three limbs involved are said to be *triplegic*. Involvement of all four limbs is termed *quadriplegia*. Monoplegia and triplegia are uncommon; most monoplegic patients have subtle signs of hemiplegia, and most triplegic patients have four-extremity involvement. *Diplegia* is a term often applied to a pattern of four-extremity involvement in which the lower limbs are more severely affected than the upper limbs. Patients with four-extremity involvement often have more sensory and intellectual impairment than patients with hemiplegia. "Total involvement" more accurately describes the condition of many of these patients than quadriplegia.

Early diagnosis of cerebral palsy is most accurately based on a high index of suspicion and careful developmental testing. Infants with significant CNS damage usually show motor abnormalities within the first few months of life if carefully tested. Consistent hypotonia or rigidity on examination are early signs of severe brain damage. In less severely involved infants, developmental delay is often first noted by parents between ages 6 and 8 months, when poor head control, lack of sitting balance, and failure to roll become apparent. Minimally affected children may escape diagnosis until age 18 to 24 months; persistent tiptoe gait or early hand dominance often are the first abnormalities noted. In an infant with a suggestive history, a tentative diagnosis of cerebral palsy is warranted when normal motor milestones are not achieved on schedule, when primitive reflexes persist, or when abnormal reflex patterns are consistently present.

Apparent neurologic abnormalities vary from day to day in young patients and are significantly affected by the infant's overall state of irritability, hunger, and fatigue. Gentle, repeated examinations in a warm and quiet setting should be conducted before a tentative diagnosis of cerebral palsy is made. Parents should be informed of the examiner's suspicions; most often they are aware of subtle developmental delay before the physician. Open discussion should be encouraged, but care must be taken to avoid presenting either too negative or too positive a prognosis. Developmental delay, retardation, and cerebral palsy are frightening terms, and physicians often discount or minimize significant abnormal findings in an attempt to allay parental anxiety. Such support is fragile and misleading. On the other hand, it is often difficult to fully establish the extent of CNS damage for several years, and an early bad prognosis may not be borne out later. Neurologic and orthopedic consultations should be encouraged when a diagnosis of cerebral palsy is first suspected; independent evaluations are valuable in subsequent discussions with the family and in planning long-term care.

Certain reflex patterns and developmental milestones are helpful in the early diagnosis of cerebral palsy. Careful sequential testing often permits estimation of ultimate motor function. A number of involuntary reflexes present in the infant fade with normal development. Moro's reflex is elicited by neck extension in the neonate; the normal response is abduction of both arms, initial extension of the elbows, wrists, and fingers, followed by slight elbow, wrist, and finger flexion. The response is normally present at birth and fades by age 3 to 6 months. Complete absence of Moro's reflex at birth or persistence beyond 6 months is suggestive of CNS injury. Asymmetry may indicate brachial plexus injury, fractures of the shoulder girdle or upper extremity, or infection in the upper limb.

The foot-placing response is normally present from birth. If the infant is supported by the trunk in the upright position and the dorsal surfaces of the feet are dragged along the under surface of a table, the usual response is hip and knee flexion followed by placement of the feet on the table. Complete absence of the foot-placing response indicates central lesions; asymmetry of response may indicate peripheral nerve injury, lower extremity fracture, or infection.

The asymmetric and symmetric tonic neck reflexes are occasionally present in normal infants. When the head of a supine infant is gently turned to the side, extension or lessening of flexion of the limbs on the chin side and flexion of the limbs on the occiput side constitute the asymmetric neck reflex. The symmetric tonic neck reflex can be elicited by supporting the neonate in the prone position and gently flexing and extending the neck. Neck extension produces elbow extension, and neck flexion produces elbow flexion when the response is present. The asymmetric and symmetric tonic neck reflexes may or may not be present in normal infants at birth, but when present, they should fade and disappear by age 4 to 6 months. Obligate reflex responses in the first few months or persistence after age 6 months is abnormal.

Normal infants respond to being supported in the upright position with momentary hip and knee extension and ankle plantar flexion. The response is normally brief and is followed by hip and knee flexion and ankle dorsiflexion. Persistent extension, especially when accompanied by marked hip adduction (often called scissoring) is abnormal and is a bad prognostic sign for independent walking.

The parachute response develops by age 12 months in normal infants. To elicit the reflex, the child is supported by the trunk in the standing position. Support is next momentarily relaxed, and the head and trunk are allowed to fall forward. The normal response is forward flexion of the shoulder and elbow, wrist, and finger extension, as if to protect the head when falling. Absence of the parachute response at age 12 months is a significant abnormal finding.

Persistence of one or more primitive reflexes past age 6 to 12 months is an ominous finding; failure of sitting balance to develop by 12 months or failure of the parachute reaction to appear on schedule greatly decreases the chances of eventual walking. Because of the difficulties of neonatal and infantile neurologic examina-

tions, testing should be repeated on several occasions before conclusions are reached. Neurologic consultation is indicated when available.

The goals of orthopedic care in cerebral palsy are to maximize function and prevent deformity. Even though the CNS lesion is fixed, the musculoskeletal manifestations of cerebral palsy change with growth. Progressive contractures that result from chronic muscle imbalance may make gait awkward and unstable in patients who have enough control of function and balance to walk. Contractures around the pelvis may cause obliquity, which interferes with sitting balance, or may result in limitation of hip motion, which interferes with nursing care. Although such complications are not always preventable, a combination of carefully planned physical therapy, bracing, and surgical treatment can minimize the resulting disability.

Realistic goals are a prerequisite for the long-term care of the cerebral palsy patient. Such children usually have a combination of musculoskeletal, sensory, and intellectual deficits. Surgical procedures, orthotic devices, and therapy programs designed to encourage walking are futile in children who lack necessary cortical control of muscle function. Similarly, extensive tendon transfers in the hand and wrist are of little value in children who lack sensory discrimination or voluntary muscle control. Whenever possible, a long-range plan of treatment should be established early and modified when appropriate as further growth and development occur.

In general, patients with primarily spastic involvement are easier to care for than patients with dyskinesias or ataxic disorders. Physical therapy and orthotic support can be used to inhibit increased muscle tone or overcome imbalance in some patients; surgical muscle recessions, tendon lengthenings, and neurectomies can be employed in others to compensate for abnormal tone. Pharmacologic attempts to control increased tone to date have proved disappointing; troublesome side effects have often outweighed benefits. Selective posterior rhizotomy is currently under evaluation as a means of decreasing spasticity in some patients. Initial results have been encouraging, but further followup is needed before widespread use can be recommended.

Ataxic patients respond far less predictably. Lack of central coordination interferes with attempts to train patients in activities of daily life. Bracing of one or more extremities to inhibit involuntary motion may result in increased activity in unrestrained limbs. Muscle releases and tendon transfers often compound abnormal posture. Unfortunately, pharmacologic attempts to control spasticity and dyskinesia have so far been unrewarding in most instances since drug dosages high enough to decrease abnormal tone produce undesirable sedation. Surgical attempts to decrease abnormal motion by rhizotomy or by implantation of electronic central stimulation units have been for the most part unsuccessful.

It is often possible to judge an infant's ultimate ability to walk by age 12 to 18 months from the nature and distribution of motor involvement. The prognosis in spasticity is better than in other forms of cerebral palsy, and patients with minimal involvement fare better than those with more extensive lesions. Associated intellectual retardation is a significant adverse factor, and the availability of comprehensive physical and occupational therapy services is a positive factor in marginal cases.

Spastic children with monoplegia or hemiplegia almost always become walkers, although ambulation may be delayed 3 or 4 years. Most require external supports such as handrails, walkers, or crutches for only a short time. Equinus contractures of the involved ankle are common in such patients. At first these contractures are flexible and easily corrected by gentle stretching. Physical therapy may prolong this period and delay the development of fixed contractures. In time, however, fixed contractures develop in almost all patients. One or both muscles of the gastrocnemius-soleus group are most commonly involved; hamstring and hip flexor contractures frequently are present as well. Short leg braces, sometimes preceded by casting to decrease spastic muscle tone and gain correction, are often useful when contractures are minimal. Eventually, Achilles tendon lengthening procedures are required in most patients. Postoperative support in the form of short leg braces or night splints may be required to maintain correction gained at surgery.

Ultimate ambulation in spastic children with three- or four-extremity involvement is more difficult to judge. If Moro's, symmetric, and asymmetric neck reflexes are absent at age 12 months, extensor thrust and scissoring are not prominent, and a parachute reaction is present, eventual ambulation can be reasonably expected. The persistence of one or more infantile reflexes or the absence of protective reflexes by age 12 to 18 months makes walking much less likely, as does moderate to severe intellectual retardation.

Most patients with four-extremity involvement who will become walkers do so by age 4 to 5 years. Most require crutches or a walker when first walking; many continue to require external support. Contractures around the hips, knees, and ankles often interfere significantly with gait and can be very frustrating to manage. Brace support is often necessary, and surgical correction may be required. Unfortunately, braces are often awkward to apply, heavy, and uncomfortable. Unless carefully fitted and fabricated, they may hinder rather than help the cerebral palsy patient. Surgery, too, is often unpredictable. Attempts to control contractures by muscle releases or neurectomies have, on occasion, led to overpull of antagonist muscles and new deformities. Tendon transfers are much less predictable in cerebral palsy than in other paralytic diseases. To be successful, surgery must be carefully planned, goals must be realistic, and adequate outpatient physical therapy facilities must be available.

The orthopedic management of children who will not become walkers is difficult. Goals must be realistic. Therapy programs, bracing, and surgical procedures aimed at preserving sitting balance, increasing independence, or facilitating nursing care are warranted, but unreasonable expectations must be avoided. The motor deficits in cerebral palsy patients originate from CNS damage; vigorous physical therapy or extensive surgery rarely if ever compensate for severe brain damage.

Sitting balance is essential to children who will be wheelchair patients, and every reasonable attempt should be made to obtain and preserve it. Some hypotonic, dyskinetic, and ataxic children lack the strength or control necessary to sit independently. During the first 12 to 18 months of life, such patients may be propped in a seated position with pillows. Later, however, transporter chairs with lateral supports, V-belts, and head rests may be necessary to maintain balance. Suitable portable chairs that fold to fit into automobiles are commercially available and permit parents to take their children along on trips outside the home. This is valuable both for the child and the parent. By age 8 to 10 years, many patients have outgrown such chairs, and standard wheelchairs with appropriate modifications to provide support and permit self-propulsion, if possible, are necessary.

Contractures of the hip flexor and adductor muscles may interfere with nursing care and later cause hip dislocation and pelvic obliquity. Such contractures are most common in nonambulatory spastic patients. Initially, adductor overpull may be managed by passive stretching exercises and splinting. Often, however, surgical intervention is required. A variety of surgical procedures have been developed, including release of the adductor muscle origins with or without division of the obdurator nerve, adductor origin recession, and femoral shortening osteotomy. Unfortunately, no surgical procedure has been uniformly successful. In general, surgical procedures designed to compensate for adductor overpull work best when performed before hip subluxation or dislocation develops.

Treatment of hip dislocation in cerebral palsy is difficult. Without treatment, dislocation produces a flexed, adducted posture of the lower extremity, which makes sitting and perineal care difficult. Pain is often a problem, and many such patients become bedfast. Decubitus ulcers, atelectasis, aspiration, and pneumonia often follow. Surgical treatment is often frustrating. Open reduction with femoral and/or pelvic osteotomy is sometimes required but may be complicated by redislocation, hip stiffness, or deep infection. Resection of the proximal femur is at times performed to gain motion and relieve pain, but it, too, may be followed by hip pain and stiffness. At present, there is no universally accepted answer to the problem of spastic hip dislocation.

Pelvic obliquity and spinal muscle imbalance may lead to scoliosis in cerebral palsy patients. Such curves are often progressive and, if untreated, lead to sitting imbalance and respiratory compromise. Nursing care becomes difficult, and pain may be severe. The communicative difficulty that many severely involved patients experience often makes interpretation of their symptoms difficult, and their pain may be unintentionally ignored.

Brace treatment is often impossible in such patients. They cannot cooperate with the active exercise programs that are an integral part of nonoperative treatment, and they tolerate the constant pressure of conventional orthoses poorly. Custom-molded total-contact braces and specially fabricated seat inserts can sometimes be employed for less severe curves, but they are not as predictably successful in cerebral palsy as in idiopathic scoliosis. Operative treatment is often required to halt progression and relieve pain. Frequently both anterior and posterior spine fusion with internal fixation devices are required. In carefully selected patients, such procedures improve balance, relieve pain, facilitate nursing care, and free the patient's upper extremities for the activities of daily life. The magnitude of the procedures is great, however, and not all cerebral palsy patients are appropriate candidates.

MYOPATHIC AND NEUROPATHIC DISEASES

A number of disorders cause progressive weakness in childhood and adolescence. They vary widely in age at onset, clinical course, and prognosis, but most are first manifested by weakness in infancy or childhood. The diseases can be divided into two main groups on the basis of clinical and laboratory investigations: primary disorders of muscle (myopathic diseases or muscular dystrophy) and primary diseases of the CNS or peripheral nerves (neuropathic diseases).

Muscular Dystrophies

The muscular dystrophies are a group of genetically transmitted primary diseases of muscle that were first described in the 19th century. They vary in age at onset, hereditary pattern, and distribution of weakness, but most begin during childhood or early adolescence and are characterized by progressive muscle weakness. They are generally presumed to be the result of a genetic deficiency of an enzyme necessary to maintain the integrity of muscle cells. The muscular dystrophies can be subdivided into several varieties, based on clinical course and genetic patterns.

Duchenne type muscular dystrophy is the most common primary myopathic disorder. In fact, the term "muscular dystrophy" is often used synonymously with Duchenne type dystrophy. The abnormal gene responsible for the condition has been localized on the short arm of the X chromosome, but its product or precise effect on muscle cells has not yet been identified. Although the condition was named for Duchenne after his published descriptions in 1861, Little and Meryon noted the clinical picture in 1853. These early descriptions of a familial, slowly progressive disease affecting boys and characterized by weakness, intellectual slowness, and inevitable fatal progression remain accurate.

Duchenne type dystrophy is a sex-linked recessive disorder with a high spontaneous mutation rate. Approximately 1 in 3,000 male children are affected. As many as one third of new cases have no family history and are presumed to represent mutation. As in other sex-linked recessive disorders, boys are predominantly affected. Since the abnormal gene is carried on one maternal X chromosome, 50% of a carrier mother's male children can be expected to develop the clinical disorder. On occasion, girls may develop the clinical findings of classic Duchenne type dystrophy. This may occur in Turner's syndrome (XO) or in the Turner mosaic disorders (X/XX) or may be the result of autosomal translocation of the short arm of the X chromosome that permits the abnormal trait to be manifested.

Although the exact biochemical effect of the abnormal gene in Duchenne type dystrophy is not known, the histologic and biochemical alterations produced in affected patients have been well documented. Skeletal muscle is most severely involved, but cardiac muscle is affected as well. Muscle fiber necrosis, macrophage infiltration, and disorganized attempts at regeneration are characteristic microscopic findings. Histochemical studies show alterations in glycogen content and muscle enzyme function. Ultrastuctural studies show defects in muscle plasma membrane that probably result in alterations in calcium metabolism and lead to death of muscle cells.

The most consistent laboratory finding in affected individuals is elevation of serum creatine kinase (CK). Levels may be elevated 10 to 100 times normal in early childhood and then begin to fall during the juvenile period, perhaps as a result of decreasing muscle mass. Affected patients show increased urinary excretion of creatine and decreased excretion of creatinine. Creatine kinase levels two to three times normal have been reported in sisters of Duchenne patients early in childhood and may be a reflection of the carrier state in girls. Creatine kinase levels fall at puberty in these patients, and after puberty, CK levels are no longer reliable manifestations of the carrier state.

Mild motor and intellectual developmental delay and inability to keep up with peers are often the first signs of Duchenne type dystrophy reported by parents. The onset of weakness in affected males usually begins before age 5 years and may be noted shortly after a child begins to walk. The muscles of the shoulder girdle and pelvis are involved first; affected children are clumsy and often have difficulty climbing stairs. Diffi-

culty in rising to a standing position from a seated position on the floor (Gowers' sign) is a classic finding. Because of weakness of hip extensor and knee extensor muscles, affected children must use one or both hands to brace the lower extremities when rising.

Distal progression of the disease is often marked by apparent hypertrophy of the calf muscles and equinus contracture of the ankles. At times, this may lead to an incorrect diagnosis of idiopathic toe walking, clubfoot, or cerebral palsy. In reality, fatty degeneration of the gastrocnemius-soleus muscles occurs, leading to heel cord contracture and progressive disability. Deep tendon reflexes are normal or only slightly diminished early in the course of Duchenne type dystrophy. Eventually, deep tendon reflexes become depressed or disappear because of muscle weakness or tendon contracture. No loss of sensation occurs, and muscle fasciculation, a sign of denervation, is rarely seen. Motor and sensory nerve conduction studies are normal.

The usual course of Duchenne type dystrophy is steady progression and increasing disability. Hip and knee extensor weakness and heel cord contractures make standing balance difficult. Most affected patients lose the ability to walk early in the second decade. As trunk muscle involvement progresses, collapsing neuromuscular scoliosis often develops, and sitting balance deteriorates. Frequently patients must use their upper extremities for support, further compounding their disability. Respiratory impairment secondary to thoracic muscle weakness and progressive scoliosis usually leads to pneumonia and death late in the second decade.

There is no cure for Duchenne type dystrophy. The goals of orthopedic treatment are to maintain function as long as possible and to prevent progressive deformities, which further handicap the involved child. Tendon lengthenings and lower extremity bracing are useful to preserve the ability to stand and walk early in the course of the disease. Physical therapy programs can help maximize a patient's potential, but unfortunately, aggressive muscle strengthening programs have not been demonstrated to compensate for progressive myopathy.

The spinal deformity that accompanies Duchenne type dystrophy is deforming, disabling, and painful. Scoliosis usually develops shortly after the patient stops walking and is insidiously progressive. Nonoperative management is usually unsuccessful. Commercially available canvas corsets are of little or no help. Specially fabricated plastic body jackets can be useful in slowing progression of some curves. Seating modifications and lateral wheelchair supports are occasionally helpful in maintaining balance. Neither bracing nor seat modification prevents progressive deformity in most patients.

The role of surgical intervention in the management of scoliosis in Duchenne type dystrophy has become more clear in the past 5 years. It has been repeatedly demonstrated that muscular dystrophy patients can safely tolerate correction and stabilization of severe deformity even when significant decreases in pulmonary function are present, as long as certain guidelines are followed. Spinal instrumentation rigid enough to permit immediate mobilization is necessary to prevent further loss of strength during the postoperative period. Ventilatory assistance must be used with caution in patients with severe diminution in pulmonary function to minimize the risk of ventilator dependency. Meticulous hemostasis during surgery is essential. Results of correction of spinal deformity are dramatic. Pain relief, improved sitting balance, and increased functional capability are immediate benefits. Many patients report improved respiratory function, most

probably from the mechanical effect of stabilizing the trunk. To provide the most benefit with the least risk, spinal instrumentation and fusion should be performed as soon as spine deformity becomes apparent in the sitting muscular dystrophy patient.

A number of less common forms of muscular dystrophy have clinical signs and genetic transmission patterns significantly different from those of Duchenne type dystrophy. In many of these syndromes, major muscle involvement is confined to the trunk and either the upper or lower limbs, with facial muscle sparing. In other varieties, facial muscle involvement occurs as well. In most, progression is not as rapid as in Duchenne type dystrophy, and prolonged survival is the rule. Collectively, these disorders have been termed the limb-girdle syndromes. The most common of these rarer forms of muscular dystrophy is often referred to as limb-girdle dystrophy, or autosomal recessive muscular dystrophy of childhood. Unlike Duchenne type dystrophy, it is transmitted as an autosomal recessive trait and characterized by pronounced weakness in the pelvic and shoulder girdle musculature. The distal muscles of the limbs are less severely affected. Serum creatine kinase levels are elevated in involved patients, and muscle biopsy findings resemble those of Duchenne type dystrophy. Initial symptoms develop slowly in either the muscles of the pelvis or the shoulder girdle, and distal involvement occurs later. Its course is variable. In a few cases, rapid progression similar to that of Duchenne type dystrophy occurs, but more often the disease is much more slowly progressive. Many of the same deformities of the trunk and limbs as in Duchenne dystrophy develop with the passage of time, but the disease course usually extends over 10 to 20 years. Most affected patients usually die in young to middle adult life of respiratory disease, which may be compounded by severe spine deformity.

Fascioscapulohumeral dystrophy is a form of progressive muscle weakness that affects primarily the muscles of the face and the shoulder girdle. It is transmitted as an autosomal dominant trait and tends to be much less severe than either Duchenne type dystrophy or limb-girdle dystrophy. The clinical onset may occur from midchildhood through early adult life. Progression may be very slow, and aborted cases are common. Weakness of the facial muscles and of the deltoid, trapezius, and scapular muscles are the chief clinical findings. Distal involvement and lower extremity involvement is uncommon. Most affected patients have a normal life span.

The orthopedic management of patients with slowly progressive forms of muscular dystrophy is aimed at preserving function and preventing disabling contractures. Walking is the best physical therapy for most patients, and every effort should be made to maintain ambulatory function. Spine deformity should be treated aggressively in patients with slowly progressive muscular dystrophies. The disability and pain of progressive scoliosis can be minimized or prevented with careful orthotic management and surgical intervention. Total-contact bracing may be employed in the early phases of the disease, and posterior spine fusion with internal fixation is often indicated later. Preoperatively and postoperatively, aggressive physical therapy and respiratory therapy programs are necessary to minimize the weakness that may result from prolonged postoperative immobilization.

Neuropathic Diseases

A number of hereditary diseases of the lower motor neuron and peripheral nerves produce progressive weakness of the trunks or limbs. The patterns of involvement, rate of progression, severity, and age at onset vary widely. In some disorders, such as the spinal muscle atrophies, the disease process appears to arise primarily in the anterior horn cells of the spinal cord. In other diseases, such as Charcot-Marie-Tooth disease, the disorder may involve peripheral nerves primarily. Rapidly progressive, severe neuropathic disorders are often confused with Duchenne type muscular dystrophy because of the severe proximal muscle weakness that develops. They are, however, distinct pathologic entities. Muscle degeneration in the neuropathic disorders is secondary to denervation. Serum creatine kinase levels may be normal or only mildly elevated in contrast to the extraordinarily high levels found in the muscular dystrophies. Electromyographic studies demonstrate primarily neuronal disease rather than myopathic disease.

The spinal muscle atrophies are a spectrum of diseases characterized by progressive anterior horn cell degeneration, resulting in trunk and limb weakness. The diseases have been divided into subgroups based on age at onset and rate of progression, but often the distinction between types is blurred. It has been common practice to refer to infantile onset spinal muscle atrophy as Werdnig-Hoffmann disease and to later onset spinal muscle atrophy as Kugelberg-Welander disease. More recent classifications of spinal muscle atrophy do not employ the eponyms. Characteristic differences in prognosis among the various forms of spinal muscle atrophy justify separation into separate groups.

In the most severe form of spinal muscle atrophy, known as spinal muscle atrophy 1 (SMA 1), weakness develops in utero or within the first month of life. Decreased fetal movement in the third trimester may be noted. Generalized hypotonia is present on examination on neonatal examination. Head control is often poor, and affected children may have difficulty in sucking and swallowing. The intercostal muscles and accessory muscles of respiration are weak, and coughing and crying may be impossible. Shoulder girdle muscles and pelvic muscles may be weak or paralyzed. Distal muscle function may not be so severely affected. Deep tendon reflexes are absent, but sensory nerve function is spared. Death often occurs within the first year of life from respiratory infection.

In spinal muscle atrophy 2, onset of symptoms occurs between the 2nd and 12th month. This form of spinal muscle atrophy has occasionally been called chronic Werdnig-Hoffmann disease. It progresses less rapidly, and survival into midchildhood is common. Muscle fasciculation and deep tendon reflex absence are more noticeable than in SMA 1. A few involved patients can sit without support early in the course of the disease; none can walk independently. Scoliosis and increased lumbar lordosis develop in nearly all patients.

Patients with spinal muscle atrophy 3 develop symptoms after the first year of life. Delay in achieving motor milestones is common. Distal weakness develops first and is followed by proximal limb and trunk weakness. Deep tendon reflexes are decreased or absent. Sensation is normal and no pathologic reflexes are present. Bladder and bowel function are normal. As the disease progresses, the ability to walk independently is lost, and scoliosis frequently develops. Prolonged survival is common.

The principles of orthopedic management of patients with spinal muscle atrophy are similar to those of patients with muscular dystrophies. Every effort must be made to maintain function and prevent painful and disabling deformities. In many cases, little can be done to aid children with severe forms of infantile muscular atrophy. Patients with more moderate degrees of involvement usually can be braced to a sitting position with total-contact orthoses and made mobile with specially modified wheelchairs. Light-weight bracing may aid in keeping patients with mild forms of spinal muscle atrophy ambulatory. Spine deformity is a serious complication of all forms of the disease. Total-contact bracing can provide temporary support for affected patients, but progression is the rule despite bracing in most cases. Patients with moderate and mild forms of the disease may require spine fusion to halt progression and correct deformity.

Inherited Disorders of Motor, Sensory, and Autonomic Neurons

A number of hereditary disorders of peripheral sensory and motor nerves are characterized clinically by atrophy of distal limb musculature and abnormalities of nerve conduction velocities. Recent studies indicate that the disorders are the result of a number of different pathophysiologic processes. Symptoms, signs, genetic patterns, and prognosis vary with type. Involvement may be primarily sensory (e.g., congenital insensitivity to pain), primarily motor, primarily autonomic (congenital dysautonomia), or mixed. Musculoskeletal involvement is most prominent in patients with mixed involvement.

The terms Charcot-Marie-Tooth disease and peroneal muscle atrophy have been applied to that subgroup with mixed motor and sensory involvement. The entire group is sometimes referred to as the *hereditary sensory and motor neuropathies*. In these patients, muscle atrophy is distal and symmetric. Cavus and varus deformity of the ankle and foot are common presenting complaints. Lower extremity reflexes tend to be depressed or absent, and decreases in sensory, position, and vibratory senses may be present. Later in the disease course, clawing of the hands develops from paralysis of intrinsic musculature. Muscle fasciculation secondary to denervation may be present. Decreased peripheral nerve conduction velocity is the diagnostic finding on electromyography.

Peroneal muscle atrophy has been subdivided further based on hereditary patterns and nerve conduction studies. Two genetic transmission patterns have been noted. Patients with autosomal dominant varieties tend to be less severely involved than patients with autosomal recessive disease. In patients with severe forms of the disease, onset may begin early in childhood, while in less severe forms onset may be noted later in adolescence or in early adult life.

The orthopedic management of affected patients depends on the severity of the disease. When cavus and varus deformities of the foot and ankle become severe, surgical correction by osteotomy and fusion of the midfoot are necessary to relieve pain and preserve function. Surgical correction of the frequent claw-toe deformities may also be necessary. Older patients with contractures of the hands may benefit from extrinsic tendon transfers to restore balance. Spine deformity has been noted in some patients with Charcot-Marie-Tooth disease. Brace treatment may be used early in the course of the disease, but progression must be treated by surgical stabilization.

Arthrogryposis Multiplex Congenita

Arthrogryposis multiplex congenita is an uncommon musculoskeletal disorder characterized by multiple joint contractures present at birth that respond poorly, if at all, to manipulation, range of motion exercise programs, or serial casting. There is a broad spectrum of involvement; in the most severe cases, rigid extension contractures of knees and elbows,

clubfeet, wrist and finger flexion contractures, and neck hyperextension are present. Medial rotation deformities of the shoulders and flexion contractures of the hip are common in the most severely involved patients. In less extreme cases, rigid contractures of one or more peripheral joints may be the only clinical manifestations of the disorder. Often there is no function in the major motor groups around the involved joint. There is no sensory deficit, and affected patients usually have normal intelligence. Life span is not affected in most patients; individuals with marked restriction of ventilatory function are at risk for pulmonary disease and may not survive into adult life.

The etiology of arthrogryposis is not known. Pathologic studies of the spinal cord at autopsy in affected patients show decreased numbers of anterior horn cells. This may be the result of failure of formation of the anterior cord or of an intrauterine disorder affecting the developing spinal cord. Unlike the spinal muscle atrophy states, however, the neurologic process is nonprogressive. Joint contractures are presumed to result from the absence of normal fetal movements. It is possible that the clinical features of arthrogryposis are the result of a variety of pathologic processes.

Marked restriction of motion of involved joints is the hallmark of arthrogryposis. Clubfeet, when present, are severe and respond poorly to nonoperative and operative treatment. The total arc of motion present in involved knees or elbows may be less than 30 degrees. Scoliosis is not common at birth but may develop later in childhood and may interfere with sitting balance.

Children with arthrogryposis often have suprisingly good function in spite of significant loss of motion. Treatment is directed toward maximizing the child's potential. In the newborn period, frequent gentle range of motion exercises and serial splintage are sometimes helpful and should be employed even though gains are often temporary. Clubfoot should be repaired in patients who are potential walkers, and an attempt should be made to correct knee flexion contractures when present, since knee flexion interferes with ambulation. Range of motion exercises and splintage are sometimes useful in decreasing wrist and hand contractures.

It is usually not possible to increase range of motion in an involved joint significantly through physical therapy or surgery. Sometimes, however, surgical realignment of a limb can permit full use of the limited motion that may be present in an extremity. A range of elbow motion from full extension to 45 degrees flexion may be of little use to a severely involved child. Osteotomy and realignment to permit an arc of motion from 45 degrees flexion to 90 degrees flexion may permit independent feeding and self care. Tendon transfers are sometimes employed to power limbs in which a satisfactory arc of motion has been achieved but no motor function is present.

Recurrence of deformity is common in patients with arthrogryposis, and initially good results may deteriorate with time. Fortunately, remarkable adaptive mechanisms sometimes permit even children with the most extreme joint stiffness to perform many activities of daily life. Parents of involved infants will need support and reassurance throughout growth and development.

BRACHIAL PLEXUS INJURIES

Birth injuries of the brachial plexus were described during the last half of the 19th century by Duchenne, Erb, and Dejerine-Klumpke. Most commonly they are the result of traction on the nerve roots and trunks that compose the plexus during difficult deliveries. Affected babies are often large, and shoulder dystocia frequently complicates delivery. Approximately 10% of involved infants present in the breech position. The upper portion, lower portion, or both portions of the plexus may be involved; clinical signs depend on the pattern of neurologic involvement.

The extent of damage to individual nerves varies. At times, true avulsion of nerve roots may occur, but in other instances, compression or stretch injuries may leave the nerve intact within its sheath. In such cases, secondary hemorrhage and edema may compound the initial injury. Recovery potential depends on the extent of injury; incomplete injuries have a better prognosis than complete injuries.

Affected neonates have decreased or absent active motion in the involved limb or limbs. Moro's reflex will be asymmetric in unilateral cases and diminished in bilateral cases. When the upper plexus is involved (Erb's palsy, C5–C6 nerve roots), the affected limb will be adducted and medially rotated, the elbow extended, and the forearm pronated. In lower plexus injuries (Klumpke's paralysis, C8–T1 nerve roots), the wrist and fingers are flexed as a result of paralysis of extrinsic and intrinsic extensors. Upper plexus injuries are most common, followed by injuries of the entire plexus. Isolated lower plexus injuries occur much less commonly.

Brachial plexus injury is one of a number of problems that result in decreased active motion in the upper limb in the neonatal period. Septic arthritis or osteomyelitis in the upper limb and birth fractures of the clavicle or proximal humerus must be considered in the differential diagnosis. A suggestive history, decreased muscle activity, and lack of roentgenographic signs of skeletal injury imply neurologic damage rather than fracture or sepsis. Joint aspiration may be necessary in some cases to exclude infection. Careful documentation of findings at first examination is necessary to permit evaluation of recovery. Litigation often follows brachial plexus injury, and early neurologic and orthopedic consultation is justified.

When brachial plexus injury has been confirmed, the affected arm should be immobilized at the infant's side for 2 to 3 weeks to prevent further damage and to permit early repair to occur. Range of motion exercises and abduction splintage is not appropriate in the neonatal period. At 2 to 3 weeks, a program of gentle abduction and lateral rotation excercises can be started. These should be repeated several times daily during the first 2 to 3 years of life. At no time should the arm be forced into extreme positions of lateral rotation and abduction. Abduction splintage has fallen into disfavor in the primary treatment of brachial plexus injuries; abduction contracture may complicate its use.

Partial recovery of function is common in all but the most severe cases of brachial plexus injury. The potential for recovery is greatest during the first 2 years of life; significant recovery is unusual after age 2 years. Estimation of residual disability and long-range treatment plans should be delayed until maximum spontaneous recovery has occurred.

SPINAL DYSRAPHISM

Developmental defects of the spinal cord and posterior elements of the vertebral column range in severity from asymptomatic spina bifida occulta to complex myelomeningocele. The resulting musculoskeletal involvement and the nature of associated abnormalities vary with the extent and location of the neural defect. Lesions of the spinal cord and vertebral column are classified by the extent of involvement of the vertebral arches, meningeal tissues, and underlying neural elements.

Spinal dysraphism is the term applied to any defect in the formation of the spinal cord or the posterior elements of the vertebral column. *Spina bifida occulta* is the simplest form of spinal dysraphism (Fig 9–1,A and B). In this condition, the lamina of the involved vertebral segment fail to meet in the midline, and a resultant

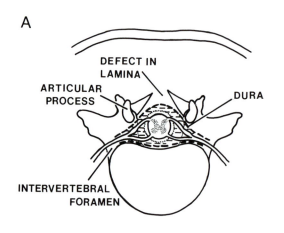

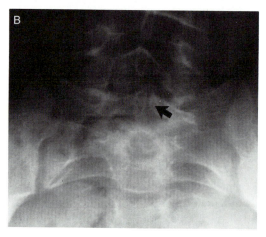

FIG 9–1.
A, spina bifida occulta. (Redrawn after Curtis BH: Classification of myelomeningocele and congenital spinal defects, in American Academy of Orthopaedic Surgeons: *Symposium on Myelomeningocele.* St Louis, CV Mosby Co, 1972, Chapter 1. Reproduced by permission.) **B,** roentgenographic appearance of spina bifida occulta. Note failure of lamina to meet in midline *(arrow).*

bony defect overlies the spinal canal at that point. *Meningocele* exists when there is protrusion of a cerebrospinal fluid–filled pouch of meningeal tissue through a defect in the posterior vertebral elements and overlying skin (Fig 9–2). In pure meningocele, underlying neural tissue is not involved, and no neurologic deficit is present. When neural tissue is involved, the defect is termed *myelomeningocele* (Fig 9–3). Some degree of neurologic abnormality complicates all cases of myelomeningocele. Paralysis distal to the lesion with loss of bladder and bowel control is the most common sequelae.

The etiology of spinal dysraphism is unknown. Some experimental evidence links the disorder to abnormalities of folate metabolism. Two pathophysiologic theories are considered possible. In some

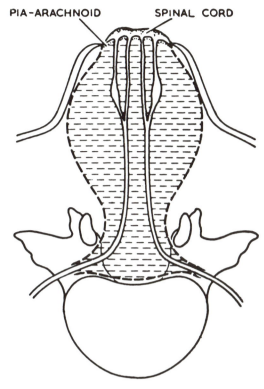

FIG 9–3.
Myelomeningocele (From Curtis BH: Classification of myelomeningocele and congenital spinal defects, in American Academy of Orthopaedic Surgeons, *Symposium on Myelomeningocele.* CV Mosby Co, St Louis, 1972, Chapter 1. Reproduced by permission.)

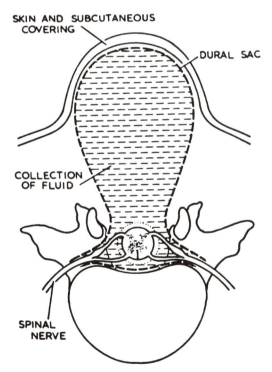

FIG 9–2.
Meningocele (From Curtis BH: Classification of myelomeningocele and congenital spinal defects, in American Academy of Orthopaedic Surgeons: *Symposium on Myelomeningocele.* St Louis, CV Mosby Co, 1972, Chapter 1. Reproduced by permission.)

cases, myelomeningocele may represent a failure of closure of the neural plate early in embryonic development. In other instances, it may be the result of rupture of a previously closed neural tube later in fetal development. Abnormal formation of the ventricular system leading to increased cerebrospinal fluid pressure within the central canal of the neural tube may be responsible for such lesions.

Spina bifida occulta occurs in approximately 6% of the North American population. The fifth lumbar vertebra is most commonly involved. Most often individuals with spina bifida occulta have no associated neurologic abnormalities. Cutaneous abnormalities such as a hairy patch, dimpling, or an open sinus are signs of more significant involvement and require careful investigation. When such findings are noted on physical examination, orthopedic or neurosurgical consultation is recommended.

Myelomeningocele occurs in approximately 1 in 1,000 live births in North American infants of European descent. It is more common in Great Britain and less common in black infants and in infants of Jewish descent. It is probably a multifactorial genetic condition. The risks to successive pregnancies rise with increasing numbers of first-degree relatives. A mother with one affected child has approximately a 5% chance of having a second involved child. If two children are involved, the risk to a subsequent child is said to be approximately 10%.

Myelomeningocele defects may occur at any location in the spinal column. Higher defects are associated with significantly greater neurologic deficits and long-term complications. Lesions in the lumbosacral region are far less handicapping. By convention, the level of the defect is identified by the lowest functioning spinal nerve rather than by the radiographic site of the bony lesion. Although it is correct to refer to a patient who has fair quadriceps muscle function and no other distal motor function as a L-3–L-4 level myelomeningocele patient, it is simpler and functionally just as appropriate to group patients by approximate level of involvement. This is summarized as follows:

LEVEL OF DEFECT	NEUROLOGIC DEFICIT
Thoracic	No sensation or motor power below hips
Upper lumbar	Some sensation below hips; hip flexors present; knee extensors present
Lower lumbar	Knee flexors and extensors present; ankle dorsiflexors and hip abductors present
Sacral	Hip extensors and ankle plantar flexors present

It is often difficult to establish level of involvement during the first months of life. Reflex activity below the site of the spinal defect may be present and cause some confusion. Incomplete lesions occur in some cases, with resultant sparing of distal function. Repeated careful examination is essential.

Hydrocephalus occurs in 80% to 90% of patients with myelomeningocele. It is more common in high lesions than in low lesions. Hydromyelia, dilatation of the central canal of the spinal cord, has recently been noted in a number of myelomeningocele patients. When unrecognized or untreated, it can lead to progressive weakness in the upper extremities and spinal deformity.

It has become standard practice in most centers in the United States to close all but the most severe myelomeningocele defects soon after birth. With subsequent ventricular shunting and supportive pediatric care, most patients can be expected to survive the neonatal period and enter infancy. During subsequent growth and development, the musculoskeletal consequences of the spinal lesion must be addressed to allow maximum mobility and independence.

Walking ability depends in large part on the level of the neural lesion. Patients with sacral lesions almost always are functional walkers. Patients with thoracic level lesions can often be braced into an upright position in childhood and may learn to walk using conventional or reciprocating orthoses. These patients rarely maintain functional ambulation as adults. Patients with lumbar lesions may or may not maintain functional ambulation as adults. Strong quadriceps function, plantigrade foot position, avoidance of obesity, and near normal intelligence greatly increase the likelihood of functional walking as an adult.

Patients with defects in the upper lumbar and thoracic levels will spend the majority of their productive years in the sitting position, even though they may be able to walk in therapy or around the house. For these patients, supple hips and a stable and erect spine are essential. Unfortunately, the combination of structural defects of the spine and unbalanced muscle pull often result in severe secondary deformity unless detected early and appropriately treated.

The unbalanced pull of the hip flexors and adductors in myelomeningocele patients with defects at the L-3–L-4 levels leads to hip dislocation in a high percentage of patients. Hip dislocation occurs less commonly in patients with higher or lower lesions. In patients who are vigorous walkers, located hips are desirable to decrease the energy expenditure of walking, and surgical attempts to balance the muscle forces around the hips are justified. Extensive hip surgery in other patients is more controversial. No conclusive evidence indicates that hip dislocation in the myelomeningocele patient who is not a functional walker leads to painful degenerative arthritis. Surgical procedures that result in stiff but located hips decrease rather than increase function.

Spine deformity is common in myelomeningocele patients. The incidence and complexity of deformity rise with more proximal lesions. Sacral level lesions rarely cause significant deformity; severe deformity almost always develops in patients with thoracic level lesions. Deformity may be the result of mechanical instability secondary to structural abnormalities of the vertebral column or may result from muscle imbalance around the spine. Some patients appear to develop spine deformities as a result of increased pressure within the central canal of the spinal cord; the mechanism of this is not known.

In most instances, bracing is of only temporary use in the treatment of spine deformity in these patients. It is often employed in an attempt to gain time while growth of the spine occurs but rarely prevents the eventual progression of deformity. Surgical correction is necessary when progressive deformity develops. Collapsing thoracolumbar gibbus in patients with thoracic level lesions is especially difficult to manage. Early intervention and stabilization is necessary to prevent significant deformity and preserve function.

It is beyond the scope of this text to deal with the medical, social, psychological, and ethical problems involved in the care of the myelomeningocele patient. Comprehensive care is essential for successful management. This is perhaps best done in cooperation with a specialized myelomeningocele team. Unless adequate long-term outpatient support is available, medical and surgical intervention will not achieve maximum results.

SUGGESTED READINGS

Aston JW: Brachial plexus birth injury. *Orthopedics* 1979; 2:594.

Bleck EE: Locomotor prognosis in cerebral palsy. *Dev Med Child Neurol* 1975; 17:18.

Bunch W: Muscular dystrophy, in Hardy JH (ed): *Spinal Deformity in Neurological and Muscular Disorders*. St Louis, CV Mosby Co, 1973.

Curtiss BH: *Orthopedic Management of Muscular Dystrophy and Related Disorders*. American Academy of Orthopaedic Surgeons: Instructional Course Lectures, St Louis, CV Mosby Co, vol 19, p 78, 1970.

Dubowitz V: *Muscle Disorders in Childhood*. London, WB Saunders Co, 1978.

Dyck PJ: Inherited neuronal degeneration and atrophy affecting peripheral motor, sensory, and autonomic neurons, in Dyck PJ, et al (eds): *Peripheral Neuropathy*, ed 2. Philadelphia, WB Saunders Co, 1984.

Engel AG: Duchenne Dystrophy, in Engel AG, Banker BO (eds): *Myology*. New York, McGraw-Hill Book Co, 1986.

Goldner JL: *Cerebral Palsy—General Principles*. American Academy of Orthopaedic Surgeons: Instructional Course Lectures, St Louis, CV Mosby Co, 1970, vol 20.

Gomez MR: Motor neuron diseases in children, in Engel AG, Banker BO (eds): *Myology*. New York, McGraw-Hill Book Co, 1986.

Hoffer MM: *Basic Considerations and Classifications of Cerebral Palsy*. American Academy of Orthopaedic Surgeons: Instructional Course Lectures, St Louis, CV Mosby Co, 1976, vol 25.

Hoffer MM, et al: Functional ambulation in patients with myelomeningocele. *J Bone Joint Surg Am* 1983; 55:137.

Nelson KB, Ellenberg JH: Antecedents of cerebral palsy. *N Engl J Med* 1986; 315:81.

O'Reilly DE, Walentynowitz JE: Etiologic factors in cerebral palsy: A historical review. *Dev Med Child Neurol* 1981; 23:633.

Paneth N: Birth and the origins of cerebral palsy. *N Engl J Med* 1986; 315:124.

10

Children and Sports

Angela D. Smith, M.D.

Modern children participate in a wide variety of organized sports activities. Physicians involved in the care of children must be familiar with the benefits and risks of such activities for the immature athlete. The significant anatomical and physiologic differences between the child and adult competitor must be considered when counseling or caring for children involved in sports. Greenstick fractures and growth plate injuries are perhaps the most familiar examples of age-related differences, but they are by no means the only ones. Aerobic and anaerobic metabolic capabilities, response to conditioning programs, thermal regulation, and psychological adaptation to competitive sports programs differ significantly between children and adults. In this section, some basic concepts of sports medicine in the immature athlete will be presented. Research in these areas is very active, and much controversy surrounds some topics. Readers actively involved in the care of childhood athletes are encouraged to review the suggested references at the end of the chapter for more detailed information.

PHYSIOLOGIC CONSIDERATIONS

Aerobic and Anaerobic Metabolism

Energy requirements for daily life and athletic activities are met through a combination of aerobic and anaerobic metabolic pathways. In brief, energy requirements for those activites requiring endurance are met through aerobic pathways, while those activities requiring short bursts of maximum stength are powered by anaerobic metabolic pathways.

The usual index of aerobic capacity is maximal oxygen uptake. Aerobic capacity is lower in children than in adults, and correspondingly, maximal oxygen uptake is less. From ages 6 to 12 years, the maximal oxygen uptake of both boys and girls increases at similar rates. At puberty the maximal oxygen uptake begins to level off. This occurs between ages 12 and 14 years in girls; in boys maximal oxygen uptake increases up to age 18 years. Aerobic capacity is often expressed in terms of maximal oxygen uptake per kilogram of body weight. Although prepubertal girls are similar in height and weight to boys of the same age (except for 2 years around puberty when they are slightly larger), the maximal aerobic capacity of boys is greater at all ages. The aerobic capacity of girls actually decreases after puberty, as the percentage of body fat increases. When maximal oxygen uptake is related to lean body mass, however, age and sex-related differences become much less significant. The age-related changes in maximal oxygen uptake allow older children to perform better than younger ones in endurance events such as long-distance running. Apparent improvements in performance in endurance activities in younger children probably occur through increased efficiency of activity rather than through aerobic conditioning.

The anaerobic threshold is the exercise intensity level at which anaerobic metabolism largely replaces aerobic metabolism and serum lactate begins to rise sharply. Anaerobic capacity is the ability to perform work without utilizing oxidative metabolic pathways. Short-burst supramaximal bouts of exercise that last for no more than several minutes such as sprints, jumps, and vaults are primarily anaerobic activities. The anaerobic capacity of a child is much less than that of an adult, whether expressed in absolute terms or per kilogram of body weight. This appears to reflect decreased activity of glycolytic enzymes in children.

Temperature Regulation

The significant thermoregulatory differences between adults and children must be considered when planning training regimens and competitive events. In hot climatic conditions, children sweat less than adults. Heat dissipation occurs more through convection and radiation than through evaporation. In cold air, children can maintain core body temperature while running, skiing, skating, or playing hockey. The child's ability to maintain core temperature when exercising in cool water is lower than that of adolescents and adults. This seems related to their relatively higher surface area and thinner subcutaneous adipose tissue. Hypothermia is subtle; there are few warning signs of excessive cooling. Shivering, euphoria, peripheral vasoconstriction, disorientation, and increasing lethargy are highly suggestive. Situations in which hypothermia may arise should never be permitted to occur.

Children and adolescents exercising in warm and hot environments should be encouraged to drink fluids since they, like adults, cannot be relied on to replace water loss by voluntary drinking. Dehydration and heat exhaustion are marked by decreased sweating, lethargy, tachycardia, and peripheral vasoconstriction. Gradual cooling and rehydration are the key points in treatment, but prevention is more important. Deliberate water restriction, practiced by some wrestlers to qualify for lower weight classes, must be strongly discouraged.

Strength and Endurance Training

The effects of supervised training on strength and endurance in children have not yet been fully investigated, but the results of available studies are of great interest. Prepubertal children show virtually no increase in maximal oxygen uptake after training, in contrast to older adolescents and adults. Performance often improves, however, probably as a result of increased skill. Studies of 11- and 12-year-old Japanese boys suggest that with training an increase in the anaerobic threshold occurs. Studies of prepubertal boys and girls in the United States have suggested a relationship between anaerobic threshold and athletic performance, but further longitudinal controlled studies of the aerobic and anaerobic capacities of children are needed before definitive recommendations can be made for effective and safe endurance training. If the recommendations for adults are extrapolated, a safe training program for endurance activities for older children and adolescents should consist of a 5- to 10-minute warm-up period, 20 to 30 minutes of activity to maintain heart rate at 70% maximum (maximum heart rate = 220 − athlete's age), and a 5- to 10-minute cool-down period. Long-distance running should be discouraged until children are well into adolescence. An upper limit of 10 km is appropriate for most younger athletes.

Strength training for prepubertal children remains controversial despite clinical evidence that gains in strength can be obtained safely with appropriate weight-training regimens. Small controlled studies of boys and girls 10 to 11 years old demonstrated increases in strength in specific muscle groups without injury under a supervised program of progressive resistance and flexibility exercises. Significant improvements in strength are possible, probably through changes in neuro-muscular recruitment patterns, even though muscle bulk increases very little in the absence of androgenic hormones.

The keys to safe strength training programs in prepubertal athletes are close supervision, low weight, high repetition activities, and stretching exercises. Most weight training is best done on machines appropriately adjusted for size (Fig 10–1). If these are not available, or if children are too small, free weights may be used under careful supervision. Two or three sets of ten repetitions using approximately 60% of the child's maximum lifting ability

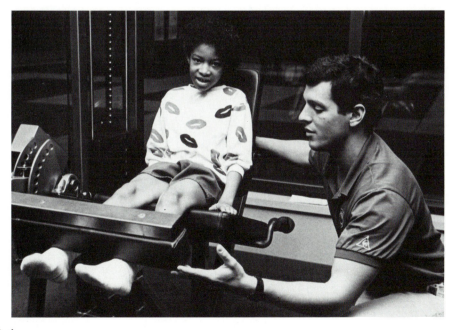

FIG 10–1.
Weight training machines can be safely used for children if properly adjusted for size and if proper supervision is available. (Courtesy of Division of Sports Medicine, Al DuPont Institute, Wilmington, Del.)

for each muscle group are sufficient. As strength increases, resistance can be gradually increased. Strength training sessions should be repeated no more frequently than every other day.

Flexibility training should be incorporated into strength training programs (Figs 10–2 and 10–3). Stretching exercises are best done one or two times daily, rather than every other day, and should be done slowly in a warm and comfortable environment. Together, strength and flexibility training may prove important in the prevention of injuries among prepubertal children and adolescents.

A review by the President's Council

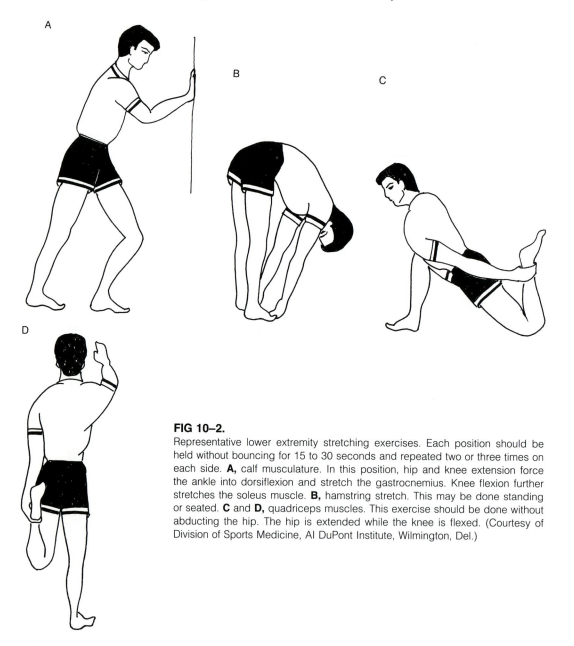

FIG 10–2.
Representative lower extremity stretching exercises. Each position should be held without bouncing for 15 to 30 seconds and repeated two or three times on each side. **A,** calf musculature. In this position, hip and knee extension force the ankle into dorsiflexion and stretch the gastrocnemius. Knee flexion further stretches the soleus muscle. **B,** hamstring stretch. This may be done standing or seated. **C** and **D,** quadriceps muscles. This exercise should be done without abducting the hip. The hip is extended while the knee is flexed. (Courtesy of Division of Sports Medicine, AI DuPont Institute, Wilmington, Del.)

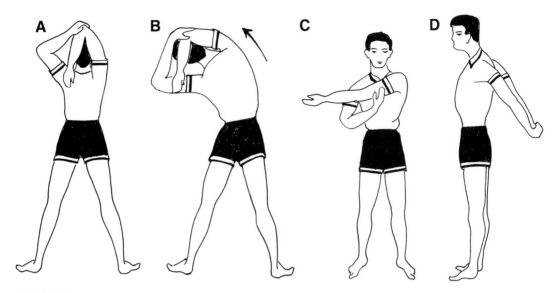

FIG 10–3.
Representative trunk and upper extremity stretching exercises. These are especially useful for athletes participating in overhand sports such as tennis, swimming, and pitching. **A,** one arm is used to pull the other behind the head across the midline and passively flex the elbow as much as possible. This stretches the triceps muscles as well as the muscles that control the scapula. **B,** lateral trunk flexion stretches the muscles of the back and chest wall. **C,** assisted adduction of the arm further stretches scapular musculature. **D,** extension of the shoulder stretches the anterior shoulder muscles. (Courtesy of Division of Sports Medicine, Al DuPont Institute, Wilmington, Del.)

on Physical Fitness found boys' strength to be slightly greater than girls' at all ages. However, the consensus among fitness experts is that prepubertal children of similar ages may safely participate even in contact sports together. After puberty, the determination of size and strength is more important than the child's sex in choosing groups for athletic competition. As adolescent males increase muscle mass with maturity, coeducational contact sports become more dangerous. Even among adolescent males, the safest method of team assignment for contact sports is by size and strength since boys mature at markedly different rates.

Menarche

The occurrence of menarche may be influenced by the intensity of exercise of a prepubertal girl. Any female athlete who participates at a high level of athletic activity may experience delayed menarche. Delay is more frequent in athletes with lower percentages of body fat, such as runners, gymnasts, and ballet dancers. Menarche delayed past 14 years of age in ballet dancers has been associated with an increased incidence of scoliosis and stress fractures. Menarche delayed past age 16 years should not be presumed to result solely from athletic participation. Careful investigation is generally indicated.

The relationship between delayed menarche and future osteoporosis in the female athlete is of theoretical concern. Females increase the mineral content of their bones only until early in the third decade of life. From that time, bone mineral is continuously lost. Athletic females do seem to form more bone in the weight-bearing regions than sedentary females do, but the lack of normal estrogen cycling in amenorrheic athletes may negate this usual increase of mineral content. Additional study is necessary to provide better information for appropriate counseling of amenorrheic active adolescents and young women.

ATHLETIC INJURIES

General Principles

Prevention is the key word in childhood sports injuries. This requires a combination of careful supervision, proper training, good equipment, skilled officiating, and common sense. Training sessions of gradually increasing length and intensity reduce the likelihood of stress fractures and overuse syndromes. Adequate time for stretching and cooling down must be provided. Periods of rest must be provided between practice sessions, and fluid replacement should be enforced. Adequate time for heat acclimation must be permitted when necessary. A cool mist spray should be available in hot climates and should be used liberally. Practice sessions should place at least as much emphasis on technique as on endurance training in the preadolescent athlete.

Young athletes engaged in noncontact sports such as running, swimming, and tennis, like adults, may develop overuse syndromes. These can usually be prevented by ensuring necessary flexibility and strength training, replacing worn equipment promptly, and increasing the training regimen slowly. All activity sessions should begin with a brief warm-up, generally to the point of perspiration. Once the muscles are warm, a set of stretching exercises should be done before actual play begins. After the game or event is over, a cool-down set of stretching exercises should be done, and ice packs should be applied to painful areas if necessary.

Baseball is probably the most popular children's team sport in North America. The frequency of chronic and acute injuries in baseball is very low, but a few precautions are necessary to keep the sport safe for children. Little League pitchers should be rotated to other positions when possible to avoid overuse injuries of the elbow. Limits should be placed on the length of practice sessions and on the number of innings that a child may pitch in a game. It is not wise to permit a child to pitch for extended periods in successive games or on multiple teams. Batting caps should be worn to reduce the possibility of head injuries.

Serious injuries are uncommon in young children who participate in football, hockey, and soccer. The frequency of injury rises as children approach adolescence and increase in size and strength (Fig 10–4). Football and wrestling have especially high injury rates. Athletes who

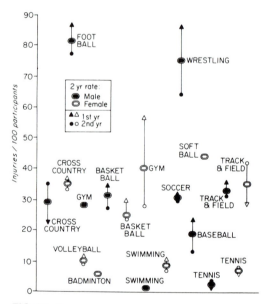

FIG 10–4.
Injury rates for 2 years of selected high school sports; injury rate was 10% lower during second year of study. (From Garrick JG, and Requea RK: Injuries in high school sports. *Pediatrics* 1987; 61:465. Reproduced by permission.)

participate in these sports should maintain the best possible condition. Unfortunately, many of the more serious injuries sustained in competition are not easily preventable. Proper coaching, good equipment, and strict enforcement of rules are necessary to keep the incidence of injury in these sports low.

The efficacy of prophylactic knee bracing in football and soccer is controversial. Although braces designed to protect the anterior cruciate ligaments are probably valuable after injury and subsequent repair, no evidence attests to their usefulness in decreasing the injury rate in healthy individuals. There are anecdotal reports that the rate of injury may in fact be higher in players who use knee braces, perhaps because they play more aggressively, or because the braces preload the cruciate ligaments. At this time, the author does not recommend prophylactic knee bracing for adolescent football players.

Return to Participation After Injury

Two major criteria must be met before an athlete returns to play after sustaining a musculoskeletal injury. Strength of all major muscle groups must be normal, and flexibility should be excellent. The athlete who returns to full participation inadequately rehabilitated is frequently reinjured. Restricted alternate activities are usually possible before return to full participation. A figure skater with a back injury, for example, may maintain aerobic endurance and lower extremity strength by bicycling. Whenever possible, alternate activities should be designed to utilize the same sport-specific muscle groups necessary for the athlete's primary sport.

Specific Musculoskeletal Injuries

Although children have always been at risk for fractures, sprains, and lacerations while playing, they have begun to sustain the overuse injuries common in adults only recently. This change has occurred as many children have moved from the intermittent and varied games of the playground to year-round organized single-sport athletics. Children who participate daily in a single sporting activity place the same stresses on their musculoskeletal systems each session without allowing sufficient time for recovery. In adults, such repetitive activity may lead to stress fractures or tendinitis, and both of these problems occur in the child. The immature athlete has the additional risk of developing avulsion fractures of the tendinous insertions at apophyses.

Stress Fractures

Stress fractures occur rarely in the very young child, but they are occasionally seen in athletes 10 years of age and older. Stress fractures in younger or less active children may be secondary to metabolic bone disease, which should be ruled out if atypical history or radiographic findings are noted. Most stress fractures occur soon after a change in some part of a training regimen. The change may be obvious, such as increasing daily running mileage from 2 to 5 miles. However, subtle changes can lead to the onset of symptoms, such as beginning the indoor track season and running on a different type of surface, or even using a new brand of athletic shoes. Initially, the pain of a stress fracture is usually worse during and immediately following activity. Eventually, the pain may become constant. On physical examination, there is point tenderness at the site of fracture. Local swelling and even palpable healing callus may be apparent. Radiographs obtained within the first 2 to 3 weeks after onset of pain may be negative, but later radiographs demonstrate periosteal new bone formation and often show a well-defined fracture line (Fig 10–

5). Radioisotope bone scans have been employed to aid in early diagnosis and to distinguish stress fractures from other pathologic changes in bone.

Stress fractures may ordinarily be treated by restriction of activity until symptoms subside and there is radiographic evidence of new bone formation. For stress fractures involving the metatarsals, a brief period of partial weight bearing on crutches or immobilization in a short leg cast may be necessary to control pain. Stress fractures of the tibia can usually be managed by restriction from weight bearing until symptoms subside. If the patient is unreliable, immobilization in a long leg cast may be necessary to prevent a nondisplaced fracture from becoming a more serious problem. Stress fractures of the proximal femur, common in young military recruits as a consequence of prolonged marches under pack, are uncommon in young athletes. Because the potential for displacement in these fractures is great, immobilization in a spica cast or operative fixation is sometimes considered.

Apophyseal avulsion fractures are stress fractures unique to immature patients. Although avulsion fractures may result from a sudden single acute force, most avulsion fractures of adolescence are related to recurrent stress injuries. A tendon inserts into bone through a traction apophysis, which is connected to the remainder of a long bone by a growth plate. With the stress of repetitive microtrauma, the physeal cartilage may become disrupted and fragmented, causing activity-related discomfort. A sudden strong contraction of the inserting musculotendinous unit, or a direct blow to the area, may pull the apophysis completely free from the long bone (Fig 10–6). Avulsion fractures are especially common in the pelvis. Frequently avulsed apophyses include the anterior superior iliac spine, the anterior inferior iliac spine, the iliac apophysis, the lesser trochanter, and the ischium. Sometimes the pain is so severe that bed rest is required for several days before protected weight bearing is possible. Restriction of painful activities for 3 to 4 weeks usually allows sufficient early healing to begin gentle rehabilitation exercises of stretching and strengthening of the involved musculotendinous units. Severely displaced avulsion fractures may rarely be treated surgically in the elite athlete to avoid the minimal loss of power that might result if the fracture were allowed to heal in the displaced position. Ischial tuberosity avulsions may be complicated by myositis ossificans, causing a prominence that may be painful with sitting. Myositis ossificans of this area is difficult to treat and may recur after surgical excision.

Head and Neck Injuries

Head and neck injuries occur most often in collision sports such as football, boxing, and wrestling but may occur in

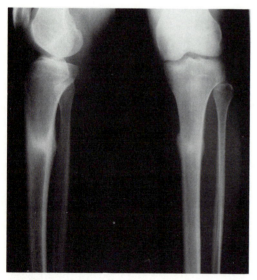

FIG 10–5.
Stress fracture of the proximal tibia. Note transverse increase in density within the shaft of the proximal third of the tibia and the subperiosteal new bone formation around the fracture site.

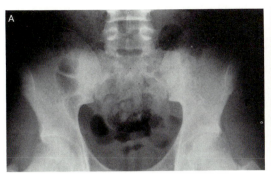
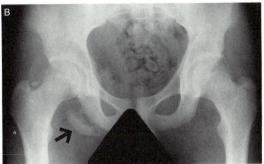

FIG 10–6.
A, avulsion of the anterior superior iliac apophysis *(arrow).* (Courtesy of Stuart Morrison, M.D.) **B,** avulsion of the ischial apophysis *(arrow).* (Photograph courtesy of Division of Sports Medicine, AI DuPont Institute, Wilmington, Del.)

individual sports such as gymnastics and diving as well. When head injury associated with loss of consciousness or cervical spine injury is suspected, the spine must be immobilized and primary evaluation carried out without moving the spine. Cervical spine injury must be suspected in all patients with neck pain and in all comatose patients. Thorough physical examination and careful radiographic evaluation are essential before treatment recommendations can be made or before return to activity can be permitted.

Closed Head Injury.—Concussion is the term applied to closed head injury that results in temporary loss of consciousness without focal anatomical brain injury. Loss of consciousness in these patients is probably the result of jarring of the reticular activating system. Affected children may not recall the circumstances of injury and may complain of nausea, dizziness, or headache. No focal signs are present on neurologic examination. Radiographic examination of the skull is not necessary if no pain or tenderness is noted on palpation of the head. Cervical spine radiographs should be obtained if neck pain, tenderness, or muscle spasm is present.

Children who sustain closed head in-

jury associated with loss of consciousness, no matter how brief, should be promptly removed from play and undergo evaluation in a hospital setting. If the loss of consciousness was less than 5 minutes, and if no focal neurologic abnormalities are noted on repeated examinations over a several-hour period at the hospital, adolescents may be followed at home. Children less than 12 years old and all patients who are unconscious for more than 5 minutes are best followed as inpatients. Concussion followed by a brief lucid period, and then by secondary depression of level of consciousness with localizing peripheral neurologic signs, is the hallmark of acute epidural hemorrhage. Immediate neurosurgical consultation is mandatory.

Cervical Spine Injury.—Cervical spine injuries in children and adolescents may be the result of significant injuring forces applied to a normal cervical spine, or of normal loading in a congenitally unstable spine. Symptoms and signs vary widely. Acute spine injury with immediate loss of distal neurologic function following a severe blow to the head or neck, an improper tackle, a fall, or a diving mishap is the most well-recognized pattern of injury. After initial stabilization of the airway and immobilization of the spine to prevent further damage, primary documentation of the extent of neurologic compromise is essential. Sacral sensory sparing in patients with otherwise apparently complete cord transection suggests an incomplete injury and implies that some functional recovery can be expected. Complete distal loss of motor function and sensation or progressively deteriorating distal neurologic function are much more ominous signs.

A number of less serious injuries of the cervical spine occur in adolescents who participate in contact sports. "Burners" or "stingers" are really cervical nerve root or brachial plexus stretch injuries that cause a neurapraxia, a temporary loss of normal nerve conduction. Forced lateral bending of the cervical spine, often combined with some extension or flexion, causes a traction neurapraxia and results in temporary loss of sensation and strength of the upper extremity. Normal function usually returns within several days. If a deficit persists, the diagnosis of "burner" may be questioned and an electromyographic study may be indicated. Although most athletes who sustain brachial plexus traction injuries have normal spinal canals, those who sustain this type of injury should be evaluated with cervical spine radiographs to rule out the presence of a congenitally narrow spinal canal or an occult fracture. Athletes with congenital spinal stenosis should be cautioned against participating in sports that frequently lead to cervical trauma. Young athletes should not be allowed to return to contact sport participation until sensation and strength have returned to normal. Patients who experience recurrent brachial plexus neurapraxias should be discouraged from playing sports likely to cause reinjury.

Instability of the upper cervical spine has been reported in patients with Down's syndrome (trisomy 21). The exact incidence of atlantoaxial instability in Down's syndrome is not known but has been estimated by the Orthopaedic Section of the American Academy of Pediatrics as approximately 10% to 15%. Although not all patients with C-1–C-2 instability are symptomatic, they are at risk for acute injury in sports. Guidelines for evaluation of patients with Down's syndrome were developed for the Massachusetts Special Olympics program; the Orthopaedic Section of the American Academy of Pediatrics considers them applicable to all patients with Down's Syndrome:

1. All patients with Down's syndrome should have lateral roentgenograms of the cervical spine in neutral, flexion, and extension position. Children with an atlanto-dens interval of greater than 4 mm or adults with an interval greater than 3 mm require further clinical and radiographic evaluation.

2. When symptoms of neurologic compromise are present in patients with C-1–C-2 instability, surgical stabilization is necessary to prevent sudden and catastrophic spinal cord injury. Signs may be transient and subtle and include decreasing exercise tolerance, bowel or bladder incontinence, syncopal episodes, seizures, as well as pyramidal tract signs or transient flaccid paralysis.

3. When radiographic evidence of cervical spine instability is present but there is no evidence of neurologic impairment, parents should be advised that the natural history of asymptomatic instability is not known, and that periodic repeat neurologic and radiographic evaluation are necessary, probably at 6- to 12-month intervals. Such children should not be permitted to participate in contact sports or in soccer, gymnastics, and diving. The authors believe that consideration should be given to prophylactic surgical stabilization in these cases.

4. Since the developmental history of the C-1–C-2 region in Down's syndrome has not been established, immature patients with no evidence of instability at the time of first examination should be carefully followed; repeat radiographic examination may be advisable at 2- to 3-year intervals even in the absence of neurologic abnormalities during juvenile and adolescent growth and development.

Lumbar Spine

Lumbar spondylolysis, a defect of the pars interarticularis of a vertebra, is a frequent cause of low back pain in the adolescent athlete, particularly the football player, hockey player, wrestler, or gymnast. Some of these patients have a preexistent congenital defect in the pars made symptomatic by sports; others sustain a true stress fracture as a result of repetitive activities that place axial loads on the extended spine. Low back pain, occasionally radiating down the posterior aspect of the thighs, hamstring muscle spasm, and loss of lumbar lordosis are the main findings in symptomatic patients. Neurologic deficits, common in adults with degenerative spondylolisthesis, are uncommon in adolescents.

Primary treatment is nonoperative and consists of hamstring stretching and abdominal strengthening exercises. At times, brace immobilization is necessary. If the defect is a recent stress fracture, it may heal with conservative treatment. If the defect is congenital and has become symptomatic because of activity, it is not likely to heal. Surgical stabilization may be necessary when symptoms persist in spite of nonoperative management. Immature patients with spondylolysis and spondylolisthesis are at risk for progression of slip with further growth, whether or not they are symptomatic, and they must be followed radiographically until mature. When progression occurs, surgical treatment is indicated.

Shoulder

Overuse injuries of the shoulder occur most often in athletes involved in throwing sports, racket sports, and swimming. The two most common categories of overuse injuries around the shoulder are impingement injuries and injuries related to recurrent minor subluxation of the shoulder. Mild rotator cuff strains may occur in adolescents, but true rotator cuff tears are rare. More serious injuries of the shoulder, including true dislocation and fractures through the growth plate of the proximal humerus, have been discussed in Chapter 2. Differentiation of impingement syndromes from subluxation may be difficult and requires careful review of the patient's history and thorough physical examination. Roentgenograms are often not helpful except in extreme or long-standing cases.

Impingement syndromes result from chronic contact of the greater tuberosity of the humerus and its attached musculotendinous cuff against the overlying acromion process of the scapula. In affected patients, tenderness is most pronounced over the subacromial bursa, the supraspinatus tendon, and the anterosuperior shoulder capsule. The biceps tendon may be tender and its sheath edematous. Passive medial and lateral rotation are painful when the humerus is abducted 90 degrees, and pain may be reproduced by adducting the forward flexed humerus across the body.

Athletes participating in swimming and overhead throwing usually have increased shoulder motion, and as a consequence, recurrent mild subluxation may be difficult to diagnose. Swimmers generally have increased sagittal plane motion of the humeral head within the glenoid. Patients who perform overhead throwing normally have increased lateral rotation of the throwing shoulder compared to the opposite shoulder. If the amount of lateral rotation only equals the opposite shoulder, then motion has usually been lost.

The initial treatment for both impingement syndromes and subluxation of the shoulder is partial or total restriction of painful activities, local application of ice, and an exercise program to restore normal motion and strength. The most important strengthening exercises are those for the lateral rotators of the shoulder. These may be performed using either an elastic band or weights for resistance and should be done at least once daily. Oral nonsteroidal anti-inflammatory drugs may be utilized for more severe or persistent cases. Recurrent subluxation that does not respond to conservative methods may require surgical repair.

Elbow

Young pitchers may develop pain in the dominant elbow after prolonged bouts of pitching without appropriate breaks from activity. The symptoms may be caused by tendinitis and respond rapidly to a conservative program of rest, ice, and stretching and strengthening exercises. However, pitcher's elbow symptoms in the young child or adolescent are frequently caused by osteochondritis dissecans of the capitellum, which may result in loose body formation and permanent disability (Fig 10–7). Early diagnosis and appropriate operative or nonoperative treatment may prevent serious articular damage.

Knee

Overuse syndromes and injuries around the knee are probably the most common sports-related problems in childhood and adolescence. These are covered in Chapter 4.

Lower Leg and Ankle

Overuse injuries of the lower leg may result in shin splints. Pain along the medial border of the tibia is frequently caused by inflammation of the perios-teum. In most young athletes, this painful periostitis is associated with weakness of the posterior tibial muscle and tenderness along its tendon. More localized tenderness of the tibia is suggestive of a stress fracture. Patients with severe pain should be managed initially by rest, with ice packs and anti-inflammatory agents as necessary. When acute symptoms subside, a program of strengthening exercises for the posterior tibial muscle should be started. Less symptomatic patients can be treated with anti-inflammatory agents and exercise, with less severe restriction of activity.

Serious injuries of the ankle ligaments and joint capsule are uncommon in children. Forces sufficient to cause damage to the ligaments of the ankle in adults usually produce fractures in patients with open physes. Ankle sprains become more common as adolescents approach skeletal maturity. The usual mechanism of injury is plantar flexion and inversion, with resultant stress on the anterior and anterolateral ligaments of the ankle. In acute injuries, the onset of pain is immediate. Swelling and discoloration develop later. In patients with recurrent more minor sprains, pain and swelling may occur after exercise and diminish with rest.

It is essential to distinguish ligament injury from ankle fracture before beginning treatment. Tenderness along the distal metaphyseal regions of either the tibia or fibula is suggestive of fracture, while tenderness anterior and inferior to the lateral malleolus is more likely secondary to soft tissue injury. Roentgenograms of the ankle should be obtained if any doubt exists at all about the nature of the injury. In patients with acute injuries, roentgenograms should be obtained before ankle stability is tested.

If there are no fractures around the ankle, the ligaments may be safely tested. The lower leg should be held firmly with one hand, while the other hand grasps

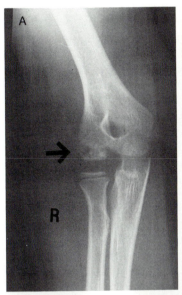
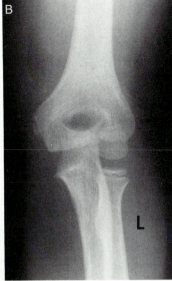
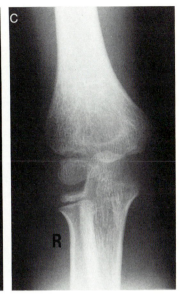

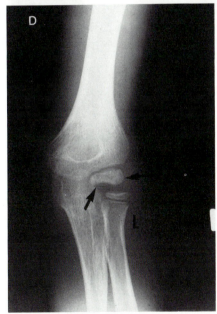

FIG 10–7.
Two cases of Little League pitchers with osteochondritis of the capitellum associated with pain while throwing and mild swelling over the radial head after playing. (Roentgenograms courtesy of Stuart Morrison, M.D.) **A** and **B,** right-handed 11-year-old boy. Note the rarefaction and fragmentation of the secondary center of ossification *(arrow)* of the right capitellum compared to the left side. **C** and **D,** left-handed 10-year-old boy. Note increase in radiodensity and apparent collapse of the secondary center of ossification *(arrowheads)* of the left capitellum compared to the right side.

the heel. Laterally directed force on the heel tests the medial collateral ligaments of the ankle; medially directed force tests the lateral collateral ligaments. Plantar flexion and inversion test the commonly injured anterolateral ligaments. Straight anterior and posterior forces test the joint capsule as well as the medial and lateral ligaments. Less than 0.5 cm of laxity should be present in any direction.

Acute ankle sprains should be treated with ice, elevation, and immobilization. Compression wraps, if used, must be carefully applied. A single elastic bandage passed in a figure-of-eight fashion around the heel and malleoli provides little support for the ankle and encourages swelling distal to the ankle. Athletic tape applied from the metatarsals to the junction of the middle and distal thirds of the lower leg provides much more effective acute immobilization and compression. An alternative means is a brace or stirrup that allows plantar flexion and dorsiflexion while preventing significant inversion and eversion.

When acute pain and swelling have subsided, ankle rehabilitation can be started. Isometric strengthening exercises for the major stabilizing muscles of the

ankle are essential to prevent recurrent injury (Fig 10–8). Under the supervision of a physician, physical therapist, or certified athletic trainer, the athlete's rehabilitation may be shortened markedly by thorough control of edema and early initiation of active exercises to restore strength and motion. Return to participation can be permitted when strength and flexibility are normal.

Pain and spasm in the invertors or evertors of the foot and ankle occur occasionally late in childhood or early in adolescence. Associated tenderness may be

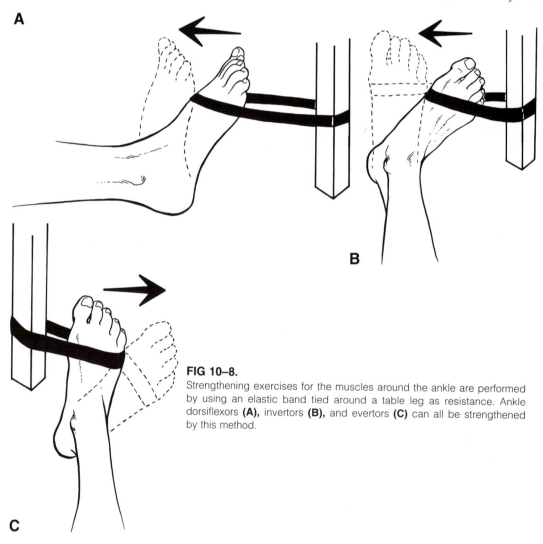

FIG 10–8.
Strengthening exercises for the muscles around the ankle are performed by using an elastic band tied around a table leg as resistance. Ankle dorsiflexors **(A),** invertors **(B),** and evertors **(C)** can all be strengthened by this method.

found on palpation over the tendon sheaths of the peroneal muscles or the posterior tibial muscle. Passive and active hindfoot motion may be markedly restricted. Such findings may indicate a congenital abnormality of the foot such as tarsal coalition or an accessory ossicle that interferes with normal function. When a brief period of rest or alterations in footwear fail to relieve symptoms, orthopedic evaluation is indicated.

Osteochondritis dissecans of the talus is an occasional cause of pain around the ankle in adolescents (Fig 10–9). Symptoms include recurrent swelling after exercise, locking, and aching, diffuse pain. It is probably traumatic in origin, although the initial episode may not be severe. As in the knee, the loose bony fragment is usually attached to the underlying subchondral bone by fibrous tissue. Unlike the knee, the etiology is probably an osteochondral fracture rather than a developmental variant. Nondisplaced osteochondral fragments may be treated conservatively, with restriction of activity but maintenance of range of motion. Acute osteochondral fractures are treated by avoiding weight bearing for 4 to 6 weeks. Minimally displaced fragments may require surgical pinning, and severely displaced avascular fragments are usually excised.

Heel pain is common in immature athletes. Most complain of tenderness overlying the posterior aspect of the calcaneus around the site of the insertion of the Achille's tendon. Pain is accentuated on exercise and relieved by rest. Squeezing the posterior aspect of the heel reproduces symptoms. Passive dorsiflexion of the foot may be limited, and a cavus configuration of the foot may be present. Radiographs may show irregularity or increased density of the calcaneal apophysis. The disorder is self limited and has been considered to be analogous to Osgood-Schlatter disease at the knee. Symptoms subside at the time of closure of the apophysis. Stretching exercises, combined with foam heel lifts, plastic or rubber heel cups, cushioned athletic shoes, ice packs, and nonsteroidal anti-inflammatory agents usually provide symptomatic relief. Brief restriction of activity may be necessary.

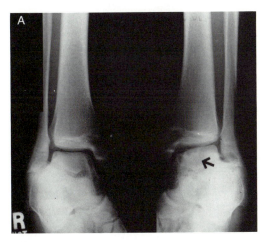 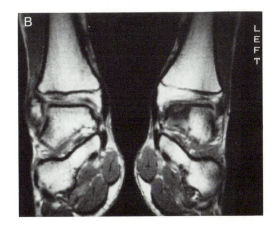

FIG 10–9.
Osteochondritis of the talus. **A,** note the radiolucent area *(arrow)* on the superior medial surface of the left talus compared to the right side. **B,** magnetic resonance imaging (MRI) scan of the talus shows a marked decrease in signal intensity from the affected region, a finding similar to that seen in Legg-Calvé-Perthes disease of the hip. (Roentgenograms courtesy of Stuart Morrison, M.D.)

Plantar fasciitis occurs most frequently in the same age brackets as Achilles tendinitis or calcaneal apophysitis. Often affected children have tight calf muscles and high arches. Affected individuals report pain on palpation over the entire plantar fascial surface. Often this is worse in the morning and subsides somewhat throughout the course of the day as affected tissues gradually stretch. Vigorous sports usually worsen the symptoms. Ice packs, stretching exercises, mild anti-inflammatory agents, and retraining usually provide relief.

PSYCHOLOGICAL CONSIDERATIONS

The child or adolescent athlete is immature psychologically as well as physically. Participation in competitive sports strongly influences the development of his or her self-image and independence. Parents and coaches should provide encouragement and guidance, enabling the athlete to achieve maximum potential. When adults forget that the young athlete needs to develop independently, and instead begin living a vicarious career through the child's athletic achievements, a variety of dysfunctional psychological patterns may develop. Even appropriately encouraging parents may unconsciously signal their children that greater achievements are expected. Coaches occasionally stress such high goals that the athlete feels personal failure if they are not met. The young athlete frequently experiences a sense of letting the coach or parent down. Sometimes the child correctly notes that a parent or coach seems to value him solely for his athletic abilities. Any of these situations may produce a psychosomatic manifestation.

Diminutive stature and extraordinary agility are characteristic attributes of many current gymnastic champions, and the late juvenile and early adolescent years are periods of peak performance for many girls who participate in organized gymnastics, figure skating, or ballet. Changes in body size and configuration at puberty may adversely affect a young woman's competitive ability. When undue emphasis has been placed on the value of successful competition in establishing the child's self-worth, a number of reactions have been documented. Anorexic behavior in an attempt to forestall weight gain and the development of secondary sexual characteristics is common. Disability out of proportion to physical findings after minor injuries has also been frequently noted. Such findings signal the need for psychological evaluation and counseling.

Although a great deal of attention has been devoted to the physical aspects of overtraining and the overuse syndromes, there has been to date much less concern about the psychological effects of overtraining. Burnout is not uncommon in elite young athletes, particularly in individual sports such as tennis, gymnastics, swimming, and track and field. Early signs include changes in eating and sleeping habits, tearfulness, and lack of desire to train. Psychosomatic symptoms may be quite bizarre, especially in very young athletes. At the earliest signs of overtraining, aggressive counseling is indicated. Often training must be cut back or stopped until goals, expectations, and fears can be carefully explored.

Early recognition and effective counseling may interrupt extreme behavior patterns. The coaches and parents should be realistic, and they must help the young athlete to set reasonable goals without overbearing pressure. The athlete needs guidance in handling performance demands and stress. Athletic participation can allow a young person to develop confidence, self-esteem, independence, and psychological strength if coaches and care givers assist the athlete in minimizing stressful situations and guilt feelings and focusing on positive experiences and attainable goals.

SUGGESTED READINGS

Atomi Y, Fukunaga T, Yamamoto Y, et al: Lactate threshold and VO_2 max of trained and untrained boys relative to muscle mass and composition, in Rutenfranz J, et al (eds): *Children and Exercise*, Human Kinetics Publishers, Champaign, Ill, 1986, vol 12.

Bar-Or: *Pediatric Sports Medicine for the Practitioner: From Physiologic Principles to Clinical Applications*. Springer-Verlag, New York, 1983.

Ogilvie B: Psychology and the elite young athlete. *Physician Sportsmed* 1983; 11:195–202.

Sewall L, Micheli L: Strength training for children. *J Pediatr Orthop* 1986; 6:143–146.

Smith N (ed): *Sports Medicine: Health Care for Young Athletes*. American Academy of Pediatrics, Evanston, Ill, 1983.

Warren M, Brooks-Gunn J, Hamilton L, et al: Scoliosis and fractures in young ballet dancers: Relation to delayed menarche and secondary amenorrhea. *N Engl J Med* 1986; 314:1348–1353.

Weltman A, et al: The effects of hydraulic resistance strength training in prepubertal males. *Med Sci Sports Exerc* 1986; 18:629–638.

Wolfe R, Washington R, Daberkow E, et al: Anaerobic threshold as a predictor of athletic performance in prepubertal female runners. *Am J Dis Child* 1986; 140:922–924.

Index